Elongate Mineral Particles

This groundbreaking book explores the complex world of elongate mineral particles (EMPs), critical occupational and environmental agents with significant public health implications. It carefully distinguishes between asbestiform EMPs, which pose serious health hazards to humans, and non-asbestiform elongate particles such as cleavage fragments, which have different characteristics and lower (or negligible) health risks. This distinction is vital for accurate risk assessment and appropriate regulatory approaches in both occupational and environmental contexts.

The comprehensive volume covers multiple scientific aspects of EMPs, including their geological origins and mineralogy, specialized analytical characterization methods, toxicological properties and carcinogenic potential, and the specific dimensional parameters that influence their toxicity. It also addresses classification methodologies for distinguishing between asbestiform and non-asbestiform particles, examines how EMPs interact with the human respiratory system, evaluates current regulatory frameworks while identifying needed improvements, and presents illuminating case studies on EMP risk assessment.

Elongate Mineral Particles: Characterization, Classification, and Risk Analysis is written for professionals across multiple disciplines. This book serves as an essential resource for health and safety specialists, industrial hygienists, toxicologists, epidemiologists, mineralogists, public health personnel, and pathologists. Its accessible yet scientifically rigorous approach makes it valuable for any scientist or practitioner interested in understanding the mineralogy and health effects of asbestos and other fibrous minerals, providing the readers with the knowledge needed to address these important public health challenges.

"*Elongate Mineral Particles: Characterization, Classification, and Risk Analysis* is the definitive text that our profession has needed for decades. It will fundamentally shape our understanding and approach to one of the most critical challenges in occupational and environmental health.

This is not just an academic exercise but also a foundation of rational risk assessment and public policy. It is certain to become the standard reference in the field."

– Shu-Chun Su, Ph.D., *Independent Researcher*

"*This outstanding text is a must read for anyone who is interested in the potential for elongate mineral particles in disease causation. The authors, who are well-recognized experts in the field, provide a thorough and mathematically rigorous analysis of the factors that are related to pathogenesis and carcinogenesis as a consequence of fiber exposures.*"

– Victor Roggli, M.D., Professor of Pathology,
Duke University Medical Center

Elongate Mineral Particles

Characterization, Classification, and Risk Analysis

Andrey Korchevskiy and Ann Wylie

CRC Press
Taylor & Francis Group
Boca Raton London New York

CRC Press is an imprint of the
Taylor & Francis Group, an **informa** business

Front cover image: Getty images. Fibrous ice crystals from Haines, Alaska, USA

First edition published 2026
by CRC Press
2385 NW Executive Center Drive, Suite 320, Boca Raton FL 33431

and by CRC Press
4 Park Square, Milton Park, Abingdon, Oxon, OX14 4RN

CRC Press is an imprint of Taylor & Francis Group, LLC

ISBN: 978-1-032-53829-7 (hbk)
ISBN: 978-1-032-54316-1 (pbk)
ISBN: 978-1-003-42427-7 (ebk)

DOI: 10.1201/9781003424277

Typeset in Times
by Apex CoVantage, LLC

Contents

About the authors

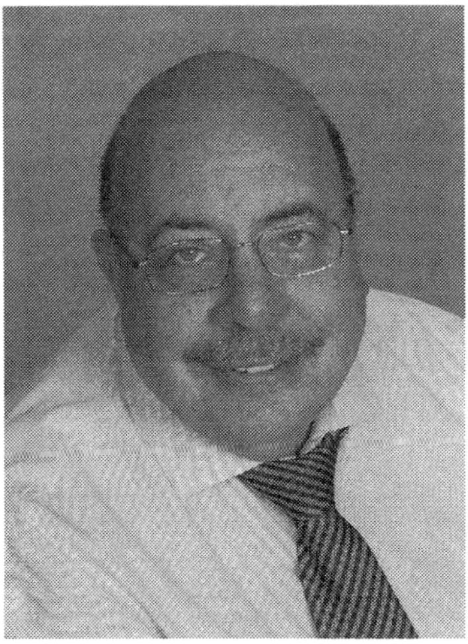

Dr. Andrey Korchevskiy, PhD, DABT, CIH, is a diplomate of the American Board of Toxicology (DABT) and a certified industrial hygienist (CIH), USA. He is the Director of Research and Development at Chemistry & Industrial Hygiene, Inc. (C&IH) (Lakewood, Colorado). Dr. Korchevskiy holds separate PhD degrees in Applied Mathematics and Biology. He has over 150 publications in various peer-reviewed journals and was a leading editor and author of a monograph on risk assessment for asbestos and other fibrous minerals. He has also published works in the area of the theory of numbers, his favorite area of mathematics.

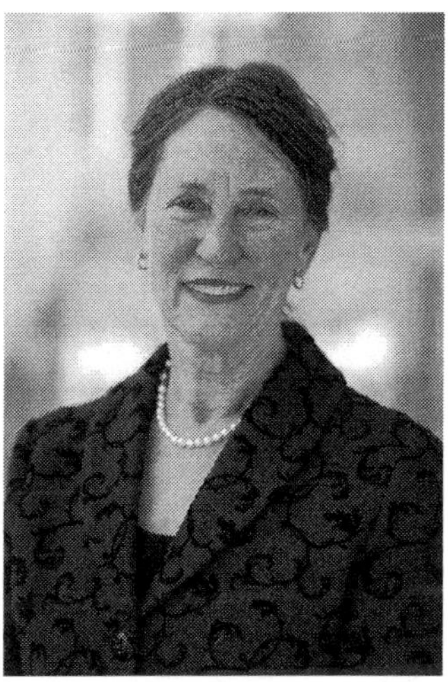

Dr. Ann Wylie, PhD, holds a BA from Wellesley College and a PhD from Columbia University, USA. She joined the faculty at the University of Maryland in 1972, where she has taught courses in optical mineralogy, mineralogy, economic geology, X-ray diffraction, and ore microscopy. She currently holds the rank of Emerita Professor and Distinguished Scholar Teacher in the Department of Geology. She is an elected fellow of the Geological Society of America and the American Association for the Advancement of Science. She is also a senior scientific advisor for Chemistry & Industrial Hygiene, Inc. Her work has been published in both the mineralogical and toxicological literature. She has served as a consultant to both government and industry.

Contributors

Richard Attanoos Consultant Pathologist at University Hospital of Wales, Cardiff, and Professor at the School of Medicine, Cardiff University UK.

Dr. Richard Attanoos qualified in Medicine at Imperial College Medical School, London University, in 1988 and holds a Fellowship of the Royal College of Pathologists, United Kingdom. He presently works as a consultant pathologist at the University Hospital of Wales, Cardiff, and is Honorary Professor at Cardiff University. Dr. Attanoos is an invited member of the United States – Canadian Mesothelioma Reference Panel, International Mesothelioma Panel, and Asbestosis Committee of the College of American Pathologists/Pulmonary Pathology Society. He is an elected International Fellow of the College of American Pathologists. Much of his research work since the late 1980s' has been in the fields of environmental and occupational lung disease, inhaled particles, asbestos, and mesothelioma. Dr. Attanoos has been a medical advisor to the United Nations European Parliament on Mesothelioma, All-Party Parliamentary Committee of the British Government, and Cross-Party Group of the Welsh Assembly Government on the Health Effects of Asbestos. Dr. Attanoos has been a contributing author to the World Health Organisation Classification of Tumours of the Lung, Pleura, Thymus, and Heart (Malignant Mesothelioma), and a contributing author to the International Committee Chemical Safety of Inhaled Silicates and Clay minerals. He has published over 200 peer-reviewed papers in the scientific literature, has more than 30 book chapters, and has one book entitled "Mesothelioma."

Kelly Bailey President at Kelly Bailey Consulting, LLC. USA.

Mr. Kelly Bailey has worked as an industrial hygienist for 50 years, with 36 years in the rock, sand, and gravel mining industry at Vulcan Materials Company, Birmingham, Alabama. He is a graduate of Lamar University in Texas with BS degrees in chemistry and human biology. He is a certified industrial hygienist from the American Academy of Industrial Hygiene and a Fellow of the American Industrial Hygiene Association. Mr. Bailey's specialty is exposure assessment and control of dust, diesel particulate, asphalt fumes, welding fumes, mineral fibers, and noise in the mining and construction industries. He has expertise in establishing occupational health programs in companies, exposure data analysis, and reporting. Mr. Bailey has published many articles on the above topics and presented them numerous times to varied audiences. Since June 2016, Mr. Bailey has been the sole owner of an industrial hygiene consulting firm, Kelly Bailey Consulting, LLC, which assists companies in their establishment of occupational health and industrial hygiene programs, assists mining trade associations in the areas of crystalline silica and naturally occurring asbestos. Mr. Bailey is also co-owner of an industrial hygiene database company, Industrial Hygiene Exposure Management Systems, LLC.

Andrey Korchevskiy Director of Research and Development at Chemistry & Industrial Hygiene, Inc. USA.

Dr. Andrey Korchevskiy, PhD, DABT, CIH, is a diplomate of the American Board of Toxicology (DABT) and a certified industrial hygienist (CIH), USA. He is the Director of Research and Development at Chemistry & Industrial Hygiene, Inc. (C&IH) (Lakewood, Colorado). Dr. Korchevskiy holds separate PhD degrees in Applied Mathematics and Biology. He has over 150 publications in various peer-reviewed journals and was a leading editor and author of a monograph on risk assessment for asbestos and other fibrous minerals. He has also published works in the area of the theory of numbers, his favorite area of mathematics.

Arseniy Korchevskiy Database specialist and statistician at Chemistry & Industrial Hygiene, Inc. USA.

Arseniy Korchevskiy is a statistician and software engineer at Chemistry & Industrial Hygiene, Inc. In recent years, he has published peer-reviewed papers and book chapters on the topics of epidemiological analysis and modeling in toxicology and public health.

Brooke T. Mossman University Distinguished Professor with the Department of Pathology and Laboratory Medicine at the UVM College of Medicine in Burlington Vermont USA.

Brooke T. Mossman, MS, PhD, is a University Distinguished Professor and Professor Emerita at the University of Vermont College of Medicine. She was the Director of the NIEHS-funded Environmental Pathology Program at UVM for 25 years. Her research on biological effects of elongated mineral fibers and silica has been supported by funding from several institutes of the NIH, the EPA, the American Cancer Society, and the Mesothelioma Applied Research Foundation (MARF). She has received a Career Achievement Recognition Award for her scientific accomplishments from the American Thoracic Society, the Wagner Award from the International Mesothelioma Interest Group, and was elected to the Plutocrat Society for excellence in pathology research. She has published more than 325 scientific articles, books, book chapters, and monographs on mineral-induced lung disease. During her research and academic career, she has been appointed to over 100 international and national scientific boards, including the Board of Counselors of the National Cancer Institute, National Institute for Occupational Safety and Health and National Academies of Science.

Dr. Ann Wylie Emerita Professor and Distinguished Scholar Teacher in the Department of Geology USA.

Dr. Ann Wylie, PhD, holds a BA from Wellesley College and a PhD from Columbia University, USA. She joined the faculty at the University of Maryland in 1972, where she has taught courses in optical mineralogy, mineralogy, economic geology, X-ray diffraction, and ore microscopy. She currently holds the rank of Emerita Professor and Distinguished Scholar Teacher in the Department of Geology. She is an elected fellow of the Geological Society of America and the American Association for the Advancement of Science. She is also a senior scientific advisor for Chemistry & Industrial Hygiene, Inc. Her work has been published in both the mineralogical and toxicological literature. She has served as a consultant to both government and industry.

Preface

This book came into existence due to the ongoing public discussions regarding mineral particles and their possible toxic effects. Humanity has been accompanied by numerous toxic agents throughout its evolution and development. Asbestos, one of the most concerning representatives of the category of elongate mineral particles, has been a mineral form known for centuries. The greatest of German poets, J.W. Goethe, related qualities of asbestos to immortality and the vulnerability of human souls:

> We bear the stains of earth,
> And flames that blessed us
> Will give us no rebirth
> As to asbestos.
>
> **(Translated by Andrey Korchevskiy)**

The discovery of asbestos toxicity, and especially carcinogenicity, raised many concerns about the safety of other minerals, especially if they somewhat resembled commercial asbestos. One of the greatest lessons of the last decades, however, is the understanding that characteristics of one toxic agent cannot be automatically transferred to others, even if the resemblance is significant. A famous example is thalidomide, which has two isomers (compounds with identical chemical structures), differing only as mirror reflections of each other. However, one of them is a pharmacological sedative, while the other causes severe birth defects. Compounds such as 1-propanol, 2-propanol, and methoxyethane differ only by arrangements of atoms. At the same time, 2-propanol (rubbing alcohol) has limited toxicity, while methoxyethane is a chronic toxicant with significant health outcomes for humans.

Mineral types of commercial asbestos were selected by geologists and industries for their specific qualities. Amosite, crocidolite, anthophyllite asbestos, chrysotile, and, less commonly, tremolite asbestos and actinolite asbestos were mined and used in various applications for their unique qualities created in nature, including tensile strength, chemical and fire resistance, and the ability to be woven. No man-made material has ever been able to replicate commercial asbestos in its characteristics. The toxicity of asbestos fibers is also unique and contrasts with that of chunky particles composed of the same minerals but produced by fragmentation of rocks, not formed by nature as fibers. Such particles cannot be woven or used for flame protection or insulation. In an old legend, both King Charlemagne and Tsar Peter the Great were presented with a beautiful tablecloth that was thrown into the fire after a lavish dinner: the kings were angered by the profligacy of their hosts but then astonished by the fact that the tablecloth was safely removed from the fire. Not even Merlin the Sorcerer would be able to create a tablecloth from the numerous elongate particles present in the human environment unless they possess the specific qualities of asbestos fibers. The same story applies to asbestos carcinogenicity: not every long mineral particle is asbestos, and not all of them are able to harm human health in the same way.

Even commercial asbestos by itself clearly demonstrates how mineralogy and geological history make various types of elongate particles different in their toxicological effects. Mesothelioma – the deadly neoplasm that remains one of the mysteries of medicine, uncurable even after the many successes of cancer treatment in the last decades – could only be caused by certain elongate mineral particles (asbestos or its close relatives) and not by others. Tobacco smoking does not increase the risk of mesothelioma; crystalline silica is a carcinogen but does not cause cancer of the pleural mesothelial tissue. This means that the body treats elongate particles differently from non-elongate ones. This transition from non-elongate to elongate effects cannot, however, happen instantly: elongate particles must have sufficient deviation from the characteristics of non-elongate structures before their toxicity becomes so different that a new type of cancer (mesothelioma) arises. The current definition of elongate mineral particles (when their larger dimension is at least three times greater than the smallest) is still an insufficient boundary between particle shapes impacting toxicological behavior; other dimensional and structural characteristics also play a role.

Shorter particles are significantly less dangerous, even if they are elongate. Particles with a length of less than 5 μm have been repeatedly demonstrated to act like dust, not like asbestos. Particles longer than 5 μm were first noticed during the analysis of human lungs, when the toxicity of asbestos was discovered. The "red line" seemed arbitrary here (why exactly 5 μm, indeed?), but in reality, this threshold of length appears to reflect the true toxicokinetics and toxicodynamics of elongate structures.

Chrysotile, the so-called white asbestos, is the most widely spread commercial type of asbestos. It is remarkable how significantly chrysotile differs from other types of commercial asbestos. White asbestos belongs to the serpentine mineral group, whereas all other asbestos types belong to the amphibole mineral group. But it is not only its name that makes chrysotile distinct from crocidolite, amosite, or tremolite asbestos. Chrysotile is low in iron by chemical formula, while many amphiboles are known for their abundant iron content. Also, chrysotile is not rigid and has been demonstrated to dissolve quickly in lung fluid or in the interior of macrophages and are readily removed from the lungs. Amphiboles, on the contrary, are generally rigid, stay in human lungs for decades, and are removed slowly by clearance mechanisms. This is why it is not surprising that chrysotile is much less potent for human mesothelioma (as has been demonstrated through human epidemiological data by various authors). These differences show how the mineralogy of particles is reflected in their toxicity.

Talc would be another good example. In some deposits, talc may exist as a fibrous component, detected as elongate particles. However, talc is not asbestos. Being the "softest mineral in earth," talc produces elongate structures of such low rigidity that they appear to be inactive in many biological reactions. Talc structures are not expected to penetrate cell membranes. Even elongate talc is much closer to chrysotile in its biopersistence than to long-lived amphiboles. This is why elongate talc particles cannot increase the risk of mesothelioma in humans, and this fact is very important for risk analysis.

It is essential, therefore, to develop a scientific basis for the analysis of elongate mineral particles. This is the reason this book has been written.

The authors of this book met for the first time in 2019 when they started collaborating on their first paper in co-authorship. Professor Ann Wylie had a long-term career in the geology and mineralogy of asbestos at the time of the meeting. Andrey Korchevskiy was a mathematician and toxicologist with keen interest in quantitative structure-activity relationship (QSAR) modeling, as well as in elongate particles and their complex behavior in the environment and enigmatic biological modes of action. After the publication of their paper in 2020, Ann Wylie and Andrey Korchevskiy published more than 15 peer-reviewed papers together, prepared numerous presentations, and collaborated with scientists from around the world, studying the important topic: mineralogical principles of the toxicology of elongate mineral particles. In 2024, work on this book started, bringing a new level of understanding to the toxicology of elongation.

The authors hope that the book will find its readers, but also that some of the ideas in the book will result in practical applications. As emphasized above, elongate particles are abundant in nature. If every elongate structure were to be regulated as asbestos, there would be no human activity that could proceed given the high carcinogenic potential of asbestos. The best public policy should focus on establishing strict regulations for dangerous agents in the environment. But these agents should be evaluated properly and excluded from regulations if the facts regarding their toxicity are not substantiated. The scientific results in this book, as the authors believe, fully support the current understanding of the existence of two categories of elongate particles – asbestiform and non-asbestiform – that has been developed by regulators. In particular, the International Agency for Cancer Research (IARC) clearly stated that their conclusion regarding asbestos carcinogenicity does not relate to the non-asbestos habit of particles. In the United States, the Occupational Safety and Health Administration (OSHA) has also deregulated non-asbestiform mineral particles in their standards. Our book should bring additional arguments to support the steps taken by IARC and OSHA and demonstrate that they remain scientifically valid even after decades of toxicological studies.

The authors acknowledge the National Stone, Sand, and Gravel Association (NSSGA) for their support in creating the dimensional database used for the preparation of this book. It should be noted that NSSGA has never impacted the database and was not consulted on any aspects of its use in our studies. NSSGA never provided a single dataset for inclusion in the database, and the content of this book was never reviewed by NSSGA prior to publication. No money was received by the authors from NSSGA or other sources for writing chapters of this book.

Also, although the authors have participated in litigation matters as consultants or experts, they declare that this work did not affect the preparation of this book. The scientific truth and knowledge-based protection of public health were the only driving forces for the authorship team.

The authors would like to emphasize the great contributions made by several renowned collaborators who prepared chapters included in the book. In particular, Dr. Brooke T. Mossman wrote a review of toxicological mechanisms defining the role of various dimensional characteristics in the development of asbestos-related cancers. Kelly Bailey co-authored a chapter on the Boulder City Bypass project, providing a unique vision on the topic from the environmental and occupational hygiene points of view. Dr. Richard Attanoos contributed to the chapter on asbestos lung concentrations. Arseniy Korchevskiy supported database development and statistical modeling.

The authors would also like to thank the National Institute of Occupational Safety and Health (NIOSH), fellow scientists, and students whose time was spent on the laborious task of measuring elongate particles by electron microscopy. Without their willingness to share their data, this book would not have been possible.

Dr. David Weill was also instrumental in advising the authors on topics related to the human respiratory system and approaches to its modeling.

Debbie Vaughan made a significant contribution in preparing the book materials for publication and supporting the authors in their work. In general, Chemistry & Industrial Hygiene, Inc. provided comprehensive support and assistance for the development of this book, remaining one of the best think tanks in toxicology and industrial hygiene in the USA and internationally. We also acknowledge the Geology Department of the University of Maryland, where Dr. Wylie continues to serve as Professor Emerita.

Also, the authors are grateful to Taylor & Francis and specifically to James Hobbs and Becky Lane for recognizing the importance of this topic and making this publication possible.

The authors are specifically grateful to our families, who were a source of incredible support for our work, extending far beyond the regular daily hours.

The book is intended for industrial hygienists, toxicologists, epidemiologists, mineralogists, attorneys and paralegals, public health professionals, pathologists, and every scientist and practitioner interested in the health effects of asbestos and other fibrous minerals. The authors believe that the book will be relevant for the efforts of public health risk assessment, regulatory policy, and for determining the mode of action of asbestiform fibers in producing mesothelial cancer as a possible key to improving medical treatment approaches and for finding a cure for mesothelioma.

Andrey Korchevskiy, PhD, DABT, CIH

Ann Wylie, PhD, Professor Emerita

Dimensions matter! Introduction

Mineral fibers are a natural component of the physical environment in many places in the world. For thousands of years, humans have utilized mineral fibers for their amazing characteristics. They are called "fibers" because of their specific shape – long, thin, and strong, resembling organic fiber. Asbestos is a major example of the fibrous form.

It took decades for people to realize that commercial asbestos was not only a valuable commodity but also a significant hazard to human health. Several decades of studies were required to reach the understanding that various subtypes of mineral fiber express very different qualities, some of which are highly relevant for toxicological impact in animals and humans. This led scientists to the idea of distinguishing between naturally grown asbestiform fibers and mechanically generated elongate particles, named "cleavage" or non-asbestiform fragments.

For a better understanding of the types of particles that will be discussed in this book, we prepared the following chart demonstrated in Figure 0.1. (The authors are grateful to Monica McGrath-Koerner for her participation in the creation of the chart.)

The chart shows that elongate mineral particles coexist in the environment with non-asbestiform particles. The category of elongate mineral particles includes asbestiform particles and elongate cleavage fragments, produced by fragmentation (comminution), as well as a third category represented by elongate single crystals. Asbestiform particles include asbestos and other mineral types of elongate structures. Cleavage fragments, in turn, can be elongate and non-elongate. Non-asbestiform particles comprise cleavage fragments and other types of dust unrelated to asbestos.

When considering the health effects of inhaled mineral particulates aerosolized by the disturbance of rock or soil, the minerals most often studied are quartz for silicosis and elongated particles of amphibole and serpentine for asbestos-related diseases. By the very use of the term "elongate," dimensions become central to the study of the carcinogenicity of asbestos.

One of the most important examples can be made based on the studies of amphiboles. Amphiboles are a group of common rock-forming minerals found in rock covering vast expanses of Earth's crust. Amphibole is common in the waste rock of metal and industrial mineral mines alike. Amphibole is an excellent mineral group for studying the health effects of silicate mineral aerosols because it can accommodate by substitution all the major elements that make up Earth's crust, presenting a broad range of chemical variability among occurrences. In dusts, it is found as elongate particles, also in a wide range of sizes and shapes, often designated by "aspect ratio," defined as length divided by width. Some variation in morphology is

DOI: 10.1201/9781003424277-1

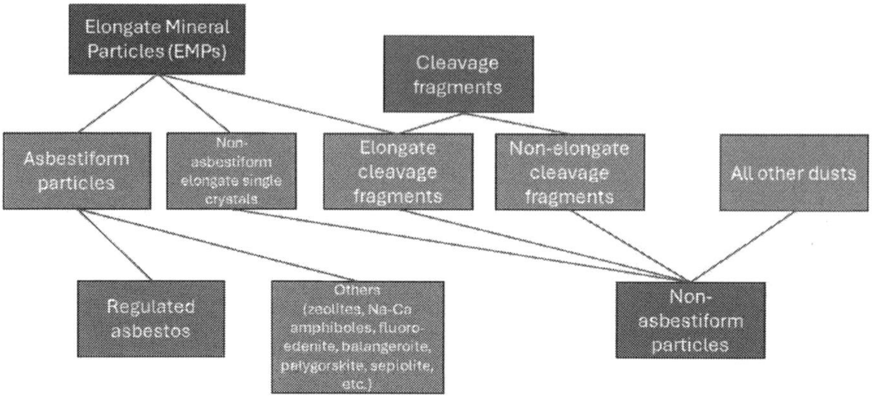

FIGURE 0.1 Different types of mineral particles

related to chemical variability, but almost any composition can be found somewhere on Earth both as asbestiform fiber and as massive rock that forms elongated particles when crushed. The double-chain silicate structure is rigid and durable, and, although there are variabilities in solubility rates with composition, which may affect potency, dissolution rates overall are slow enough in the human lungs that once deposited in the alveolar regions, their impact can continue for much of a person's life, as reflected in the long latency period for mesothelioma. The fact that these are very common minerals and that they occur naturally with a large range in physical form (with variable health outcomes following exposure) makes them ideal for understanding the role of dimensions in the carcinogenesis of rigid, durable silicate and oxide minerals generally. For example, from what we now know about the carcinogenic properties of amphibole asbestos, it is obvious why Wagner et al. (1985) found wooly erionite from Turkey and Oregon to be so potently mesothelioma-genic: it is durable, asbestiform, and the fibers are narrower than 0.2 μm.

Serpentine, on the other hand, is a sheet silicate of very restricted chemical composition. In its massive form, it is valued as a road aggregate because of its uniformity and toughness. Serpentine fibers are formed from silica and magnesium hydroxide sheets rolled into tubes, forming the serpentine mineral chrysotile. The fibers formed are not rigid, and they are soluble enough in the lung that their impact on a healthy lung is short-lived. Because the health effects observed following inhalation of serpentine asbestos are different from those of amphibole asbestos, differences in their physical and chemical properties provide insight into the mechanisms of fiber carcinogenesis. Other sheet silicates are known to form fibers (halloysite, talc, attapulgite, and sepiolite), but we will not discuss them in this book in detail because they do not appear to have health effects comparable to asbestos.[1]

It should be noted that the dimensions of elongate mineral particles have been implicated as the primary reasons for their carcinogenic potency. Numerous studies have addressed the dimensional characteristics of fibers to assess their toxicity in general and carcinogenicity in particular (Timbrell, 1965; Timbrell et al., 1971, 1988;

Stanton et al., 1981; Berman et al., 1995; Oberdörster et al., 2005; Berman & Crump, 2008b; Lippmann, 2009; Loomis et al., 2010; Barlow et al., 2017; Asgharian et al., 2018; Di Giuseppe et al., 2021; Militello et al., 2021). There is general agreement among these researchers that it is the long, narrow fibers in the dust exposure that are the carcinogens. By long, these researchers generally mean L > 5 μm or L > 10 μm or more, and by narrow, W ≤ 0.1 μm to W ≤ 0.5 μm.

The authors would like to emphasize that the work included in this book has a significant difference from many other studies in the field because of the significant role that has been given to human epidemiological data. Most previous works in the field were based on animal experiments, and the question of direct applicability to humans remains. Our approach should provide more specificity in what "long, narrow" really means for the carcinogenic potency of durable mineral fiber in humans, because we prioritized the data on mesothelioma potency in human cohorts. The groundbreaking work of Hodgson and Darnton (2000) (updated by Darnton in 2023, 2024) showed that the risk for mesothelioma and lung cancer varies among asbestos occurrences at the same exposure level. The results of Hodgson and Darnton were confirmed by similar meta-analyses performed later by Berman and Crump (2008a, 2008b) and by Garbrant and Pastula (2018). This information is critical in understanding the carcinogenic potential of elongate minerals. We specifically addressed the issue of "epidemiology first" in mesothelioma studies in our letter to the editor published in 2022 (Wylie & Korchevskiy, 2022). At the same time, we demonstrate in this book that epidemiological data are supported by other sources of information; in particular, by a theoretical model of asbestos toxicity, by experimental data on carbon nanotubes, and by quantitative structure-activity modeling (QSAR) that includes dimensions, chemical composition, and other characteristics of EMPs to establish essential differences between their subtypes.

In general, the toxicity of asbestos is considered to be related to its peculiar mineralogical qualities. As we noted previously in our paper (Wylie & Korchevskiy, 2023), in the first publication on lung fibrosis caused by inhalation of asbestos dust, Cooke (1924) noted various sizes and shapes of asbestos particles in the lung sections of exposed workers, emphasizing that "the size varies from 393.6 to 3 microns in length." King et al. (1946) first reported that the effect of asbestos in laboratory animals depends on the length. In particular, the author suggested that the fibers with low length (< 2.5 μm) were expected to be fully removed from the lungs, while longer fibers cause the fibrotic reaction. Wagner et al. (1960) in their pioneering paper on the asbestos-related etiology of mesothelioma emphasized that the suspected agent was the "fibrous" form. Timbrell (1965), exploring the deposition of asbestos fibers in the lungs and the reasons why longer fibers can be found in the human alveoli vs. spherical particles that usually are limited in size, stated that "[t]he fibers most likely to be retained are those fibers that penetrate deeply before being deposited, namely those fibers most likely to escape deposition by inertial precipitation and sedimentation, namely those fibers of lowest falling speed, or smallest diameter."

Various experimental studies have been performed exploring the dependence of the toxicity of elongate particles on their size, shaping the overall idea that long, thin particles are more toxic. Timbrell et al. (1971) proposed that the lower incidence of mesothelioma among those exposed to amosite ore and milled products compared to the overwhelming number among those similarly exposed to crocidolite was due to the narrower width of most crocidolite fibers.

Association of toxicity with dimension has been known since the 1970s. For example, based on experiments on animals, in estimates published by Pott (1978), the most biologically active fibers were those with L > 10 µm, W ≤ 0.25 µm, and Stanton et al. (1981) associated maximum potency for carcinoma with particles with L > 8 and W < 0.25µm. Several later analyses of the Stanton studies pointed out that dimensional variability alone could not fully explain the observations (Dunnigan, 1984; Kane, 1991; Wylie et al., 1987). Stanton et al. (1981) also noted that some of the implanted fibrous samples resulted in highly unexpected outcomes, showing both higher and lower tumor responses than their model predicted, and suggested that rigidity and chemical composition might be important components of toxicity.

The length of fibers has been treated as the main predictor of toxicity in various studies (see the review in Barlow et al., 2017), in particular because of the ability of longer structures to produce so-called macrophage frustration (with alveolar macrophage size in humans estimated as 21.2 ± 0.3 µm) (Krombach et al., 1997) that relates to the inability of the pulmonary macrophages to fully engulf them. Tilkes and Beck (1980) demonstrated by *in vitro* and *in vivo* tests that the toxicity of asbestos and man-made mineral particles increased with increasing length. At the same time, Bertrand and Pezerat (1980) earlier argued that the predictor of fiber carcinogenicity is actually the aspect ratio, and it is "not possible to separate the effects of the two variables, length and diameter." Bonneau et al. (1986) also named aspect ratio, along with the "nature of the mineral," as two parameters defining the carcinogenic potency of a solid particle.

The small diameter of fibers, however, was found to impact fiber potency significantly. Muhle et al. (1987) pointed out that long, durable fibers (including man-made varieties) with a diameter of less than 1 µm are the most potent for cancer after intraperitoneal injection. Wylie et al. (1993) reviewed the available dimensional information and demonstrated that width is an important variable for determining the potency of asbestos fibers for mesothelioma. Recent work has also shown that specific surface area (per unit of weight or volume), which in general terms can be considered as negatively proportional to the diameter of fibers, correlates strongly with cellular reaction and cancer potency (Oberdörster et al., 2005; Korchevskiy & Wylie, 2022). The biological nature of this relationship could be twofold: the fibers with small widths are more potent (for example, because particles with smaller widths have smaller aerodynamic diameters to penetrate deeper into the respiratory system), and they also have the highest specific surface area as a secondary characteristic; or fibers with large specific surfaces are more reactive and therefore potent, but they also have smaller widths.

Berman and Crump (2008b) performed a study to evaluate cancer potency for selected "protocols," or dimensional categories of chrysotile and amphibole fibers. Berman and Crump concluded that fiber size and mineral type impact their potency. The average amphibole potency derived from the model decreased with increasing fiber width cutpoints for mesothelioma and lung cancer. The "long, lowest width" category had the highest average cancer potency. It was suggested that fibers longer than 10 μm are predictive of cancer potency, and the difference in potency of the shorter fibers (5 μm < length < 10 μm) is highly statistically significant. Fibers shorter than 5 μm were not considered to be carcinogenic. The mesothelioma potency of chrysotile was found to be not significantly different from 0. It is noteworthy that Berman and Crump used very limited dimensional information for the fiber exposure in the epidemiological cohorts. For the 16 cohorts considered in their study, Berman and Crump used 9 size distributions of asbestos fibers, often not specifically corresponding to the exposure of a specific cohort but assessed as fitting the best according to the information available. Berman and Crump emphasized the limitation of their study caused by a lack of dimensional information, especially regarding the distribution of fiber width.

The lung fiber burden of the general population, as well as of persons with disease, also provides information about the dimensionality determinants of cancer potency. Lung burden is a function of the exposure and clearance mechanisms, and it allows for a retrospective reconstruction of the retained portions of exposure and prediction of risks. Also, the fiber burden results from the dimensions of the fibers that make it up, though no consistent length- and width-dependent models for toxicity have been proposed based on lung burden (Rasmuson et al., 2014; Moolgavkar et al., 2001; Rodilla et al., 2022).

One important aspect of the studies on dimensionality and cancer risk is the recognition of the differences in cancer potency between asbestiform and non-asbestiform particles at the same level of exposure, as measured in f/cc-years. Asbestiform habit refers to the morphology of minerals that have been naturally crystallized to be easily separated into long, thin, flexible, and durable fibers, whose narrow widths and other physical and chemical characteristics make them biopersistent and toxic (Veblen & Wylie, 1993). Although some wide, brittle cleavage forms exist in nature, the elongate non-asbestiform particles of concern in inhalation are produced by mechanical forces during mining and comminution from massive minerals – the same minerals that can form as asbestos elsewhere; however, non-asbestiform mineral particles do not have the characteristics associated with the adverse health effects of asbestos, and they resemble nuisance dust more than asbestiform fibers (NRC, 1984). Non-asbestiform particles have been demonstrated to be significantly less toxic than asbestiform particles and apparently non-carcinogenic. For example, asbestiform particles were shown to be more cytotoxic in a recent NIOSH study (Khaliullin et al., 2020). Mossman (2008) suggested that the available studies concluded that non-asbestiform elongate particles (cleavage fragments) are less bioreactive and cytotoxic than asbestiform fibers. Gamble and Gibbs (2008) demonstrated that exposure to non-asbestiform amphiboles is not associated with elevated cancer risk. Garabrant and Pastula (2018) showed in their epidemiological study that non-asbestiform elongate mineral exposures are likely of low or non-existent mesothelioma potency.

We have recently published several new studies focused on the dimensionality of elongate mineral particles in relationship to their toxicity. In particular, a unique database of dimensional parameters for elongate mineral particles was assembled. The representativeness of the database is characterized in Wylie et al. (2022). The relationships between mesothelioma and lung cancer potency factors and several dimensional predictors, including fiber width and specific surface area, have been determined (Wylie et al., 2020; Korchevskiy & Wylie, 2021, 2022; Wylie & Korchevskiy, 2023). Recently, a new metric (dimensional coefficient of carcinogenicity) was proposed to predict mesothelial potency of elongate mineral particles (Korchevskiy & Wylie, 2025a, 2025b). Korchevskiy et al. (2019) demonstrated that mesothelioma potency factors of amphibole and chrysotile fibers can be modeled as a function of their chemical composition (iron, magnesium, and silicon oxide content) and aspect ratio. We will discuss these findings throughout the book.

This book is intended to lead the reader through various aspects of the dimensionality of elongate mineral particles as one of the major predictors of their toxicological potential. The first important question of what a fiber is will be addressed. Confusion and misunderstanding in the use of this term have introduced an unnecessary problem into the asbestos literature, and a thorough discussion of this term will be provided. Different dimensional definitions of a fiber will be compared and evaluated to introduce difficult issues of setting up a criterial base for determining the mineralogical and toxicological properties of elongate mineral particles.

The origin of "elongation" in minerals will be discussed, including ideas about how and where fibrous minerals form in nature. The reader will find out what "fibrous ice" is and will be able to understand how amphibole, serpentine, and zeolite mineral fibers were formed, producing the outcrops of asbestos and other asbestiform minerals, and, in general, where such occurrences might be expected to be found.

The book will lead readers through the basics of risk assessment for asbestos and other elongate mineral particles. A state-of-the-art description will be given regarding the approaches for hazard identification, exposure assessment, dose-response assessment, and risk characterization for asbestos. It will be demonstrated how epidemiological data can be utilized for risk quantification in applications not only to different mineral types of fibers but also to their dimensions. Several practical examples will be given to help readers better understand the modeling approach, risk quantification, and interpretation of the risk evaluation results.

The dimensional characteristics of various mineral fibers will be described in detail. Readers will learn how to interpret major dimensionality metrics such as length, width (diameter), specific surface area, aerodynamic diameter, fibrosity index, and others. Various central tendency dimensional characteristics of fibers will be provided for different mineral types, habits, and occurrences of EMPs.

The authors will demonstrate how dimensional metrics of elongate mineral particles correlate with their mesotheliogenic potency. Unique data on the correlation between dimensional characteristics and the carcinogenicity of fibers will be demonstrated. It will be shown how the strongest predictors of potency can be selected and used to characterize the toxicity of fibers.

Quantitative structure-activity relationship (QSAR) modeling will be used to develop regression equations that allow for the prediction of the toxicity of elongate mineral particles (EMPs) with various characteristics. Readers will see how unknown toxicological information can be reconstructed for fibers lacking toxicological data.

Methods of classification for elongate mineral particles will be explored. It will be shown that the dimensions of particles can be used to effectively distinguish between samples with asbestiform and non-asbestiform habits.

The authors will also discuss the habit of mineral particles as one of the important predictors of potency. It will be shown that the non-asbestiform type of elongate particles (resembling their asbestiform counterparts by mineral composition) is not expected to produce elevated rates of cancer in laboratory animals or in humans. This important conclusion has clear implications for many industrial areas where elongate particles are produced by mechanical forces, rather than by long-term geological growth.

The behavior of elongate mineral particles in the lungs will be discussed from the position of their dimensions. The clearance models will be demonstrated to show how the size of elongate mineral particles impacts their lung distribution.

Epidemiological aspects of fiber mineralogy will be discussed. It will be shown how mixtures of different types of fibers can change their combined potency. The example of elongate mineral particles at the Boulder Bypass project will be used to show the effects of mixed exposure to workers and communities, as well as the practical application of risk-based analysis.

The authors will also describe the implications of their findings for the regulations regarding elongate mineral particle exposure. To fully protect workers, it is important to distinguish extremely dangerous types of EMPs (like asbestiform crocidolite) from those with limited carcinogenic potency (like non-asbestiform riebeckite) and to design monitoring systems that can detect and measure carcinogenic EMPs.

Is exposure to just one fiber able to cause mesothelioma in humans? The authors will show how this question can be answered from the position of risk assessment science. Recommendations to make the regulatory environment more scientific and more protective for workers will be provided in the final chapter of the book.

The authors would like to emphasize that they specifically focused on mesothelioma (pleural or peritoneal) as a toxic endpoint for risk analysis. There are other cancers potentially caused by elongate particles, and there are non-malignant conditions (like pleural plaques or asbestosis) that can be explored separately. It might be a topic for another study that is yet to be planned.

There are obvious limitations in the studies included in this book. The information on epidemiology related to cancer in workers and populations exposed to elongate mineral particles is very limited. It is remarkable that various approaches yield similar conclusions, even if data are scarce. Also, one of the purposes of the overall study comprised in this book was to create a better source of data for current and future studies in the area of mineralogy, toxicology, and risk assessment for elongate particles.

The authors intend to express various approaches to the interpretation of the available data on asbestos toxicity. In particular, Chapters 4 and 5 provide apparently different explanations of asbestos mode of action in mesothelioma. It can be seen, however, that current theories on mesothelioma induction are not contradictory. All of them require the involvement of several counteracting factors (like, mutagenesis vs. repair mechanisms or cytotoxicity vs. immortalization of cells), explaining why the probability of mesothelioma is comparatively low even in individuals historically exposed to high concentrations of commercial asbestos.

We perceive a new outburst of scientific developments for the risk analysis of elongate mineral particles. A better terminological basis will help to understand the classification of elongate particles. New methods and standards for the classification of particles will be developed. Toxicological studies of asbestiform particles will become better designed and focused on the drivers of differences in carcinogenicity among various types of elongate structures.

The results of lung burden analysis will be widely published to demonstrate the mechanisms of deposition and clearance of elongate mineral particles. We hope that this book will provide a basis and potential guidance for multi-disciplinary studies in this area.

We also anticipate that the regulatory environment for all kinds of mineral particles will be significantly improved. The situation in which all types of asbestos are regulated in a similar way is clearly counterproductive. There is a trend to indefinitely expand the list of carcinogens, forgetting that quantitative assessment is the essence of risk assessment and solid toxicological science. Instead of unqualified lists of human carcinogens, international organizations should start publishing risk analyses of various agents, where quantitative information on their relative potency will be provided for decision-makers. Otherwise, in the end, every molecule of a chemical agent and every dust particle can be announced carcinogenic. No science can support such an approach.

We envision a future where the cure for the most serious respiratory diseases, like mesothelioma, will be found. To make this possible, it is essential to understand why various particles have different potencies to produce adverse health outcomes. Even if our book makes a very small step in this direction, we would be grateful to take this road.

NOTE

1 Oxides also form respirable fibers, as can the framework silicate zeolites such as erionite. Models to include other mineralogical characteristics that could extend potency modeling across silicate fibers generally are needed.

REFERENCE LIST

Asgharian, B., Owen, T. P., Kuempel, E. D., & Jarabek, A. M. (2018). Dosimetry of inhaled elongate mineral particles in the respiratory tract: The impact of shape factor. *Toxicology and Applied Pharmacology*, *361*, 27–35. https://doi.org/10.1016/j.taap.2018.05.001

Barlow, C. A., Grespin, M., & Best, E. A. (2017). Asbestos fiber length and its relation to disease risk. *Inhalation Toxicology*, *29*(12–14), 541–554. https://doi.org/10.1080/08958378.2018.1435756

Berman, D. W., & Crump, K. S. (2008a). Update of potency factors for asbestos-related lung cancer and mesothelioma. *Critical Reviews in Toxicology*, *38*(Suppl 1), 1–47. https://doi.org/10.1080/10408440802276167

Berman, D. W., & Crump, K. S. (2008b). A meta-analysis of asbestos-related cancer risk that addresses fiber size and mineral type. *Critical Reviews in Toxicology*, *38*(Supp 1), 49–73. https://doi.org/10.1080/10408440802273156

Berman, D. W., Crump, K. S., Chatfield, E. J., Davis, J. M. G., & Jones, A. D. (1995). The sizes, shapes, and mineralogy of asbestos structures that induce lung tumors or mesothelioma in AF/HAN rats following inhalation. *Risk Analysis*, *15*(2), 181–195. https://doi.org/10.1111/j.1539-6924.1995.tb00312.x

Bertrand, R., & Pezerat, H. (1980). Fibrous glass: Carcinogenicity and dimensional characteristics. *IARC Scientific Publications*, *30*, 901–911.

Bonneau, L., Malard, C., & Pezerat, H., 1986. Studies on surface properties of asbestos. II: Role of dimensional characteristics and surface properties of mineral fibers in the induction of pleural tumors. *Environmental Research*, *41*(1), 268–275. https://doi.org/10.1016/s0013-9351(86)80188-8

Cooke, W. E. (1924). Fibrosis of the lungs due to the inhalation of asbestos dust. *British Medical Journal*, *2*(3317), 147. https://doi.org/10.1136/bmj.2.3317.147

Darnton, L. (2023). Quantitative assessment of mesothelioma and lung cancer risk based on phase contrast microscopy (PCM) estimates of fibre exposure: An update of 2000 asbestos cohort data. *Environmental Research*, *230*, 114753. https://doi.org/10.1016/j.envres.2022.114753

Darnton, L. (2024). The Hodgson and Darnton approach to quantifying the risks of mesothelioma and lung cancer in relation to asbestos exposure. In A. Korchevskiy, J. Rasmuson, & E. Rasmuson (Eds.), *Health risk assessment for asbestos and other fibrous minerals* (pp. 233–269). John Wiley & Sons, Inc. https://doi.org/10.1002/9781119438397

Di Giuseppe, D., Perchiazzi, N., Brunelli, D., Giovanardi, T., Nodari, L., Della Ventura, G., Malferrari, D., Maia, M., & Gualtieri, A. F. (2021). Occurrence and characterization of tremolite asbestos from the Mid Atlantic Ridge. *Scientific Reports*, *11*, 6285. https://doi.org/10.1038/s41598-021-85576-w

Dunnigan, J. (1984). Biological effects of fibers: Stanton's hypothesis revisited. *Environmental Health Perspectives*, *57*, 333–337. https://doi.org/10.1289/ehp.8457333

Gamble, J. F., & Gibbs, G. W. (2008). An evaluation of the risks of lung cancer and mesothelioma from exposure to amphibole cleavage fragments. *Regulatory Toxicology and Pharmacology*, *52*(1 Suppl), S154–S186. https://doi.org/10.1016/j.yrtph.2007.09.020

Garabrant, D. H., & Pastula, S. T. (2018). A comparison of asbestos fiber potency and elongate mineral particle (EMP) potency for mesothelioma in humans. *Toxicology and Applied Pharmacology*, *361*, 127–136. https://doi.org/10.1016/j.taap.2018.07.003

Hodgson, J. T., & Darnton, A. (2000). The quantitative risks of mesothelioma and lung cancer in relation to asbestos exposure. *Annals of Occupational Hygiene*, *44*(8), 565–601.

Kane, A. B. (1991). Fiber dimensions and mesothelioma: A reappraisal of the Stanton hypothesis. In R. C. Brown, J. A. Hoskins, & N. F. Johnson (Eds.), *Mechanisms in fibre carcinogenesis*. NATO ASI Series (Vol. 223). Springer. https://doi.org/10.1007/978-1-4684-1363-2_14

Khaliullin, T. O., Kisin, E. R., Guppi, S., Yanamala, N., Zhernovkov, V., & Shvedova, A. A. (2020). Differential responses of murine alveolar macrophages to elongate mineral particles of asbestiform and non-asbestiform varieties: Cytotoxicity, cytokine secretion and transcriptional changes. *Toxicology and Applied Pharmacology*, *409*, 115302. https://doi.org/10.1016/j.taap.2020.115302

King, E. J., Clegg, J. W., & Rae, V. M. (1946). The effect of asbestos, and of asbestos and aluminum, on the lungs of rabbits. *Thorax*, *1*(3), 188–197. https://doi.org/10.1136/thx.1.3.188

Korchevskiy, A. A., Rasmuson, J. O., & Rasmuson, E. J. (2019). Empirical model of mesothelioma potency factors for different mineral fibers based on their chemical composition and dimensionality. *Inhalation Toxicology*, *31*(5), 180–191. https://doi.org/10.1080/08958378.2019.1640320

Korchevskiy, A. A., & Wylie, A. G. (2021). Dimensional determinants for the carcinogenic potency of elongate amphibole particles. *Inhalation Toxicology*, *33*(6–8), 244–259. https://doi.org/10.1080/08958378.2021.1971340

Korchevskiy, A. A., & Wylie, A. G. (2022). Dimensional characteristics of the major types of amphibole mineral particles and the implications for carcinogenic risk assessment. *Inhalation Toxicology*, *34*(1–2), 24–38. https://doi.org/10.1080/08958378.2021.2024304.

Korchevskiy, A. A., & Wylie, A. G. (2025a). Habit of elongate amphibole particles as a predictor of mesothelial carcinogenicity. *Toxicology Reports*, *14*, 101908. https://doi.org/10.1016/j.toxrep.2025.101908

Korchevskiy, A. A., & Wylie, A. G. (2025b, April 24). The empirical metric of mesothelial carcinogenicity for carbon nanotubes and elongate mineral particles. *Inhalation Toxicology* (online). https://doi.org/10.1080/08958378.2025.2486087

Krombach, F., Münzing, S., Allmeling, A. M., Gerlach, J. T., Behr, J., & Dörger, M. (1997). Cell size of alveolar macrophages: An interspecies comparison. *Environmental Health Perspectives*, *105*(Suppl 5), 1261–1263. https://doi.org/10.1289/ehp.97105s51261

Lippmann, M. (2009). *Environmental toxicants: Human exposures and their health effects* (3rd ed.). John Wiley & Sons, Inc.

Loomis, D., Dement, J., Richardson, D., & Wolf, S. (2010). Asbestos fibre dimensions and lung cancer mortality among workers exposed to chrysotile. *Occupational & Environmental Medicine*, *67*(9), 580–584. https://doi.org/10.1136/oem.2009.050120

Militello, G. M., Gaggero, L., & La Maestra, S. (2021). Asbestiform amphiboles and cleavage fragments analogues: Overview of critical dimensions, aspect ratios, exposure and health effects. *Minerals*, *11*, 525. https://doi.org/10.3390/min11050525

Moolgavkar, S. H., Brown, R. C., & Turim, J. (2001). Biopersistence, fiber length, and cancer risk assessment for inhaled fibers. *Inhalation Toxicology*, *13*(9), 755–772. https://doi.org/10.1080/08958370121106

Mossman, B. T. (2008). Assessment of the pathogenic potential of asbestiform vs. non-asbestiform particulates (cleavage fragments) in in vitro (cell or organ culture) models and bioassays. *Regulatory Toxicology & Pharmacology*, *52*(Suppl 1), S200–S203. https://doi.org/10.1016/j.yrtph.2007.10.004

Muhle, H., Pott, F., Bellmann, B., Takenaka, S., & Ziem, U. (1987). Inhalation and injection experiments in rats to test the carcinogenicity of MMMF. *Annals of Occupational Hygiene*, *31*(4B), 755–764. https://doi.org/10.1093/annhyg/31.4B.755ell

National Research Council, Committee on Nonoccupational Health Risks of Asbestiform Fibers (NRC). (1984). Asbestiform fibers: Nonoccupational health risks. In *Asbestiform fibers: historical background, terminology, and physicochemical properties* (Vol. 2). National Academies Press (US). https://www.ncbi.nlm.nih.gov/books/NBK216753/

Oberdörster, G., Oberdörster, E., & Oberdörster, J. (2005). Nanotoxicology: An emerging discipline evolving from studies of ultrafine particles. *Environmental Health Perspectives*, *113*(7), 823–839. https://doi.org/10.1289/ehp.7339

Pott, F. (1978). Some aspects on the dosimetry of the carcinogenic potency of asbestos and other fibrous dusts. *Staub-Reinhaltung der Luft*, *38*, 486–490.

Rasmuson, J. O., Roggli, V. L., Boelter, F. W., Rasmuson, E. J., & Redinger, C. F. (2014). Cumulative Retrospective Exposure Assessment (REA) as a predictor of amphibole asbestos lung burden: Validation procedures and results for industrial hygiene and pathology estimates. *Inhalation Toxicology*, *26*(1), 1–13. https://doi.org/10.3109/08958378.2013.845273

Rodilla, J., Cerrada, B., Pujadas, C., Delclos, G., & Benavides, F. (2022). Fiber burden and asbestos-related diseases: An umbrella review. *Gaceta Sanitaria*, *36*(2), 173–183. https://doi.org/10.1016/j.gaceta.2021.04.001

Stanton, M. F., Layard, M., Tegeris, A., Miller, E., May, M., Morgan, E., & Smith, A. (1981). Relation of particle dimension to carcinogenicity in amphibole asbestos and other fibrous minerals. *Journal of the National Cancer Institute*, *67*(5), 965–975.

Tilkes, F., & Beck, E. G. (1980). Comparison of length-dependent cytotoxicity of inhalable asbestos and man-made mineral fibres. *IARC Scientific Publication*, *30*, 475–483.

Timbrell, V. (1965). Human exposure to asbestos: Dust controls and standards. The inhalation of fibrous dusts. *Annals of the New York Academy of Sciences*, *132*(1), 255–273. http://dx.doi.org/10.1111/j.1749-6632.1965.tb41107.x

Timbrell, V., Ashcroft, T., Goldstein, B., Heyworth, F., Meurman, L. O., Rendall, R. E. G., Reynolds, J. A., Shilkin, K. B., & Whitaker, D. (1988). Relationships between retained amphibole fibres and fibrosis in human lung tissue specimens. *Annals of Occupational Hygiene*, *32*, 323–340. https://doi.org/10.1093/annhyg/32.inhaled_particles_VI.323

Timbrell, V., Griffiths, D. M., & Pooley, F. D. (1971). Possible biological importance of fibre diameters of South African amphiboles. *Nature*, *232*, 55–56. https://doi.org/10.1038/232055a0

Veblen, D. R., & Wylie, A. G. (1993). *Mineralogy of amphiboles and 1:1 layer silicates* (OSTI ID: 47843). Mineralogical Society of America.

Wagner, J. C., Skidmore, J. W., Hill, R. J., & Griffiths, D. M. (1985). Erionite exposure and mesotheliomas in rats. *British Journal of Cancer*, *51*(5), 727–730. https://doi.org/10.1038/bjc.1985.108

Wagner, J. C., Sleggs, C. A., & Marchand, P. (1960). Diffuse pleural mesothelioma and asbestos exposure in the North Western Cape province. *British Journal of Industrial Medicine*, *17*, 260–271. https://doi.org/10.1136/oem.17.4.260

Wylie, A. G., Bailey, K. F., Kelse, J. W., & Lee, R. J. (1993). The importance of width in asbestos fiber carcinogenicity and its implications for public policy. *American Industrial Hygiene Association Journal*, *54*(5), 239–252. https://doi.org/10.1080/15298669391354621

Wylie, A. G., & Korchevskiy, A. (2022). Letter to the editor: Epidemiology holds a key to the validation of toxicological models for elongate mineral particles. *Current Research in Toxicology*, *3*, 100062. https://doi.org/10.1016%2Fj.crtox.2021.100062

Wylie, A. G., & Korchevskiy, A. A. (2023). Dimensions of elongate mineral particles and cancer: A review. *Environmental Research*, *230*, 114688. https://doi.org/10.1016/j.envres.2022.114688

Wylie, A. G., Korchevskiy, A. A., Segrave, A. M., & Duane, A. (2020). Modeling mesothelioma risk factors from amphibole fiber dimensionality: Mineralogical and epidemiological perspective. *Journal of Applied Toxicology*, *40*(4), 515–524. https://doi.org/10.1002/jat.3923

Wylie, A. G., Korchevskiy, A. A., Van Orden, D. R., & Chatfield, E. J. (2022). Discriminant analysis of asbestiform and non-asbestiform amphibole particles and its implications for toxicological studies. *Computational Toxicology*, *23*, 100233. https://doi.org/10.1016/j.comtox.2022.100233

Wylie, A. G., Virta, R. L., & Segreti, J. M. (1987). Characterization of mineral population by index particle: Implication for the Stanton hypothesis. *Environmental Research*, *43*(2), 427–439. https://doi.org/10.1016/s0013-9351(87)80043-9

1 Definition of a mineral fiber

How do the science and regulations approach asbestiform fibers and non-asbestiform fragments?

A. Korchevskiy & A. Wylie

ELONGATE MINERAL PARTICLES

In 2011, the National Institute of Occupational Safety and Health (NIOSH) introduced the term "Elongate Mineral Particles" (EMPs) to account for the types of particles that meet the regulatory definition of fiber but are not asbestos as defined by law (NIOSH/USPHS, 1979). The term refers to particles of naturally occurring chemical elements and compounds in a rectangular or rod-like shape that are three times longer than they are wide (3:1). Under U.S. regulatory policy, the membrane filter method is used to assess asbestos exposure. By this method, EMPs longer than 5 μm captured on air filters and visible by phase contrast microscopy are referred to as "**fibers**" (Leidel et al., 1979). The World Health Organization (WHO) adds an upper limit of width of 3 μm (WHO, 1997). In proposing the term EMP, NIOSH recognized that because of the broad and nonspecific criteria for "fibers" under regulatory protocols, elongated particles of almost any mineral may be **true mineral fiber**; that is, they form in nature, like asbestos. They may be pieces of broken rock elongated during fragmentation, called **cleavage fragments**, or they may be brittle acicular single crystals sometimes referred to as **byssolite** (Verkouteren & Wylie, 2000). Utilizing this simple definition of what should be counted as a fiber may have been appropriate when it was used to assess occupational exposure to known asbestos, but in other environments, its lack of specificity is problematic. It should be noted that the Asbestos Hazard Emergency Response Act (AHERA, 1986) defines a fiber as a particle with an aspect ratio not less than 5:1 and length more than 0.5 μm, but this dimensional definition is also not specific for asbestos fibers.

Why is this fiber definition important to toxicology? It is important because applying such a broad definition of fiber to mineral dusts generally means that many particles for which no evidence of carcinogenicity exists will be considered fibers and even equated to commercial asbestos. While the existing definition apparently incorporates carcinogenic fiber, it does not define it.

 DOI: 10.1201/9781003424277-2

It should be noted that in this book, where applicable, elongate particles will be referred to according to their length and origin if known, such as **EMP-5** for EMPs longer than 5 μm; similar notation will apply for different lengths, for example, EMP-2 or EMP-4 or EMP-15. In addition, because inhalation is the method of delivery, EMPs include only particles with widths < 3 μm unless otherwise stated.

Table 1.1 contains common terms and their meanings as used in this book. The definitions for length, width, and thickness are ideal. They assume that elongate particles are enclosed by a circumscribing cuboid that is the smallest possible with the three perpendicular axes defining length (the longest), width (intermediate), and thickness (smallest). Because of the way samples are prepared for observation, thickness is normally the direction perpendicular to the field of view. Most elongate particles in the database have parallel or nearly parallel sides and blunt ends and approach this ideal shape, but for particles that do not, the ideal model for EMPs should be applied. Length and width as observed under a microscope in the field of view are then defined by the smallest circumscribing rectangle.

Mineralogists distinguish true mineral fiber from other EMPs based on properties that are derived from the unusual way mineral fiber forms: it attains its elongate

TABLE 1.1
Particle Terminology

Particle	Definition
Mineral	A naturally occurring inorganic chemical element or compound with an ordered internal atomic arrangement and defined chemical composition.
Length (L)	The longest dimension of the circumscribing cuboid for an elongate mineral particle. The length is measured by microscopy as the longest dimension of a circumscribing rectangle in the focal plane.
Width (W)	The intermediate dimension of the circumscribing cuboid for an elongate mineral particle. The width is measured by microscopy as the smallest dimension of a circumscribing rectangle in the focal plane.
Thickness (T)	The dimension of the circumscribing cuboid for an elongate mineral particle, perpendicular to the length and width plane. Thickness is normally the smallest dimension.
Aspect ratio (AR)	The ratio of length to width (L:W)
Elongate mineral particle (EMP)	Any mineral particle with a length (L)-to-width (W) ratio (aspect ratio) of 3:1 or greater. To designate the length of an EMP the following notation is used: EMP-x, where x = length in micrometers means fibers with length > x. All EMPs have widths < 3 μm unless otherwise stated.
Mineral fiber	An elongate mineral particle that attained its shape during formation in nature, with an aspect ratio sufficiently large to impart flexibility to the material in hand sample.
Fibril	A single crystal mineral fiber that cannot be further separated longitudinally into smaller components.

(Continued)

TABLE 1.1 *(Continued)*
Particle Terminology

Particle	Definition
Cleavage fragment	An elongate mineral particle created by fragmentation that is bound in whole or in part by inherent planes of weakness. A cleavage fragment may have the same chemical formula as a mineral fiber, but it is brittle and cannot separate longitudinally into fibers or fibrils.
Fibrous	The mineral habit that describes particles having the appearance of fiber or being composed of fiber.
Asbestiform	A naturally occurring, polyfilamentous mineral growth habit in which fibers are formed of parallel fibrils in bundles that can be separated into smaller fibers and fibrils with hand pressure; asbestiform minerals are flexible in hand samples and fibers have higher tensile strength than other habits of the same mineral. While fibrils are aligned nearly parallel to their common fiber axis, they are aligned randomly or semi-randomly in the directions perpendicular. Fibrils display uniform widths that change little or not at all with length. This lack of correlation makes widths and lengths independent variables. In this book, the term asbestiform may be used to describe a data set that is derived from asbestiform minerals. An asbestiform data set should have the characteristic of uniform width over a wide range in length and a low correlation between width and length.
Asbestos	A generic term applied to the asbestiform variety of serpentine (chrysotile) and the asbestiform variety of amphibole group minerals (including anthophyllite, grunerite, tremolite, actinolite, and riebeckite), that have been exploited, prospected, described in the literature, traded and sold commercially for their unique physical properties of high tensile strength, flexibility, and durability in the built environment. There is disagreement about whether the term should be applied only to the minerals first regulated as asbestos: chrysotile, tremolite asbestos, actinolite asbestos, anthophyllite asbestos, amosite, and crocidolite. To avoid confusion, in this book, and in general, the term asbestiform is preferred over asbestos unless referring to the asbestos that was in commerce in the world in the 20th century.
Non-asbestiform	Any mineral habit that is not asbestiform. Non-asbestiform may refer to brittle acicular singular crystal or simply a cleavage fragment. The most common use of the term is to draw a contrast between elongate rock fragments and mineral fibers.
Nanofiber	Any highly elongate mineral particle (or manufactured fiber such as carbon nanotubes) with parallel sides and width less than 150 nm. Given that the thickness of most mineral particles is less than the width, an orientation selected by sample preparation techniques, the thickness of mineral fibers will in most cases satisfy the normal criterion of a nanomaterial of one dimension less than 100 nm.

shape and size through crystallization from fluids in open spaces, and evidence for fluid alteration of preexisting rock can be more extensive than the localized occurrence of fiber. Fibers have distinctive physical properties such as flexibility, high tensile strength, and distinctive dimensions, and in the case of asbestos, anomalous optical properties.

TABLE 1.2
The width of all EMPs and for EMP-5 of airborne asbestos fibrils and fibers in aerosols from several mines (Gibbs & Hwang, 1980).

	Percent all EMP			Percent EMP-5		
Mineral Source	W < 60	W < 100 (nm)	W ≤ 200 (nm)	W < 60	W < 100 (nm)	W ≤ 200 (nm)
Chrysotile asbestos Quebec, Canada	61	86	96	0	14	28
Crocidolite Cape, South Africa	37	77	93	9	29	75
Amosite Transvaal, South Africa	15	25	52	0	1	18

The smallest single fiber-forming crystal is called a **fibril**. Fibrils together form the fibers one sees in a hand sample. Fibers have a silky luster, are flexible in hand samples, and usually occur in nature in veins of parallel fibrils from millimeters to meters in width. Normally, the widths of fibrils from a single occurrence vary within narrow limits. In certain rock types, especially in mountainous and volcanic regions of the world where hydrothermal fluids have been at work, small amounts of mineral fiber can be found in many locations. Some large mineral fiber occurrences, where the fibrils are very narrow and strong, have been mined, and the fiber sold as **asbestos**. The U.S. Geological Survey maintains worldwide production data for asbestos by country (https://www.usgs.gov/publications/mineral-commodity-summaries-2024).

Fibril sizes of three major worldwide types of asbestos are reflected in the narrow widths of particles found in mining aerosols (Gibbs & Hwang, 1980) (see Table 1.2). This is just one example, and the proportions of narrow fibers vary among mines, but in all cases, fibrils with widths less than 150 nm are abundant, making them **nanofibers**.

In the case of asbestos, it is likely that most EMP fibers, especially EMP-5 fibers with widths > 200 nm are a composite of multiple fibrils. For chrysotile, with unit fibril width of 10–40 nm, all of the long fibers measured are composite since all are much wider than 40 nm (Chisholm, 1983). Cape and Hammersley crocidolite, Transvaal amosite, and occurrences of other types of asbestos have more variable fibril sizes, but asbestos, especially asbestos mined in very large deposits, is dominated by fibrils that are 20–200 nm in width, irregular in cross-section, with a thickness that is less than width. Long asbestos fibers are commonly composite, and the longest, rare fibrils are on the order of 100 μm in length; most fibrils are less than 20 μm in length with the most abundant on the order of 2–3 μm. The term "short" refers to EMPs with L ≤ 5μm and "long" to those with L > 5 μm.

Adhesion between fibrils varies among occurrences. Composite fiber bundles may disaggregate readily after inhalation, enhancing dose if binding forces are small. Adhesion between fibrils of Transvaal amosite is slightly greater than between Cape or Hammersley crocidolite fibrils, as reflected in the slightly fewer amosite EMPs of the narrowest widths in mine air. Processing of mined ore to break up fiber bundles, so-called **fiberization,** may increase the proportions of long single fibrils.

Respirable EMP cleavage fragments form when humans break certain types of rock, creating dust. While fragmented particles may be elongate, they do not regularly attain aspect ratios (length/width) in excess of 20:1, although the specific dimensions of EMP fragments vary among occurrences. Rather than a uniform width, the width of fragments increases significantly as their length increases. EMP-5 fragments with widths < 200 nm are uncommon and are not present in statistically significant quantities in the large EMP database we have compiled (see Chapter 2.) EMP fragments are very common in rock dust from many areas of North America. For example, they can be formed from rock units found throughout the Appalachian and the Rocky Mountains. As such, they can occur in the dust resulting from mining, building excavations, road construction, etc. in many parts of the U.S., and the potential for occupational exposures abound. There is no compelling evidence to support the designation of cleavage fragments as carcinogens, and they are not regulated as asbestos under U.S. regulatory policy governing occupational exposure. However, asbestiform mineral fiber can occur in the same types of rock from which EMP fragments are derived and, in some cases, fiber presents the potential for significant occupational exposure during mining or excavation.

In general, elongate mineral particles, formed as fibers or fragments, will carry a surface charge that will vary among minerals and occurrences as composition, structural defects, and shape vary. Particles carrying surface charge interact with cells with which they come in contact in different ways depending on charge and charge strength (Augustine et al., 2020), solubility, and metal cation. A discussion of surface-mineral interactions can be found in Chapter 4.

The term "fibrous" is a term describing mineral habit, but its formal meaning contains ambiguity, because a material described as fibrous may or may not be mineral fiber. The term is qualitative, like other habit terms. It means to mineralogists "has the appearance of being composed of fibers"; in other words, it might or might not be composed of mineral fibers that can be separated readily. A good example is cat's eye in which mineral fiber has been replaced and cemented by quartz. It has been sometimes used in the health and environment related literature to refer to EMPs or EMP-5, but this use is not consistent with the mineralogical meaning, contributing to confusion about what is and is not a mineral fiber.

There is a third perspective on EMPs that should be considered and which this book will frame. For the protection of public health, health policy should be focused on the specific characteristics of mineral particles that can be correlated with disease excess so that **carcinogenic mineral fiber** populations **(CMF)** can be defined. CMF includes all mineral EMPs that when inhaled at certain exposure levels can be expected to contribute significantly to elevated levels of mesothelioma, lung cancer, or other asbestos-related cancers. Such an outcome directed designation for "fiber" would also address the current confusion about what do we mean by the term fiber and make it clear that EMP-5 does not define the CMF set. To define CMF populations, we must study carefully exposures that have resulted in disease.

OCCURRENCES OF KNOWN OR SUSPECTED CMF

Table 1.3 provides a list of places in the world where excess mesotheliomas have been identified and related to exposures of asbestiform mineral fiber. While lung cancers have been associated with occupational and environmental exposures other than to asbestos, occupational pleural mesothelioma excesses are almost exclusively related to exposure to asbestiform mineral fiber (although different agents were also reported as producing mesothelioma in animals and humans, and a baseline rate of spontaneous mesothelioma exists for non-exposed populations as well). In some cases, the dimensional parameters EMPA (percent of EMP-5 that have widths < 0.15 μm) and EMPB (percent of EMP-5 that have width ≤ 0.25μm) have been determined and are provided, emphasizing the long-standing recognition that size is a major factor in mineral fiber carcinogenicity (see Chapter 3 of this book). Actually, EMPA is the nanofiber component of EMP exposure. Widths of 0.15–0.25 μm within the EMPB component could consist of single wider fibrils or bundles of a few nanofibers in the case of amphibole, or, in the case of chrysotile, bundles of 25-nm fibrils.

The term *asbestiform* describes a habit of growth or growth form. Habit descriptions are qualitative and describe the way a mineral appears in hand specimens, in both its physical form and in its response to light, for example, prismatic, platy, waxy, silky, or fibrous. In hand specimen, asbestiform mineral fiber is strong and flexible, with tensile strength approaching that of steel wire. Fibrils occur in bundles that are readily separable by hand pressure. In some cases, the fibrils can combine to form fibers long enough to be woven. Under the optical microscope, the fibrillar structure of fibers is evident in both the physical form of the fibers and their optical properties.

When looking only at the dimensions of an airborne or lung burden asbestiform populations measured by transmission electron microscopy (TEM), some properties such as tensile strength and flexibility cannot be directly determined. Therefore, the term asbestiform, when applied to mineral populations derived from mineral material that is fibrillar but described only by mineral composition and particle dimensions, means high aspect ratio, uniformly very narrow widths of EMPs that are single crystals (fibrils) or bundles of fibrils, and fibril dimensions that resemble asbestos aerosols, as shown in Table 1.3 and Table 1.4. Asbestiform minerals may not always be characterized by fibrils as narrow as asbestos, and, if not, they will lack its tensile strength because tensile strength is inversely proportional to width (Griffin, 1921); sepiolite is a good example of an asbestiform mineral that is not asbestos. In some samples, fibrils may vary in size, from flexible narrow crystals to wider, glassy acicular crystals with resulting lowered tensile strength. This is typical of the asbestiform minerals found in the vermiculite mine at Libby Montana. In addition, fiber bundles vary in friability. Sometimes fibrils adhere slightly to one another due to interfibrillar secondary mineralization or in some cases, some structural conformity, as is the case for Transvaal amosite (Cressey et al., 1982), while in other cases fibril width distributions show that they readily disaggregate when disturbed or following inhalation and deposition, as is typical of Cape and Hammersley crocidolite and Canadian chrysotile.

TABLE 1.3

Asbestiform mineral locations associated with elevated incidence of mesothelioma among exposed individuals. Formal human epidemiological studies support the Darnton estimates of R_M, while other estimates of R_M are predictions based on dimensional similarity to asbestos. The lack of R_M means that an excess risk is suspected, but data are lacking for the calculation of R_M.

Asbestiform Mineral (ideal composition)	Source	EMPA (%)	EMPB (%)	R_M (%)
Amphibole				
Anthophyllite (asbestos) $Mg_7Si_8O_{22}(OH)_2$	Finland	6.85[a]	19.18[a]	0.04[c]
	Ekaterinburg, Russia	19.5[a]	38.01[a]	0.06[c]
Fluoro-edenite (asbestiform) $NaCa_2Mg_5Si_7AlO_{22}(F,OH)_2$	Biancavilla, Italy	4.59[a]	21.10[a]	0.12[c]
Grunerite (amosite asbestos) $Fe_7Si_8O_{22}(OH)_2$	Transvaal, South Africa	8.0[a]	25.3[a]	0.06[b]
	Fiberized amosite, New Jersey, U.S.A.			0.12[b]
Riebeckite (crocidolite asbestos) $Na_2Fe^{3+}{}_2Fe^{2+}{}_3Si_8O_{22}(OH)_2$	Cape, South Africa	51.6[a]	79.5[a]	0.59[b]
	Hammersley, Australia	46.8[a]	71.1[a]	0.51[b]
Tremolite (asbestiform) $Ca_2Mg_5Si_8O_{22}(OH)_2$	Metsovo, Greece	35.9[a]	68.8[a]	0.3[g]
	New Caledonia			
	Central Turkey (white soil)			
	Cyprus			
	Corsica			
Winchite $\left(CaNaMg_4\left(Al,Fe^{3+}\right)Si_8O_{22}(OH)_2\right)$, richterite (NaCaNaMg,$Fe_5$ $Si_8O_{22}(OH)_2$, and tremolite $\left(Ca_2Mg_5Si_8O_{22}(OH)_2\right)$ (asbestiform)	Libby, Montana U.S.A.	2.1[a]	18.4[a]	0.03[b]

TABLE 1.3 ***(Continued)***

Asbestiform mineral locations associated with elevated incidence of mesothelioma among exposed individuals. Formal human epidemiological studies support the Darnton estimates of R_M, while other estimates of R_M are predictions based on dimensional similarity to asbestos. The lack of R_M means that an excess risk is suspected, but data are lacking for the calculation of R_M.

Asbestiform Mineral (ideal composition)	Source	EMPA (%)	EMPB (%)	R_M (%)
Serpentine				
Chrysotile (asbestos) $Mg_3Si_2O_5(OH)_4$	Quebec, Canada			0.0009[b]
	Balangero, Italy			0.0018[d]
	Sivas, Turkey			
	Central Turkey (white soil)			
	Asbest, Russia			0.0034[f]
	Cyprus			
Antigorite (asbestiform) $(Mg,Fe)_3Si_2O_5(OH)_4$	New Caledonia			
Zeolite				
Erionite (asbestiform, aka wooly) $(K_2,Ca,Na)_2Al_4Si_{14}O_{36}.15H_2O$	Cappadocia, Turkey	43.7[c]	50.3[e]	
	Central Mexico			
Other				
Balangeroite (asbestiform) $Mg_{42}Si_{16}O_{54}(OH)_{40}$	Balangero, Italy	5.2[a]	8.7[a]	0.045[d]
Fibrous industrial talc	Gouverneur, New York, U.S.A.	17.9[a]	31.1[a]	
	Cyprus			

[a] Latest EMPA/B data (from the dimensional database)
[b] Darnton, 2023
[c] Korchevskiy et al., 2019
[d] Korchevskiy and Wylie, 2023
[e] Wagner et al., 1985
[f] Schüz et al., 2024
[g] Korchevskiy and Wylie, 2025a, 2025b

Occurrences of asbestiform minerals with known or suspected excess in mesothelioma among dust-exposed individuals and measures of fibril widths, EMPA and EMPB, are shown in Table 1.3. In some locations, sufficient information is available to estimate R_M, the potency factor for mesothelioma measured as the percent increase in the incidence of mesothelioma for each EMP-5-cc-year exposure (Hodgson & Darnton, 2000; Darnton, 2023). The highly uneven potencies (varying over four orders of magnitude) among the minerals listed demonstrate clearly the uneven potency for EMP-5, which is strong evidence for the impact of differing characteristics among EMP-5 in the exposures.

PROPERTIES OF CARCINOGENIC MINERAL FIBER

While all the occurrences listed in Table 1.3 contain carcinogenic mineral fiber, not all the mineral fibers making up the EMP-5 populations are equally potent. The search to understand the toxicology of elongated mineral particles rests on finding those properties that vary among the exposures in ways that impact potency and correlate with, and can ultimately predict, carcinogenic risk. Responses cannot be understood when the dose is based on EMP-5 only, which is equalized in the calculation of R_M. To estimate elongate mineral particle potency for asbestos-related cancers, we must characterize the EMPs in each exposure, including mineral makeup (mineral identity and chemical composition), solubility, rigidity, dimensional parameters (length, width, thickness, from which an aspect ratio, volume, and specific surface area can be derived), particle habit (composite or single crystal), surface charge, and perhaps others. In later chapters, these parameters will be discussed in more detail.

MINERAL MAKEUP OF KNOWN CMF

Amphibole

The minerals listed in Table 1.3 belong to a number of different mineral groups that are named according to the presence of common structural elements. The largest group of minerals in Table 1.3 belongs to the silicate mineral supergroup called **amphiboles,** which contains about 100 minerals differing only in chemical composition or by a very slight structural change (Deer et al., 1997). The first 13 locations given in Table 1.3 are for asbestiform amphiboles.

Asbestiform occurrences of five of the amphibole group members have been mined and sold as asbestos. Of these, only three had worldwide distribution: riebeckite forming **crocidolite asbestos**, grunerite forming **amosite asbestos**, and anthophyllite forming **anthophyllite asbestos. Anthophyllite asbestos** was mined in Finland and Russia, where its association with mesothelioma is known, and in North Carolina where no association has been established. **Tremolite asbestos** normally occurs in deposits too small for large-scale mining, but there were small mines in California, Maryland, and elsewhere in the Appalachian Mountains, as well as in India, Pakistan, and Korea. In Turkey, Greece, and elsewhere around the Mediterranean, it occurs as a component of soils used for domestic applications such as whitewash (Constantopoulos, 2008). **Actinolite asbestos** is found in Italy, where it was mined during the Roman Empire, and it is common in many small occurrences throughout the Alps and the Appalachian Mountains; however, human exposures to this mineral alone are insufficient to establish R_M at any location.

Whether or not an occurrence of an asbestiform amphibole qualifies as asbestos under the compositional constraints of federal or state law, and whether or not it has been directly linked to excess mesothelioma, it should be considered a CMF if its physical properties are the same (within limits) as the regulated commercial forms of amphibole asbestos. For example, magnesio-riebeckite can form blue asbestos, ferro-actinolite asbestos has been found associated with amosite in the Transvaal, and the literature reports asbestiform winchite (Wylie & Huggins, 1980), asbestiform magnesio-arfvedsonite (Deer et al., 1997), and asbestiform richterite (Gunter et al., 2011).

The experience of the miners and millers of vermiculite from Libby, Montana, is a case in point. The most common asbestiform mineral fiber occurring with vermiculite at Libby is the amphibole winchite. The second most common is the amphibole richterite, and the third is tremolite. Neither winchite nor richterite is listed in U.S. federal law defining the types of asbestos, although the exposures to mineral fiber at Libby have resulted in excess mesothelioma, and they are noted in administrative law by the EPA. Given the right conditions of pressure, temperature, fluid composition, and a place where fiber can form, almost any amphibole, except perhaps the most aluminum-rich varieties (tschermakite, pargasite), can be asbestiform, and if so, could be carcinogenic.

Serpentine

The second largest group represented in Table 1.3 is the **serpentines**, which include chrysotile, antigorite, and lizardite. The three serpentine minerals have essentially the same chemical composition $\left(Mg_3Si_2O_5\left(OH\right)_4\right)$ but slightly different atomic structures. All serpentine structures are built on polymerized sheets of Si-O tetrahedra. In **chrysotile**, the sheets are rolled to form a tube. The tube diameter is quite uniform across occurrences but averages range among occurrences from about 10 to 40 nm with a 5-nm central canal.

Serpentine occurs in large masses in most of the world's mountain chains in a rock called serpentinite. **Chrysotile asbestos** is found as veins in massive serpentine, although the serpentine itself may have different origins. It was the most widely used form of asbestos in the 20th century; it is still mined in some parts of the world. Fibrous **antigorite** has been identified in New Caledonia (Petriglieri et al., 2021), where an excess of mesothelioma has been reported but where tremolite-asbestos is also known (Constantopoulos, 2008; Baumann et al., 2011).

It is widely accepted that chrysotile has a much lower potency for mesothelioma than asbestiform amphibole, and some have argued that it cannot cause mesothelioma at all. The observed lower potency is not explainable by size because chrysotile closely resembles crocidolite in many dimensional aspects (although fibrils of crocidolite are slightly wider). Chrysotile is known to be leached of Mg when retained in the lung, and experimental data predict that the lifetime of a chrysotile fibril within the human lung is measured in weeks to months. To the contrary, amphibole can exist almost unaltered for many years. The solubility of chrysotile in biological fluids has been offered to explain the relatively low potency (R_M) of chrysotile. It is also known that chrysotile has a low rigidity, which also may play a role in its lower potency (see Chapter 7). In addition, chrysotile asbestos of all grades may contain EMP-fibers of the amphibole tremolite (Berman & Crump, 2008b). A recent study of many chrysotile mine products by Chatfield (2025) examined 20 samples of chrysotile from eight Canadian mines, five samples from Coalinga, California, four samples from Balangero, Italy, and two each from Brazil (Minacu), Zimbabwe, and Vermont. He found tremolite asbestos at some level from all locations, with individual sample variation from 0 to over 10,000 ppm. The lowest concentrations were from Balangero, Coalinga, and in UICCa chrysotile. He reports amosite contamination in both UICCa and UICCb chrysotile and diopside fibers from Balangero.

Also, commercial chrysotile existed in several grades, apparently having different cancer potencies. For example, Darnton (2023) demonstrated that statistically significant potency factors for chrysotile can be determined only if the textile variety of chrysotile is separated from mining/friction products grades. See Chapter 12 for analysis of different sources and potency of chrysotile fibers.

Zeolite

Zeolites are a large group of almost 100 minerals that are frequently found in surface or near-surface deposits associated with volcanic activity and in some metamorphic zones, defining a pressure/temperature zone of low-grade metamorphism. Skinner et al. (1989) list 20 that may be fibrous in appearance. They are common in the United States in the western states, especially in the altered volcanic tuffs in Nevada, Arizona, and Oregon, and in the volcanic region of central Turkey.

Zeolites are low-density aluminosilicates built on a highly polymerized Si-O tetrahedra structure that contains openings large enough to act as molecular sieves for organic compounds. They also have excellent ion exchange capacities. Both natural and synthetic zeolites are used in a wide variety of industrial applications, such as water purification and petroleum refining.

In the Cappadocia region of Turkey, elevated mesothelioma is reported from several towns where the local rock, an altered volcanic tuff, contains mineral fiber composed of **erionite**. The host rock is easily broken, and it was commonly fabricated and excavated to form dwellings. Asbestiform erionite, described by mineralogists as **woolly erionite** when it occurs as asbestiform fiber, is thought to form during the devitrification of volcanic glass. The type locality is Rome, Oregon. Rome erionite (along with the Karain, Turkey, variety) was demonstrated by Wagner et al. (1985) to be a potent animal carcinogen. Woolly erionite from Lander Co., Nevada, has also been described and is very similar to the Rome occurrence (Shedd et al., 1982). In these two locations, fibrils are narrower than crocidolite. In all other reported occurrences in the U.S., erionite is not asbestiform, although it may appear fibrous.

Pyroxenoids

Balangeroite is an uncommon silicate built on single chains of polymerized Si-O tetrahedra; it is known only from a few locations in Italy. The mineral was first identified in the chrysotile asbestos quarry in Balangero, Italy, in an asbestiform habit.

Here, balangeroite fibrils are intergrown with chrysotile fibrils in portions of the mine. Given the higher-than-expected mesothelioma incidence among the exposed cohort from the Balangero mine, Korchevskiy and Wylie (2023) suggested that if the mineral is durable, the dimensional characteristics of balangeroite are similar enough to asbestos to be responsible for some of the excess mesothelioma. Chatfield (personal communication) found balangeroite to be soluble, but it masked a highly durable fiber of diopside, a pyroxene and also a single-chain silicate.

MINERAL COMPOSITION OF EMP-5 NOT KNOWN TO BE CMF

There are more than 4000 minerals, many of which are known from only a few locations. These are not only silicate minerals but also sulfates, oxides, carbonates, phosphates, etc. Roggli (2018) has recorded EMP-5 particles that he has found in lung tissue by SEM over four decades. In addition to asbestos and erionite, his data show a wide variety of oxides, phosphates, metal whiskers, and other silicates. The discussion that follows covers the more common minerals that could be found in EMP aerosols depending on source rocks.

Table 1.4 contains locations where minerals and/or millers have been exposed to EMPs either in the waste rock or as a component of the ore, and where there have been epidemiological studies to assess lung cancer and mesothelioma incidences in an exposed cohort that do not show a correlation between exposure and risk.

TABLE 1.4
Exposures to EMPs that are not asbestiform and health studies are negative for cancer

Source	EMP Mineral	EMPA	EMPB	R_M
Homestake, South Dakota, U.S.A.	Grunerite fragment	0	0	0
Italian talc	Tremolite fragment	NA	NA	0
Wollastonite miners[a]	Wollastonite fragments			0
New York tunnel workers[b]	Hornblende fragments			0
Taconite workers[c]	Actinolite and grunerite fragments[1] and asbestiform ferro-actinolite	3.2[d]	5.[d]	0 (at the eastern part of the Mesabi range where amphibole fragments were found, but no excess mesothelioma apparently occurred)[e]

[a] Maxim and McConnell, 2005
[b] Selikoff, 1978
[c] Mandel and Odo, 2018
[d] Data from Dr. Yuan Shao (personal communication, 2021)
[e] Shao et al., 2025

Asbestiform minerals other than asbestos

There are common occurrences of asbestiform silicate minerals other than those listed in Table 1.3. Sheet silicates that belong to the clay mineral group and are not known to be associated with asbestos-related diseases include sepiolite and palygorskite (attapulgite), which are asbestiform, although their fibril widths are larger than asbestos and the fibers lack high tensile strength, as well as halloysite, which has a tubular structure like chrysotile but is composed of Al rather than Mg; fibrils of halloysite are usually quite short (Deer et al., 1962). Antigorite, a form of serpentine, occurs in an asbestiform habit in South Australia (Keeling et al., 2008). Other minerals described in the literature as asbestiform include carlosturanite, a complex chain silicate from Italy (Compagnoni et al., 1985), offretite, a zeolite (Mattioli et al., 2018), manjiroite and todorokite, Mn oxides (Gutzmer & Beukes, 2000), hydromuscovite (guembelite), a mica (Tsipuroky, 1993), and bustamite, a single chain pyroxenoid silicate (Binns, 1968). The biopyriboles jimthompsonite, clinojimthompsonite, and chesterite may be fibrous and could be asbestiform (Veblen et al., 1977). Given the right conditions, many other minerals would likely also occur in an asbestiform habit, but almost all of them occur in a non-asbestiform habit, and most will form elongate particles when fragmented.

Fibrous talc is a term used to describe asbestiform fiber that is composed of the mineral talc alone, **or** fiber that is an intergrowth of talc with other minerals, including amphiboles and biopyriboles (Stemple & Brindley, 1960; Virta, 1985; Felius, 1986). The proportion of talc in a fibrous talc fiber can be highly variable, from 100%, the most common talc fiber, to as little as 50% (uncommon). Fibers of pure talc can be found in most talc ores, both cosmetic and industrial, but intergrowth with amphiboles is known only from a few places in the world. Epidemiology does not support an association between cosmetic talc and cancer: for example, see Ierardi et al., 2022. This is important because cosmetic talc is more than 95% mineral talc and often contains fibers of pure mineral talc.

In the Gouverneur talc district of New York, in addition to fibers that are only talc, some fibrous talc fibers are composed of a talc-tremolite intergrowth, as first described by Stemple and Brindley (1960). Since about 1970, mining has been restricted to industrial talc ore in which the intergrowths consist of talc and anthophyllite, as well as other Mg-rich biopyriboles (Virta, 1985; Felius, 1986); rarely do the fibers contain small amounts of Ca, a necessary component of tremolite. Published epidemiological studies of the Gouverneur industrial talc miners and millers have been mostly negative for mesothelioma, despite exposure to mineral fiber. This may be a result of talc fibers lacking the rigidity necessary for significant biological effects or sufficient biopersistence. However, asbestiform anthophyllite has been detected in the Gouverneur talc district as a contaminant of the ore or component of the gangue in some of the mines. Asbestiform amphibole fibers present in industrial talc ores present a cancer risk for workers not seen in ores mined for cosmetic talc.

Amphibole cleavage fragments

Although the inhalation of asbestiform amphibole is implicated as the cause in many reported cases of mesothelioma, amphibole is generally not fibrous. Amphiboles are common rock-forming minerals, making up as much as 10% of rock in the U.S. (and concentrations in some rock formations are greater than 50%; only a small fraction of amphibole occurs in an asbestiform habit) (Wylie & Candela, 2015).

The atomic structure of amphibole is built with Si-O tetrahedra polymerized into double chains. The chain structure is very strong, but the bonds between the double chains are weaker. When sufficient force is applied to break a particle of amphibole, breakage occurs along two planes between the chains (referred to as prismatic cleavage), resulting in elongated fragments. Common structural defects or intergrowths, another mineral on a microscale, add a plane of weakness called **parting**, which is also parallel to the silicate chains but different from the cleavage directions, enhancing elongation during fragmentation. For these reasons, all types of amphibole will normally form EMP fragments when crushed. Amphiboles such as glaucophane and riebeckite, which have high Na (and probably those with high Li and K) content, often exhibit enhanced elongation.

The mesothelioma potency for non-asbestiform cummingtonite-grunerite exposure in the workers of the Homestake, South Dakota gold mine was estimated as zero (Garabrant & Pastula, 2018). Gamble and Gibbs (2008) argued that there was no increased risk of lung carcinoma in Homestake mine workers based on studies of Steenland and Brown (1995) and McDonald et al. (1978); it was suggested that the earlier study of miners by Gillam et al. (1976), which found elevated lung cancer risk, was not confirmed by later studies with longer follow-up. There are no studies showing an association between exposure to amphibole cleavage fragments in the absence of asbestos and excess cancer (Gamble & Gibbs, 2008).

Fragmented serpentine

In the non-fibrous form, lizardite and antigorite will not normally exhibit readily visible cleavage because of their characteristic small crystallite size, despite their layered structure, but cleavage could be expressed when particles are broken if crystals are large enough. EMPs of massive serpentine, although not formed of mineral fiber, will satisfy EMP-5 criteria.

Picrolite is a brittle, splintery form of serpentine that is composed of varying amounts of chrysotile and antigorite; although single chrysotile fibrils are not separable, the structure is not fibrillar. Picrolite occurs in veins that may have crystallized first as chrysotile, but later the fibrils annealed and antigorite formed, resulting in this brittle material that readily forms EMPs.

Common fragmented silicates other than amphibole and serpentine that form EMP-5

When some ***zeolites*** are broken, they will form EMPs. About 25% of erionite particles not of the woolly form will be EMPs (Shedd et al., 1982). Other zeolites are described as fibrous (but not asbestiform) and, because of a prismatic cleavage resembling amphibole, may form EMPs including phillipsite, paulingite, laumontite, mordenite, natrolite, mesolite, scolecite, thompsonite, ferrierite, edingtonite, natrolite, chabazite, and others.

Pyroxenes and pyroxenoids are silicate minerals built on a single chain of polymerized Si-O tetrahedra, and they exhibit prismatic cleavage much like the amphiboles. The pyroxenoids wollastonite, pectolite, and hydrotalcite, and all the pyroxenes form EMPs when crushed. Fibers of pyroxene and diopside have been reported but are extremely rare. Pyroxenes with high Na content such as aegirine or Li such as spodumene may have enhanced elongation.

Sheet silicates including members of the chlorite, pyrophyllite, talc, and mica groups, have been reported as fibrous from a few locations, and in many places, they form EMPs. While talc is known to produce elongate mineral particles (so-called fibrous talc), their habit depends on the specific locations.

The ***aluminosilicates*** are a group of minerals formed from non-polymerized Si0-O tetrahedra joined by chains of $Al(OH)_6$ octahedra. The most common of these are kyanite, sillimanite, mullite, and andalusite. Sillimanite is also known as fibrolite, in recognition of its fibrous habit. All aluminosilicates are valued for their refractory properties. The chain structure contributes to the formation of EMPs.

Biopyriboles are a group of silicate minerals that fall somewhere in structure between a double-chain amphibole and a sheet silicate like talc, but which are elongate in habit and possess prismatic cleavage. They may be occasionally found in talc ore deposits.

Almost any silicate mineral can form an EMP. Quartz does not possess prismatic cleavage and normally forms equidimensional particles. Nonetheless, it is occasionally found as EMP-5 in aerosols and lung burden.

Non-silicates

Many non-silicates would not be durable in the lung. Brucite $(Mg(OH)_2)$ is a common mineral that is known to be fibrous but soluble, and there are also carbonates, sulfates, borates, iodates, halides, nitrates, and others that would not likely be durable. While some of these minerals may be harmful, they have not been associated with mesothelioma.

Oxides such as rutile (TiO_2) are common trace minerals in lung burden studies. Rutile needles are frequently enclosed by quartz, and perhaps they are liberated when quartz is broken. Fe-rich EMPs are also common; these may be oxides of iron or metal whiskers.

UNDERSTANDING EMP TOXICOLOGY IN THE REGULATORY FRAMEWORK

When the U.S. Occupational Safety and Health Administration (OSHA) formally adopted the NIOSH membrane filter method (MFM) as the aerosol monitoring method for occupational exposure to asbestos, the criteria used to assess asbestos exposure intensity became the definition of mineral fiber, and with it, the incorrect assumption that all EMP-5s could be asbestos and all are potential carcinogens. In part to correct this assumption, NIOSH now refers to such particles as EMPs, but their designation as "fibers" remains in the methods of analyses they recommend.

The U.S. Environmental Protection Agency (U.S. EPA) has defined mineral fiber differently from OSHA, NIOSH, and the WHO. The AHERA definition for fiber is

L > 0.5 µm with an L/W of at least 5:1. This definition was to be used when clearing an indoor space for occupancy following an asbestos abatement, but it is widely accepted by the courts as a definition applicable to other analyses if TEM is used. The EPA has applied several definitions for EMPs found in water. In one method, fibers are EMP-10 (Brackett et al., 1994), and in another they are EMP–0.5 (Chatfield & Dillon, 1983). In a report to the EPA, Yamate et al. (1984) advocated for a simple 3:1 ratio with no length restriction as a fiber definition, and some studies have followed this approach.

In addition to difficulties around what counts as mineral fiber, the methods used to count will provide different data describing the same population (see Chapter 2). Exposures in the workplace are measured in EMP-5/cc following the membrane filter method (MFM), where narrow fibers are unidentifiable and, in the case of chrysotile, may be invisible. Based on the resolution of the method, NIOSH initially recommended that when particles are counted by TEM, a minimum width of 0.25 µm be used to make the counts equivalent, and a new set of counting rules was recommended. According to a recent NIOSH update to their 7400 method (NIOSH/CDC, 2019), amphibole fibers as narrow as 0.05 µm and chrysotile as small as 0.15 µm in width are visible by PCM, a recognition that the assumptions underlying the PCME methods are invalid. In addition, counting by SEM and TEM are frequently different because longer particles are visible by SEM while TEM methods focus on the shorter, narrower portions of a population. These issues are discussed in more detail in Chapter 2.

Most of the dimensional criteria used to define "fiber" require additional qualification when related to toxicological characteristics. Though initially most definitions were driven by available analytical methods and other practical considerations, they appeared to provide reasonable estimates in many instances when used in environments where asbestos was the primary elongate mineral in the aerosol.

For example, there were no specific toxicological reasons to define an aspect ratio of 3:1 (or 5:1) as a threshold for carcinogenic particles. However, non-elongate particles produce no excess mesothelioma risk in humans. There is obviously a value of aspect ratio that makes elongate particles toxicologically different from their spherical analogs. Based on our dimensional database, which will be described in detail elsewhere in this book, all particles with an aspect ratio of less than 5:1 have a dimensional coefficient of carcinogenicity (DCC) of less than 0.01, making them highly unlikely to be mesothelial carcinogens (see Chapter 4, and Korchevskiy & Wylie, 2025a, 2025b). An aspect ratio of 3:1 provides both analytical and toxicological meaning, being a conservative estimate of the category of mesothelial carcinogens, but also signifying a group of particles that can be differentiated from non-elongate particles with sufficient odds.

The cutpoint of 5 µm as an approximation for a minimum length for a CMF population is supported by many studies. Exposure to fibers shorter than 5 µm has been demonstrated to be non-predictive for mesothelioma (Roggli, 2015; Barlow et al., 2017; Bernstein, 2022). In particular, Wylie and Korchevskiy (2023), based on quantitative structure activity relationship (QSAR) modeling, demonstrated that particles shorter than 5 µm apparently do not contribute to mesothelioma risk. Berman and

Crump (2008b) suggested that only fibers longer than 10 μm appear to be carcinogenic. However, all occupational exposure estimates are based on EMP-5, so it will remain an important measure of CMF until additional work addresses the minimum length of CMF (which appears to be in the range from 5 to 10 μm but may even be longer).

Alternate definitions of "fiber" make comparing data on the nature of particle exposures difficult. The inclusion of fragments under fiber counting rules means that exposure levels of EMP-5 alone will be unreliable indicators of carcinogenic potential. For advancements in understanding the toxicity of elongate mineral particles to occur, exposure assessments must include the narrowest fibers; if overlooked, the risk will be underestimated. To the extent possible, consideration should be given to the full range in the sizes of EMPs in an exposure.

MANUFACTURED FIBERS AND MINERAL EMP TOXICITY

Different forms of elongated particles (EP) and nanofibers have been fabricated and manufactured into many products today. These EPs include metal whiskers, carbon nanotubes, ceramic fibers, and fiber glass. Researchers have found a broad range of cellular and animal responses to manufactured fibers that vary in ways that are similar to EMPs with respect to the relationship between dimensionality, tensile strength, durability, and carcinogenicity. In this book, where studies on manufactured materials are relevant, they will be discussed.

Work with manufactured fibers has shown that if inorganic fibers are not durable, they cannot be carcinogenic. The EU Scientific Committee on Occupational Exposure Limits (SCOEL) states that all inorganic manufactured fibers with critical dimensions (WHO definition of a fiber: L > 5μm, W < 3μm and L/W at least 3:1) (WHO, 1997) are suspected of having carcinogenic potential and therefore are classified a priori as category 3 carcinogens. This classification need not apply if it can be shown that the fiber fulfills one of a number of conditions including:

- a short-term biopersistence test by inhalation showing that fibers longer than 20 μm have a weighted half-life of less than 10 days; and
- a short-term biopersistence test by intratracheal instillation showing that fibers longer than 20 μm have a weighted half-life of less than 40 days.

Carbon fibers and nanotubes have been manufactured in a variety of widths, lengths, and rigidities. IARC identifies only one, MWCNT-7, as a potential carcinogen. However, some studies on carbon nanotubes are highly relevant for understanding mineral carcinogenicity, especially the importance of rigidity. We will address this issue in detail in Chapter 7 of this book.

NOTE

1 An association between EMP exposure and mesothelioma is possible but inconclusive. No association between amphibole exposure or exposure to any other specific mineral and mesothelioma risk has been shown or even suggested.

REFERENCE LIST

AHERA. (1986, October 22). *Asbestos hazard emergency response act of 1986. H.R. 5073, 15 U.S.C. 2641, public law 99-519, 99th congress (1985–1986)*. https://www.congress.gov/bill/99th-congress/house-bill/5073/text

Augustine, R., Hasan, A., Primavera, R., Wilson, R. J., Thakor, A. S., & Kevadiya, B. D. (2020). Cellular uptake and retention of nanoparticles: Insights on particle properties and interaction with cellular components. *Materials Today Communications*, *25*, 101692. https://doi.org/10.1016/j.mtcomm.2020.101692

Barlow, C. A., Grespin, M., & Best, E. A. (2017). Asbestos fiber length and its relation to disease risk. *Inhalation Toxicology*, *29*(12–14), 541–554. https://doi.org/10.1080/08958378.2018.1435756

Baumann, F., Maurizot, F., Mangeas, M., Ambrosi, J-P., Douwes, J., & Robineau, B. (2011). Pleural mesothelioma in New Caledonia: Associations with environmental risk factors. *Environmental Health Perspectives*, *119*(5), 695–700. https://doi.org/10.1289/ehp.1002862

Berman, D. W., & Crump, K. S. (2008b). A meta-analysis of asbestos-related cancer risk that addresses fiber size and mineral type. *Critical Reviews in Toxicology*, *38*(Suppl 1), 49–73. https://doi.org/10.1080/10408440802273156

Bernstein, D. M. (2022). The health effects of short fiber chrysotile and amphibole asbestos. *Critical Reviews in Toxicology*, *52*(2), 89–112. https://doi.org/10.1080/10408444.2022.2056430

Binns, R. A. (1968). Asbestiform bustamite from a cavity lining within the Broken Hill lode, New South Wales. *Journal of the Geological Society of Australia*, *15*, 1–8. https://doi.org/10.1080/00167616808728675

Brackett, K. A., Clark, P. J., & Millette, J. R. (1994). *Determination of asbestos structures over 10 micrometers in length in drinking water* (EPA Method Number 100.2, EPA-600R94134). https://ntrl.ntis.gov/NTRL/dashboard/searchResults/titleDetail/PB94201902.xhtml

Chatfield, E. J. (2025). Associated minerals in chrysotile deposits and their potential health risks. *Frontiers in Public Health*, *13*. https://doi.org/10.3389/fpubh.2025.1583469

Chatfield, E. J., & Dillon, M. J. (1983). *Analytical method for determination of asbestos fibers in water* (U.S. EPA Method Number 100.1, EPA-600/4-83-043). https://www.nemi.gov/

Chisholm, J. E. (1983). Transmission electron microscopy of asbestos. In S. S. Chissick & R. Derricott (Eds.), *Asbestos; properties, applications and hazards* (pp. 85–168). John Wiley and Sons.

Compagnoni, R., Ferraris, G., & Mellini, M. (1985). Carlosturanite, a new asbestiform rock-forming silicate from Val Varaita, Italy. *American Mineralogist*, *70*(7), 767–772.

Constantopoulos, S. H. (2008). Environmental mesothelioma associated with tremolite asbestos: Lessons from the experiences of Turkey, Greece, Corsica, New Caledonia and Cyprus. *Regulatory Toxicology and Pharmacology*, *52*, S110–S115. https://doi.org/10.1016/j.yrtph.2007.11.001

Cressey, B. A., Whittaker, E. J. W., & Hutchison, J. L. (1982). Morphology and alteration of asbestiform grunerite and anthophyllite. *Mineralogical Magazine*, *46*(338), 77–87. https://doi.org/10.1180/minmag.1982.046.338.13

Darnton, L. (2023). Quantitative assessment of mesothelioma and lung cancer risk based on Phase Contrast Microscopy (PCM) estimates of fibre exposure: An update of 2000 asbestos cohort data. *Environmental Research*, 114753. https://doi.org/10.1016/j.envres.2022.114753

Deer, W. A., Howie, R. A., & Zussman, J. (1962). *Rock-forming minerals* (1st ed.). Longmans.

Deer, W. A., Howie, R. A., & Zussman, J. (1997). *Rock-forming minerals. Vol. 2B: Double-chain silicates* (2nd ed.). The Geological Society.

Felius, R. O. (1986, July 13–18). *EM-research into the fibrous constituents of an industrial talc powder* (p. 97). Abstract 14th General meeting IMA, Stanford University, Stanford, CA.

Gamble, J. F., & Gibbs, G. W. (2008). An evaluation of the risks of lung cancer and mesothelioma from exposure to amphibole cleavage fragments. *Regulatory Toxicology and Pharmacology: RTP* (online), *52*(1 Suppl), S154–S186. https://doi.org/10.1016/j.yrtph.2007.09.020

Garabrant, D. H., & Pastula, S. T. (2018). A comparison of asbestos fiber potency and elongate mineral particle (EMP) potency for mesothelioma in humans. *Toxicology and Applied Pharmacology*, *361*, 127–136. https://doi.org/10.1016/j.taap.2018.07.003

Gibbs, G. W., & Hwang, C. Y. (1980). Dimensions of airborne asbestos fibres. In J. C. Wagner (Ed.), *Biological effects of mineral fibres* (IARC Scientific Publication No. 30, pp. 69–78). IARC Scientific Publications, Lynn.

Gillam, J. D., Dement, J. M., Lemen, R. A., Wagoner, J. K., Archer, V. E., & Blejer, H. P. (1976). Mortality patterns among hard rock gold miners exposed to an asbestiform mineral. *Annals of the New York Academy of Science*, *271*, 336–344. https://doi.org/10.1111/j.1749-6632.1976.tb23129.x

Griffin, A. A. (1921). The phenomena of rupture and flow in solids. *Philosophical Transactions of the Royal Society of London. Series A, Containing Papers of a Mathematical or Physical Character*, *221*, 163–198.

Gunter, M. E., Dyar, M. D., Lanzirotti, A., Tucker, J. M., & Speicher, E. A. (2011). Letter – Differences in Fe-redox for asbestiform and nonasbestiform amphiboles from the former vermiculite mine, near Libby, Montana, U.S.A.† *American Mineralogist*, *96*, 1414–1417. http://dx.doi.org/10.2138/am.2011.3800

Gutzmer, J., & Beukes, N. J. (2000). Asbestiform manjiroite and todorokite from the Kahahari manganese field, South Africa. *South African Journal of Geology*, *103*(3–4), 163–174.

Hodgson, J., & Darnton, A. (2000). The quantitative risks of mesothelioma and lung cancer in relation to asbestos exposure. *The Annals of Occupational Hygiene*, *44*(8), 565–601. https://doi.org/10.1016/s0003-4878(00)00045-4

Ierardi, A. M., Best, E. A., & Marsh, G. M. (2022). Updated Italian cohort data continues to confirm lack of mesothelioma in pooled cohort of international cosmetic talc miners and millers. *Inhalation Toxicology*, *34*(5–6), 135–144. https://doi.org/10.1080/08958378.2022.2053251

Keeling, J. L., Raven, M. D., Self, P. G., & Eggleton, R. A. (2008). Asbestiform antigorite occurrence in South Australia. *Australian Institute of Mines and Metallurgy*, *8*, 329–336.

Korchevskiy, A. A., Rasmuson, J. O., & Rasmuson, E. J. (2019). Empirical model of mesothelioma potency factors for different mineral fibers based on their chemical composition and dimensionality. *Inhalation Toxicology*, *31*(5), 80–191. https://doi.org/10.1080/08958378.2019.1640320

Korchevskiy, A. A., & Wylie, A. G. (2023). Toxicological and epidemiological approaches to carcinogenic potency modeling for mixed mineral fiber exposure: The case of fibrous balangeroite and chrysotile. *Inhalation Toxicology*, *35*(7–8), 185–200. https://doi.org/10.1080/08958378.2023.2213720

Korchevskiy, A. A., & Wylie, A. G. (2025a). Habit of elongate amphibole particles as a predictor of mesothelial carcinogenicity. *Toxicology Reports*, *14*, 101908. https://doi.org/10.1016/j.toxrep.2025.101908

Korchevskiy, A. A., & Wylie, A. G. (2025b, April 24). The empirical metric of mesothelial carcinogenicity for carbon nanotubes and elongate mineral particles. *Inhalation Toxicology* (online). https://doi.org/10.1080/08958378.2025.2486087

Leidel, N. A., Bayer, S. G., Zumwalde, R. D., & Busch, K. A. (1979). *USPHS/NIOSH membrane filter method for evaluating airborne asbestos fiber* (Publication No. 79-127). USPHS/NIOSH. https://doi.org/10.26616/NIOSHPUB79127

Mandel, J. H., & Odo, N. U. (2018). Mesothelioma and other lung disease in taconite miners; the uncertain role of non-asbestiform EMP. *Toxicology and Applied Pharmacology*, *361*, 107–112. https://doi.org/10.1016/j.taap.2018.04.008

Mattioli, M., Giordani, M., Arcangeli, P., Valentini, L., Boscardin, M., Pacella, A., & Ballirano, P. (2018). Prismatic to asbestiform offretite from northern Italy: Occurrence, morphology and crystal chemistry of a new potentially hazardous zeolite. *Minerals, 8*(2), 69. https://doi.org/10.3390/min8020069

Maxim, L. D., & McConnell, E. E. (2005). A review of the toxicology and epidemiology of wollastonite. *Inhalation Toxicology, 9*, 451–466. https://doi.org/10.1080/08958370591002030

McDonald, J. C., Gibbs, G. W., Liddell, F. D. K., & McDonald, A. D. (1978). Mortality after long exposure to Cummingtonite-Grunerite. *American Review of Respiratory Disease, 118*, 271–277. https://doi.org/10.1164/arrd.1978.118.2.271

National Institute for Occupational Safety and Health (NIOSH/CDC). (2019). *Asbestos and other fibers by PCM, method 7400, issue 3* (5th ed.). NIOSH Manual of Analytical Methods (NMAM). https://www.cdc.gov/niosh/nmam/pdf/7400.pdf

National Institute for Occupational Safety and Health (NIOSH/USPHS). (1979). *NIOSH membrane filter method for evaluating airborne asbestos fibers* (Publication No. 79-127). NIOSH. https://stacks.cdc.gov/view/cdc/112897

Petriglieri, J. R., Laporte-Magoni, C., Salvioli-Mariani, E., Ferrando, S., Tomatis, M., Fubini, B., & Turci, F. (2021). Morphological and chemical properties of fibrous antigorite from lateritic deposit of New Caledonia in view of hazard assessment. *Science of the Total Environment*. https://doi.org/10.1016/j.scitotenv.2021.146185

Roggli, V. L. (2015). The so-called short-fiber controversy: Literature review and critical analysis. *The Archives of Pathology & Laboratory Medicine, 139*(8), 1052–1057. https://doi.org/10.5858/arpa.2014-0466-RA. PMID: 26230599

Roggli, V. L. (2018). Measuring EMPs in the lung: What can be measured in the lung: Asbestiform minerals and cleavage fragments. *Toxicology and Applied Pharmacology, 361*, 14–17. https://doi.org/10.1016/j.taap.2018.06.026

Schüz, J., Kovalevskiy, E., Olsson, A., Moissonnier, M., Ostroumova, E., Ferro, G., Feletto, E., Schonfeld, S. J., Byrnes, G., Tskhomariia, I., Straif, K., Morozova, T., Kromhout, H., & Bukhtiyarov, I. (2024). Cancer mortality in chrysotile miners and millers, Russian FEderation: Main results (Asbest chrysotile cohort study). *Journal of the National Cancer Institute, 116*(6), 866–875. https://doi.org/10.1093/jnci/djad262

Selikoff, I. J. (1978). Carcinogenic potential of silica compounds. In G. Bendz, I. Lindqvist, V. Runnström-Reio (Eds.), *Biochemistry of silicosis and related problems*. Plenum Press.

Shao, Y., Ramachandran, G., Mandel, J. H., MacLehose, R. F., & Alexander, B. H. (2025). Mesothelioma risks and cumulative exposure to elongate mineral particles of various sizes in Minnesota taconite mining industry. *Occupational & Environmental Medicine, 82*, 7–13. https://doi.org/10.1136/oemed-2024-109647

Shedd, K. B., Wylie, A. G., & Virta, R. L. (1982). *Size and shape characterization of fibrous zeolites by electron microscopy*. U.S. Department of the Interior, Bureau of Mines.

Skinner, H. C. W., Ross, M., & Frondel, C. (1989). *Asbestos and other fibrous materials: Mineralogy, crystal chemistry and health effects*. Oxford University Press. https://doi.org/10.1093/oso/9780195039672.001.0001

Steenland, K., & Brown, D. (1995). Mortality study of gold miners exposed to silica and nonasbestiform amphibole minerals: An update with 14 more years of follow-up. *American Journal of Industrial Medicine, 27*(2), 217–229. https://doi.org/10.1002/ajim.4700270207

Stemple, I. S., & Brindley, G. W. (1960). A structural study of talc and talc-tremolite relations. *Journal of the American Ceramic Society, 43*(1), 34–42. https://doi.org/10.1111/j.1151-2916.1960.tb09149.x

Tsipuroky, S. J. (1993). *Guembelite, an asbestiform 2M (sub 2) dioctahedral Al, mg mica* (Vol. 30, p. 145). Programs and abstracts, Annual Clay Minerals Conference.

Veblen, D. R., Buseck, P. R., & Burnham, C. W. (1977). Asbestiform chain silicates: New minerals and structural groups. *Science, 198*(4315), 359–365.

Verkouteren, J. R., & Wylie, A. G. (2000). The tremolite-actinolite-ferro-actinolite series: Systematic relationships among cell parameters, composition, optical properties, and habit, and evidence of discontinuities. *American Mineralogist, 85*(9), 1239–1254. https://doi.org/10.2138/am-2000-8-917

Virta, R. L. (1985). *The phase relationship of talc and amphiboles in a fibrous talc sample.* U.S. Bureau of Mines Report of Investigation 8923.

Wagner, J. C., Skidmore, J. W., Hill, R. J., & Griffiths, D. M. (1985). Erionite exposure and mesotheliomas in rats. *British Journal of Cancer, 51*(5), 727–730. https://doi.org/10.1038/bjc.1985.108

World Health Organization (WHO). (1997). *Determination of airborne fibre number concentrations – a recommended method, by phase-contrast optical microscopy (membrane filter method).* World Health Organization. https://iris.who.int/handle/10665/41904

Wylie, A. G., & Candela, P. A. (2015). Methodologies for determining the sources, characteristics, distribution, and abundance of asbestiform and nonasbestiform amphibole and serpentine in ambient air and water. *Journal of Toxicology and Environmental Health, Part B: Critical Reviews, 18*, 1–42. https://doi.org/10.1080/10937404.2014.997945

Wylie, A. G., & Huggins, C. W. (1980). Characteristics of a potassian winchite – asbestos from the Allamoore Talc District, Texas. *Canadian Mineralogist, 18*, 101–107.

Wylie, A. G., & Korchevskiy, A. A. (2023). Dimensions of elongate mineral particles and cancer: A review. *Environmental Research, 230*, 114688. https://doi.org/10.1016/j.envres.2022.114688

Yamate, G., Agarwal, S. C., & Gibbons, R. D. (1984). *Methodology for the measurement of airborne asbestos by electron microscopy* (Contract No. 68-02-3266). Environmental Monitoring Systems Laboratory, Office of Research and Development, U.S. Environmental Protection Agency. https://nepis.epa.gov/Exe/ZyPURL.cgi?Dockey=9101KTW6.txt

2 Measuring EMPs
Analytical approaches and the development of the dimensional database

A. Korchevskiy & A. Wylie

INTRODUCTION

MEASURING CONCENTRATIONS IN AIR AND BULK SAMPLES

One of the most unusual aspects of asbestos as a carcinogen is that its amount is measured not on a weight basis, but on counting concentration principles. It is assumed that the number of fibers entering the body is more important to evaluate than their weight, contrary to many other toxicants, which are measured in terms of weight. There is a second explanation for counting fibers instead of weighing them: the early scientists who worked with asbestos toxicity recognized individual fibers in air samples and counted them to compare concentrations. Though it is often difficult to fully distinguish mineral fibers in airborne samples from other particles, the error of weighing samples was judged to be higher than fiber counting. This is why, in regulations and toxicological experiments, counting metrics are used for asbestos: it can be fibers/unit volume of air or fibers/wt if in a bulk sample. Also, in toxicology, it is important to consider the surface area of elongate particles, in conjunction with other parameters, like the surface area of particles per surface area of cells. In human lungs, asbestos concentrations are measured in units of fibers per microgram of lung tissue. These expressions of abundance are unique among carcinogens and require different analytical approaches to obtain. They are also labor-intensive to obtain and have not yet been fully automated (although attempts have been made to introduce computer-based counting procedures).

Today, most commercial laboratories in the United States that analyze airborne particles or bulk samples for asbestos follow protocols that have been developed by the United States government or by two voluntary standards organizations: the International Standards Organization (ISO) and ASTM International (ASTM). These protocols were developed by a committee of knowledgeable laboratory analysts in response to the widespread use and disturbance of asbestos-containing materials in the built environment during the 20th century. They recognized the need for reliable analytical protocols for laboratories that were forming to deal with the environmental fallout from asbestos. In particular, the history of the phase-contrast microscopy method for asbestos was recently described by Burdett (2024). Table 2.1 lists the most commonly used protocols for analysis that are followed by many laboratories

DOI: 10.1201/9781003424277-3

TABLE 2.1
Commonly used methods for establishing concentrations of fiber in air and bulk samples.

Method	Source	Comments
a. Phase contrast optical microscopy (f/cc)	**NIOSH METHOD 7400, Issue 3, April 29, 2019 - ASBESTOS and OTHER FIBERS by PCM. (NIOSH, 2019)**	This is the membrane filter method that counts EMP-5 fibers collected on air monitoring filters with phase contrast microscopy (PCM). The analysis reports f/cc. Method limits include lack of visibility established by NIOSH as 0.15 µm for chrysotile and 0.05 µm for amphibole. In the absence of other information, all fibers are considered asbestos, but the method is to be used where the presence of asbestos in the air is "known a priori."
	ISO 8672:2014. Air Quality – Determination of the number concentration of airborne inorganic fibers by phase contrast optical microscopy – membrane filter method (ISO, 2014a)	Similar to NIOSH 7400.
	OSHA ID-160 Asbestos in Air (OSHA, 1997)	Membrane filter method equivalent to NIOSH 7400 without a lower limit of width specified. Alternate discriminatory criteria can be incorporated.
b. Phase contrast optical microscopy supplemented by electron microscopy for PCME (f/cc by mineral)	**ASTM D7201 – 06 (Reapproved 2020) Standard Practice for sampling and counting airborne fibers, including asbestos fibers, in the workplace, by phase contrast microscopy (with an option of transmission electron microscopy) (ASTM, 2020)**	This is the membrane filter method based on NIOSH 7400, OSHA ID-160, and ISO 8672 that includes optional transmission electron microscopy (TEM) with two sets of counting rules to determine fiber concentration. Counting rule A is aspect ratio (AR) = > 3:1. Counting rule B is AR >= 5:1. Both counting rules specify recording the lengths and widths of EMP-5 with widths = > 0.2 < 3.0 µm, although the upper limit of 3 µm is discretionary.
c. Transmission electron microscopy for concentration in air of PCME (f/cc by mineral type)	**ASBESTOS by TEM: NIOSH METHOD 7402 Issue 3 August 1, 2022. (NIOSH, 2022)**	The stated goal is to count phase contrast equivalent fiber (PCME). The method counts and records the length and width of EMP-5, width > 0.25 µm by transmission electron microscopy (TEM) with up to 20,000x magnification from air monitoring filters with direct transfer sample preparation. Classification by SAED is limited to four categories: amphibole, chrysotile, ambiguous, none. Does not require zone axis indexed patterns. Requires Si peak to be 75% of peak height at > 500 counts/channel; specifies elemental proportions in an EDXA spectrum for 5 amphiboles and chrysotile.

	ISO 10312 Ambient air – Determination of asbestos fibers – Direct transfer transmission electron microscopy method (TEM) 2nd Edition 2019–10 (ISO, 2019a)	Counts and records the length and width of 5:1 EMP–0.5 fibers and bundles (composed of 5:1 EMP–0.5) and/or PCM equivalent fibers specified as EMP–0.5 W > 0.25 μm by TEM with direct transfer sample preparation at magnification up to 100,000x (measurement bin 10 nm for 1 mm at 100,000x). Minimum signal for EDXA 10,000 counts from Si Kα. Two indexed zone axes for mineral identification from unknown sources along with EDXA are required for enough of the fibers that EDXA becomes reliable alone. Specifies International Mineralogical Association mineral nomenclature. Separate procedure if asbestos source is known.
d. Transmission electron microscopy for concentration in air of EMPs of all widths (f/cc by mineral type)	**ISO 13794–2019 Ambient air – Determination of asbestos fibers – Indirect-transfer transmission electron microscopy method. (ISO, 2019b)**	Counts and records by TEM the length and width of 5:1 EMP–0.5 fibers and bundles composed of 5:1 EMP–0.5 at magnification up to 100,000x (Measurement bin 1 mm at 100,000x) as in ISO10312 but with an indirect sample preparation technique. Sample preparation includes oxygen plasma ashing of air monitoring filters, residue washed in acetic acid, filtered, and samples prepared following the carbon replication procedure of ISO 10312. This method is known to increase fiber number and decrease fiber size in some samples, especially chrysotile.
	ASTM D6281 – 23. Standard test method for airborne asbestos concentration in ambient and indoor atmospheres as determined by transmission electron microscopy direct transfer (TEM). (ASTM, 2023a)	This method was adapted from ISO 10312. Counts and measures the length and width of 5:1 EMP–0.5 collected on air monitoring filters by TEM with samples prepared by direct transfer. Classification of asbestos type is based on morphology, a zone axis calibrated electron diffraction pattern, and quantitative EDXA. Direct transfer with plasma etching for MCE filters. Record width and length at 20,000x; measurement bin for 1 mm would be 50 nm.

(Continued)

TABLE 2.1 *(Continued)*

Commonly used methods for establishing concentrations of fiber in air and bulk samples.

Method	Source	Comments
e. Transmission electron microscopy of bulk material (surface wipes) (f/area by mineral type)	**ASTM D6480–19 Standard test method for wipe sampling of surfaces, indirect preparation, and analysis for asbestos structure number surface loading by transmission electron microscopy. (ASTM, 2019)**	Mineral identification based on TEM, SAED, and EDXA. Cannot discriminate between fiber and fragment reliably. Counts and records the lengths and widths of AR = 5:1 EMP–0.5 at magnification 15,000 – 20,000x (measurement bin = 50 to 70 nm).
f. Polarized light microscopy for bulk materials: Electron microscopy and XRD used for confirmation (asbestos type and %)	**EPA 600 R-93/116 Test Method: Method for the determination of asbestos in bulk building materials. (EPA, 1993)**	Analysis of building materials includes stereomicroscopic examination for habit, polarized light microscopy (PLM) for mineral identification, gravimetry for separating by density, X-ray diffraction (XRD) for mineral identification, analytical transmission electron microscopy for EDXA and electron diffraction, stereomicroscope for habit, and polarized light microscopy for classification of intentionally added asbestos. Includes sample preparation, milling, ashing, and acid washing. Method describes the asbestiform habit of particles and recognizes a mineral can be asbestiform but not asbestos because it lacks important physical characteristics.
	ISO 22262 – Air Quality – Bulk Materials (ISO, 2012)	There are three parts to this ISO method, which was developed for and is restricted to use in analyzing commercial bulk materials to which mineral fiber was intentionally added. Method states that if the fiber was not commercially mined and added intentionally, including tremolite, actinolite and anthophyllite, "no assumption can be made as to whether it is asbestiform or non-asbestiform" (22262–1 7.2.3.7.1). If 20:1 particles are present, then probably so is asbestos. Fibers counted EMP–0.05. The definition of the morphological characteristics of the fibrillar structure of asbestos, e.g., fiber bundles and spayed ends, is the same as that in EPA 600.

Part 1: Sampling and qualitative determination of asbestos in commercial bulk materials. First edition 2012-17-01. Analysis by polarized light microscopy (PLM) (detection limit = 0.1% asbestos), Scanning Electron Microscopy (SEM), and TEM. For PLM. identification is based on asbestiform morphology, color, extinction angle, and index of refraction at a known wavelength parallel and perpendicular to elongation established by immersion oil technique dispersion staining; standard Becke line methodology explicitly permitted but not discussed. For SEM and qualitative analysis by TEM, classification of asbestos is based on chemical composition by EDXA. For TEM, identification is based on ISO 10312 and ISO 13794.

Part 2: Quantitative determination of asbestos by gravimetric and microscopical methods (2014). Samples can be weighed before and after being heated to 450°C, treated with hydrochloric or sulfuric acid, elutriated in water, and separated by density using heavy liquids to concentrate amphibole. Residue filtered and dispersed for examination by ISO 22262–1. Quantitative estimates of volume abundance can be based on visual estimates (comparison to known reference materials) or point counting as described. A protocol specifically for vermiculite analysis is provided.

Part 3: Quantitative determination of asbestos by X-ray diffraction (XRD) method. The method is used to confirm and quantify asbestos previously detected by ISO 22262–1. XRD cannot distinguish elongate from equidimensional forms of minerals and cannot tell asbestiform from non-asbestiform materials. It can only be used in the known absence of non-asbestiform particles of the asbestos mineral, amphibole, and serpentine. Under ideal circumstances, with sample pretreatments (ashing and acid), XRD can detect asbestos at levels approaching 0.01 wt%.

(Continued)

TABLE 2.1 *(Continued)*
Commonly used methods for establishing concentrations of fiber in air and bulk samples.

Method	Source	Comments
	ASTM D7521 – 22 Standard test method for determination of asbestos in soil (ASTM, 2022)	Asbestos is identified by PLM determined morphology and optical properties. Optional TEM identification is based on morphology, SAED, and EDXA. Fiber by TEM is EMP–0.5 with AR => 5:1. Offers optional TEM method D6281 of fine fraction to report f/gm (structures/gm).
g. Scanning electron microscopy for concentration (f/cc by chemical composition) of PCME and EMP-5 in air	**ISO 14966–2019 Ambient air – Determination of numerical concentration of inorganic fibrous particles – Scanning electron microscopy (SEM) method (ISO, 2019c)**	Counts EMP–5. Measurements of length and width are recorded and EDXA is used for classification as in other ISO methods. Magnification up to 10,000x (measurement bin = 100 nm). All particles are counted whether fiber or fragment. In reporting, fibers with width < 0.2 μm are reported separately from those > 0.2 μm in width (PCME).
h. Scanning electron microscopy for bulk materials (surface wipes)(f/area by chemical composition)	**DIN ISO 16000-27-2014 Indoor air – Part 27: Determination of settled fibrous dust on surfaces by SEM (scanning electron microscopy) (direct method) (ISO, 2014b)**	Counts EMP-5 W > 0.2 μm and classifies based on major element ratios as seen on EDXA. Recognizes that talc and anthophyllite cannot be distinguished based on EDXA alone.
i. Transmission electron microscopy for carbon nanotubes (f/cc)	**ASTM D8526 Standard test method for analytical procedure using transmission electron microscopy for the determination of the concentration of carbon nanotubes and carbon nanotube-containing particles in ambient atmospheres (ASTM, 2023b)**	Counts tubes longer than 250 nm. Direct transfer sample preparation.

throughout the world. The short description that follows each describes some of the boundaries of each method.

Methods that rely on the membrane filter method and phase contrast optical microscopy determine airborne fiber concentration; two of them listed include supplemental mineral identification by electron microscopy. The membrane filter method is used for occupational exposure monitoring, and it is the method used to establish exposure levels for all epidemiological studies of asbestos. The analysis of bulk building materials relies primarily on polarized light microscopy (PLM), which, along with X-ray diffraction, provides observations by which fibrous minerals can be identified. In general, the methods are only applicable to building materials to which asbestos has been intentionally added and are too simplistic as described for identification of fibrous minerals generally. (Identification by PLM of naturally occurring fibers requires complex procedures not described in the methods of Table 2.1.) Electron microscopy has also been used for bulk materials. Transmission electron microscopy (TEM) offers the advantage of enabling precise dimensional measurements, chemical composition by energy-dispersive X-ray analysis (EDXA), and d-spacing measurements from zone axis selected area electron diffraction (SAED) patterns. Scanning electron microscopy (SEM) examines a larger amount of sample on a single mount than TEM and can provide chemical information for classification.

This maze of methods complicates studying the carcinogen significantly because the methods look at different portions of the sample and what is counted as fiber varies among the methods. For example, all TEM methods require measurement of the length and width of fibers counted, except for NIOSH 7402. ISO and ASTM methods use a 5:1 ratio to identify fibers by electron microscopy but a 3:1 ratio by optical microscopy. ISO and ASTM specify an upper limit of fiber width of 3 μm, but NIOSH has no upper limit. ISO and NIOSH use a minimum width of 0.25 μm (ISO 10312, NIOSH 7402), ASTM D7201 uses a minimum width of 0.2 μm,[1] and ISO 13794 and ASTM D6281 specify no lower limit. When the sample is characterized in so many ways, toxicological comparisons among them can be difficult, especially when the differences affect those very parameters that control carcinogenic potency on a scale that matters.

There are many factors that go into sample collection and preparation. A recent review by Malinconico et al. (2022) provides a comprehensive discussion of the analytical techniques that have been used in the analysis of soils and air for asbestos.

In this book, the data we rely on most heavily are the identification and measurement of dimensions of EMPs in images created by various microscopic techniques. Each method of measurement and its applications will be described. At the end of the chapter, we will return briefly to review the utility of the methods in Table 2.1.

MEASURING AIRBORNE OCCUPATIONAL EXPOSURE

PHASE CONTRAST MICROSCOPY

The measurement of exposure to airborne fibers for purposes of worker protection is based on Phase Contrast Microscopy (PCM) and the membrane filter method (NIOSH 7400; ISO 8672; OSHA ID-160; ASTM 7200; ASTM 7201). The membrane filter method specifies that asbestos fibers with a length-to-width ratio of at least 3:1

and a length greater than 5 μm (EMP-5) be counted as fibers (see Table 2.1.) PCM is a method in which part of the light is treated differently from the rest so that interference between the two paths takes place. The details of PCM are described by Longhurst (1957). Interference microscopy (Dodgson, 1963) is similar to PCM.

Without the addition of polarized light, the properties of minerals measurable by PCM are normally restricted to length (also limited by light microscopy generally, as discussed below), color, and average index of refraction relative to the surrounding medium. Index of refraction differences are such that specimens with a higher refractive index will appear dark, and those with a lower refractive index will appear bright, unless the particles are very thick, but relative differences are hard to quantify. Because most of the optical properties necessary for the identification of a mineral fiber are unavailable, PCM may not be useful for distinguishing among mineral types or for distinguishing manufactured from naturally formed particles. PCM offers slightly enhanced resolution over ordinary light microscopy and is particularly useful when the matrix has an index of refraction close to that of the particle of interest.

The resolution of an optical system is generally defined as the minimum distance by which two adjacent points can be separated. There are several different equations given for the resolving power of a light microscope, but they all depend on the numerical aperture (NA) of the objective and the wavelength of the illumination. The most common formulas are

$$d = \lambda/2NA$$

and

$$d = 0.61\ \lambda/NA$$

where d is the resolving power, λ is the wavelength of illumination, and NA is the numerical aperture of the objective (Longhurst, 1957).

In phase contrast microscopy and interference systems, the resolution may be enhanced somewhat, and the formula for resolution for the most commonly used optical system is

$$d = 0.4756\ \lambda/NA.$$

The NIOSH 7400 method for PCM specifies an objective with a NA of 0.65–0.75. Taking a wavelength in the center of visible light at 589 nm, the reference wavelength for optical properties, the resolving power of phase contrast microscopy will be about 0.4 μm. Were the object illuminated in blue light with $\lambda = 450$ nm, the resolving power would be closer to 0.3 μm.

Resolution and visibility are not the same thing, however. When counting fibers on an occupational monitoring filter, one counts what one can see, and what one can see is a function of the difference in the index of refraction of the object and the immersion medium used to render the filter "invisible" in the membrane filter method. If the difference is high, fibers much thinner than the resolution of the system can be visible. NIOSH 7400 specifies that chrysotile fibers as small as 0.15 µm and amphibole fibers of 0.05 µm are visible and will be counted.

PCME

In 1994, NIOSH introduced the concept of a PCM equivalent fiber (PCME), which would allow identification of the type of mineral by TEM, with its enhanced resolution and ability to determine chemical composition and structure, as revealed by electron diffraction, but at the same time, provide an exposure estimate of fibers that would be "equivalent" to the exposure determined by PCM (NIOSH, 1994). The NIOSH 7402 method incorporated this concept, and NIOSH recommended it for determining airborne concentration and identification of mineral particles that could be used for risk assessment. In this method, particles with a diameter greater than 0.25 µm that meet the definition of a fiber under NIOSH 7400 (EMP-5) are considered equivalent to what would be observed by PCM and are labeled PCME.

On June 14, 2019, NIOSH issued a third version of their 7400 method that provides "more accurate values for the minimum width limits for asbestos fiber detection," which they set as 0.15 µm for chrysotile and 0.05 µm for amphibole asbestos, based on published research and their own internal analysis. However, NIOSH has not yet withdrawn NIOSH 7402 or adjusted it to reflect this knowledge, despite a technical update to the method issued in August 2022, which still retains the following contradictory information: "Count all particles with diameter greater than 0.25 µm that meet the definition of a fiber (aspect ratio ≥3:1, longer than 5 µm). Use the guideline of counting all fibers that would have been counted under phase contrast light microscopy." This direction directly contradicts the information on visibility provided by NIOSH in their updates on 7400 PCM. Many electron microscopy methods described in Table 2.1 still assign lower width limits for counting fibers, usually about 0.2 µm, in an attempt to duplicate (incorrectly) PCM visibility.

Limitations of PCM and PCME

While visibility by PCM is mainly dependent on the contrast in the index of refraction between the particle and the medium in which it is immersed, precision in the measurement of particle dimensions depends on the resolution of the optical system. Visible particles with widths less than about 0.4 µm cannot be measured precisely by PCM. Generally, a length limit is imposed in PCM fiber counting. Early work on occupational monitoring methods demonstrated non-reproducibility if particles less than 5 µm in length were counted in exposure assessments, so 5 µm is the usual limit.

Given that PCM does not utilize polarized light and cannot identify most fibrous materials, it provides a reliable exposure estimate for asbestos only when the elongate particles being counted can be determined to be asbestos by some independent means, generally based on a priori knowledge of the source material of the dust. It is on PCM exposure estimates from cohort exposure in asbestos mines, manufacturing facilities, and elsewhere where this condition was met that asbestos risk assessments are based and on which permissible exposure limits (PEL) have been established by regulatory agencies in the U.S. and elsewhere. In an environment where dust components are unknown or there are many EMP-5s, PCM alone would have limited value.

Because the dimensions of asbestos have long been thought to be, along with durability, the major driver of carcinogenicity, eliminating fibers with widths ≤ 0.25 μm (NIOSH 7402) or < 0.2 μm (ASTM D7201, NIOSH 7402, and ISO 10312) removes those very fiber sizes that have been implicated most strongly in their potency for carcinogenicity, both in animal experiments (Stanton et al., 1981; Pott, 1980) and by human epidemiology (Wylie & Korchevskiy, 2023). It is our view that PCME, as defined by NIOSH 7402 (and others), provides data that are unreliable indicators of carcinogenicity and, as such, can underestimate the risk of airborne asbestos while overestimating risk from particles with limited carcinogenicity. In our opinion, NIOSH 7402 and other methods that impose a lower limit on width measurements should not be relied on to estimate toxicity or risk unless and until they are revised. It should be noted that many commercial laboratories currently modify the NIOSH 7402 method to count all fiber widths that can be practically seen in PCM-based epidemiological studies.

The overall controversy around PCM and PCME fibers has implications for risk assessment. For example, Darnton (2023, 2024) determined that the potency of chrysotile in producing mesothelioma can be estimated by a slope factor R_M, with an average of 0.0014%. This coefficient is supposed to be applied to PCM cumulative exposure values in f/cc-years, because all studies included in the epidemiological meta-analysis included exposure data measured by PCM. If cumulative exposure of chrysotile were to be measured by TEM with the width cutpoint of 0.15 μm, the risk estimation might be overestimated because every chrysotile fiber in the range of width from 0.15 μm to 0.2 μm might not be counted by all analysts. As NIOSH (2019) states in Issue 3: "However, not all microscopists can see finer chrysotile fibers between 0.15 μm and 0.2 μm without adequate training." Based on the dimensional data on chrysotile, the fraction of fibers with a width between 0.15 and 0.2 μm comprises 21 % of all PCM-visible chrysotile fibers.

If TEM were used for risk assessment purposes, here are several steps that should be taken for better characterization of fibers: (1) the size distribution of the fibers should be measured over the full range of width, (2) the distribution of measured fibers should be compared to the historical data on chrysotile as measured by phase contrast optical microscopy with the lower limits of visibility as indicated by NIOSH, (3) sample-specific correction factors can be used based on risk assessment models, including those from this book.

POLARIZED LIGHT MICROSCOPY (PLM) AND MINERAL HABIT

Whether or not bulk mineral samples are to be examined by TEM or SEM, they should first be examined by polarized light microscopy (PLM) to identify the mineral makeup and habit. Several standard methods are available for the analysis of building materials for intentionally added asbestos (EPA 600 R-93, ISO 22262, D7521), but for finding asbestos in rock and mineral products, more information must be gathered than these methods recommend because of the high likelihood of false positives. Effectively, all bulk mineral material will contain more than one mineral, regardless of what a label may say. By carefully choosing the immersion medium, the minerals that make up the sample can be identified by a skilled mineralogist.

Polarized light microscopy has been the most important method for the identification of minerals for over 200 years, and extensive references on the optical properties of every mineral are available.

Polarized light microscopy enables the observer to look at mineral properties that vary with crystallographic direction within the mineral. The vibration direction of the incident light is constrained to a single plane by a polarizer, and a rotating stage enables the particle to change orientation with respect to the vibration direction of the light. Most minerals are birefringent, such that light enters the crystalline mineral and, in most orientations, it follows two paths with perpendicular vibration directions, each with its own ray path. The rotation of the stage and sample enables each of these two rays to be observed independently. A second polarizer, referred to as an analyzer, when inserted into the system, enables observations on the interference of the two rays that are useful in identifying minerals and mineral habits.

By using PLM immersion oils, the optical properties, including principal indices of refraction (there will be two or three for most minerals), birefringence (the difference between the largest and smallest principal index of refraction), optic sign, the relationship between optic and cleavage directions, and other properties derived from "interference figures," such as the size of the optic axial angle and its dispersion, can be determined independently. For most silicate minerals, the set of properties is unique for each.

The asbestiform habit imparts high tensile strength and flexibility to normally rigid and brittle minerals, and it affects certain optical properties. Single crystals called fibrils, with widths smaller than a wavelength of light, form in groups with their long directions parallel or near-parallel to a common fiber axis direction in the asbestiform habit (Figure 2.1). The widths of fibrils vary among occurrences, ranging from 10 nm to about 200 nm. The lengths can range over orders of magnitude, from

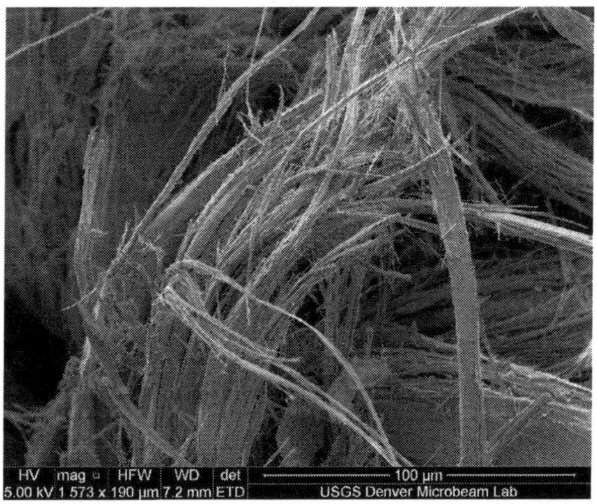
HV | mag | HFW | WD | det
5.00 kV | 1 573 x | 190 µm | 7.2 mm | ETD
100 µm
USGS Denver Microbeam Lab

FIGURE 2.1 The asbestiform habit: woolly erionite. Photo courtesy of Bradley van Gosen, United States Geological Survey.

a few hundred nanometers to a few hundred micrometers or more. In a hand specimen, in bright light, asbestos fibers appear silky. Visible fibers are composite, and the silky luster arises from these "bundles of fibrils." Anomalous properties observable by PLM are described by Verkouteren and Wylie (2002) and include parallel or near-parallel extinction when a characteristic oblique extinction is expected; two measurable principal indices of refraction when three are characteristic of the mineral; uniaxial-like interference figures; and lower than characteristic birefringence. These anomalous properties are indicative of fiber bundles and should alert to the potential for the presence of fibrils (Coffin et al., 1983). Bundles of fibrils often splay at the ends, demonstrating their composite nature.

The methods for the analysis of asbestos by polarized light microscopy listed in Table 2.1 (EPA 600 and ISO 22262) provide useful morphological descriptions of the asbestiform habit as follows:

a. The average aspect ratios in the range of 20:1 or higher for fibers longer than 5 μm.
b. Splitting of fiber bundles into fibrils that are generally less than 0.5 μm in width.
c. One or more of the following:

    1. Parallel fibers occurring in bundles.
    2. Fiber bundles displaying splayed ends.
    3. Fibers in the form of thin needles.
    4. Matted masses of individual fibers.
    5. Fibers showing curvature.

The optical properties of byssolite, a wide, glassy, brittle type of fiber, can also be anomalous because byssolite fibers are single crystals that are twinned on a sub-light scale. However, twinning does not mean the twins can readily separate into narrower fibrils along twin planes, although under pressure, they may fracture preferentially parallel to the twinning direction, a process called parting. Elongated cleavage fragments that exhibit normal optics have no potential for longitudinal splitting unless there has been incipient growth of secondary mineralization.

Minerals in asbestiform habit are the only ones known from human epidemiology to result in mesothelioma following airborne exposure (see Chapter 9). The identification of habit is best evaluated by polarized light microscopy, and mineral material should be confirmed by PLM examination if possible before accepting the designation as asbestos.

Estimating abundances by point counting

Point counting is a technique used by geologists to estimate the relative abundances of minerals in a thin slice (30 μm) of rock. The object is moved in set increments using a mechanical stage, and the mineral in the center of each field of view is identified and recorded. Abundances are then based on the number of points for each mineral.

Point counting is recommended by EPA Method 600 (Perkins & Harvey, 1993) for bulk samples of asbestos-containing building materials. For point counting to produce a reliable and reproducible estimate of abundances, however, two principles must be adhered to. First, the thickness of all components must be the same. For this reason, rocks are always cut in sections of equal thickness (30 μm). Second, the incremental movements between points must be larger than the largest particle being counted. In the case of building materials, the first principle is rarely adhered to, and for this reason, point counting may have significant errors. A visual estimate based on comparison to materials with known abundances may be equally valid, is accepted in ISO 22262–1 and is often used in determining small amounts of a mineral in a thin section of rock.

ELECTRON MICROSCOPY: ANALYSIS OF AEROSOL-SIZED EMPS

All forms of electron microscopy have a higher resolution than light microscopy and are equipped to gather both structural and chemical data from individual particles. Electron microscopy enables greatly enhanced precision in dimensional measurements over optical microscopy. Analytical electron microscopy can place constraints on mineral identification from structural information obtained by selected area electron diffraction on transmission electron microscopy (TEM) and on the relative abundances of major elements (EDXA) normally available on both TEM and scanning electron microscopy (SEM). Table 2.1 lists methods that use PCM for exposure concentration but enable TEM or SEM for confirmation of fiber identity, as well as methods for direct estimates of fiber concentration.

Sample preparation

There are many reasons for different outcomes of an electron microscopic analysis of supposedly the same material, but an important one is sample preparation, for which there are few standard methods. In this section, we will describe steps commonly used in the preparation of material for examination by electron microscopy.

Air filters

Two general methods have been used to prepare samples collected on air monitoring filters for examination by electron microscopy. One is referred to as direct transfer; the other, indirect. NIOSH 7402, ISO 10312, and ASTM D6281 use the direct method, while ISO 13794–2019 uses the indirect method for the TEM. For the SEM, only direct methods are found in Table 2.1. By direct transfer, the particles collected on an air monitoring filter are first coated, the filter dissolved, after which the particles are transferred intact to a TEM grid. The filters with particles intact may be etched in a plasma asher prior to examination by SEM stub. By indirect methods, the filters are ashed by heating or by low-temperature oxidation in an oxygen-rich environment, after which the particles are collected and redeposited to the appropriate substrate, such as coated TEM grids, smooth filters, or directly on an SEM stub. For risk assessment, the direct transfer method is most reliable, as the indirect transfer method has been demonstrated to increase the number of fibers in certain cases and decrease average lengths and widths (Chesson et al., 1990; Chatfield, 1999). While the effects may be small, they are variable and introduce uncertainty not present if the direct transfer method is used.

Tissue

Minerals have been recovered from animal and human tissue by three basic methods: acid digestion, low-temperature ashing, and freeze drying. Today, most laboratories use acid digestion because studies have shown that there is a likelihood of changing the dimensional characteristics of the mineral particles by ashing (see Chapter 6 for a more detailed discussion.) There are no universally standardized methods for the preparation of lung burden for analysis by TEM. The materials may be collected, a known weight dispersed on a filter, and direct transfer methods used to prepare samples for examination by electron microscopy.

Bulk samples

When disturbance of rock during mining, road construction, or excavations is to be undertaken, bulk samples of the rock or overburden may be taken to evaluate the potential for fiber release during comminution of the materials. Building materials that have incorporated mineral material may also become a target for analysis to determine the potential toxicity of dusts that are or could be generated from these sources. Consumer products such as play sand, cosmetics, and garden soil have all been analyzed for possible traces of asbestos. These are not the types of materials that the methods from Table 2.1 were designed for, and their use to study them has led to many of the issues that still surround our understanding of carcinogenic fibers.

Examination by low-power binocular microscopy

Bulk samples are generally first examined by binocular microscopy at low magnification for the presence of fibers. If fibrous minerals are present, they can be hand-picked for a more detailed examination. If the relative abundance of a fibrous component is the objective, bulk samples must first be crushed and then subsampled to obtain a small representative volume of material that can then be prepared for examination.

Particle size reduction and estimating volume or weight percent

Size reduction can be accomplished by using a variety of mills or by hand grinding in a mortar and pestle. The goal is to reduce the size of particles (or break up fiber bundles) so that they can be viewed by electron microscopy.

It is generally assumed that all particle sizes resulting from sample size reduction methods will have abundances of the mineral components that are in the same proportions as the original bulk material. However, minerals fragment differently, with some producing a very large number of small particles proportionally to a larger size, while for others, this ratio will be smaller. Turcotte (1986) demonstrated that particles will fragment according to a fractal model that demonstrates a linear relationship between the log number of particles and log size ($\log N = -D \log R + C$), where N is the number of particles, R is the radius, C is a constant, and D is the fractal dimension. Among the materials he studied, D varied from 1.44 to 3.54. Wylie (1993) showed that his model holds for asbestos, with D varying from 3.34 to 0.37 depending on the sample. A range in D of this magnitude among mineral components in a bulk sample can produce significant errors in weight percent or volume percent abundances, especially from TEM observations, which look at a very restricted size range of particles. Where possible, therefore, weight or volume percent abundances are best estimated from polarized light microscopy (see the section above), which can examine a wide range of particle sizes because mass and volume are concentrated in the largest, least abundant particles. If abundances are based on particle number, the TEM, in most cases, is the best instrument because the number of small particles is often several orders of magnitude greater than the number of the largest particles.

Heavy liquid separation

Heavy liquid separation can be used to separate the mineral components of a powdered sample according to density, thereby concentrating components for easier analysis and more accurate abundance estimates, especially when the component is not very abundant. This method has long been employed by geologists to separate heavy minerals such as magnetite, garnet, and olivine from lower-density silicates and oxides, or low-density minerals like zeolites from other silicates. The methods work well when there is a large difference in density among the components, and a number of different liquids are available for this purpose. However, when the minerals are close in density, such as talc (density = 2.6 gm/cm3) and chrysotile (2.55 gm/cm3), the methods are not very useful and are not recommended for this purpose by ASTM or ISO. In addition to density, these minerals may behave in water-based heavy liquids differently because talc is strongly hydrophobic while chrysotile is strongly hydroscopic. On the other hand, heavy liquids including those that are water-based, may be quite effective in separating an amphibole such as tremolite (D ≈ 3.0 gm/cm3) from talc.

Sonication

For bulk samples, solids recovered from tissue, or particles taken from a filter, it is a normal step in most laboratory procedures to disperse the material in water by sonication, sometimes adding a surfactant. Because fibrils are not normally "glued" to each other, both sonication and a surfactant enhance their separation, increasing fiber number count and providing a more complete picture of the potential for fibril release (Lee et al., 1995).

Samples from several of the mineral locations in the database have been analyzed by different labs using TEM, one of which incorporates sonication and one that does not, as shown in Table 2.2.

TABLE 2.2
Effects of sonication on anthophyllite and tremolite asbestos

Mineral	With Sonication	Without Sonication
	(% EMPA)	(% EMPA)
UICC anthophyllite asbestos	6.8	0.9
Tremolite asbestos (Korea)	39.3	14.0

Acid treatment

Prior to dispersal, sometimes bulk samples are subjected to acid treatment to remove carbonates. Cook et al. (2016) provided the dimensional data from characterization in their laboratory of a set of samples that included those used by Stanton et al. (1981). From the raw data published by Cook et al., dimensional parameters were calculated for a set of samples that were both treated and untreated with acid, as shown in Table 2.3. Very little difference in average length and width was observed.

Elutriation

To collect a sample that can be examined by TEM or SEM, the sample must be composed only of very small particles. The analysis is not of the entire bulk material, but ideally, the goal is to measure particles that can be released, become airborne, and inhaled. For water elutriation, a sample is dispersed in a column of water and allowed to settle for a fixed period of time according to Stokes' law, when a sample is withdrawn from a predetermined depth for the target size. The TEM or SEM mount is prepared from this aliquot. For air elutriation, a dust is created by mechanical disturbance of the material. The dust is collected and treated like an occupational monitoring filter. A method to detect erionite in soil developed by Berry et al. (2020) uses air elutriation to separate fibers from mineral particles with higher aerodynamic diameter, with an effective detection limit of 0.003 wt %.

Water vs. air elutriation

In 2021, Eric Chatfield published a study on the equivalence of air and water elutriation of amphibole elongate mineral particles (Chatfield, 2021). The samples chosen were not asbestiform. TEM specimens were prepared from the aqueous suspension following ISO 13794 and from polycarbonate filters by following ISO 10312. Chatfield found that air elutriation underestimates mean width (for a given length) and

TABLE 2.3
Effects of leaching on the dimensions of asbestos (Cook et al., 2016)

Mineral	Average length (μm)	Average width (μm)	EMPA fraction	EMPB fraction	Criteria particle fraction
Tremolite unleached	13.99	0.63	0.033	0.195	0.74
Tremolite leached	13.97	0.61	0.05	0.19	0.724
Crocidolite unleached	15.8	0.29	0.23	0.58	0.96
Crocidolite leached	13.06	0.3	0.26	0.56	0.95
Amosite unleached	21.8	0.57	0.03	0.2	0.84
Amosite leached	27.6	0.57	0.01	0.14	0.867
Non-fibrous grunerite unleached	7.91	1.1	0.01	0.04	0.263
Non-fibrous grunerite leached	7.19	1.03	0	0.04	0.33

that water elutriation overestimates it. This would also mean that the aspect ratio of particles separated by water elutriation would be lower than those collected from air elutriation.

Chemical analysis

Both SEM and TEM utilize energy-dispersive X-ray analysis (EDXA) to provide a chemical signature. For reasons such as particle shape, size, and variation in thickness, which are beyond the scope of this discussion, a qualitative chemical analysis rather than a quantitative analysis is normally obtained. (TEM can provide a quantitative chemical analysis of thin particles, and SEM can provide a quantitative analysis of larger particles if they are flat.) For quantitative analyses, both approaches require the use of standards with compositions similar to those of the particles being analyzed, a condition rarely encountered in the analysis of aerosols by commercial laboratories. Unfortunately, this means that minerals with compositions that are close, such as sepiolite $\left(\left(Mg_4Si_6O_{15}(OH)_2\,6H_2O\right)\right.$, talc $\left(Mg_3Si_4O_{10}(OH)_2\right)$, jimthompsonite and clinojimthompsonite $(Mg,Fe)_5\,Si_6O_{16}(OH)_2$), chesterite $(Mg,Fe)_{17}\,Si_{20}O_{54}(OH)_6$), and anthophyllite $\left((Mg,FE)_7\,Si_8O_{22}(OH)_2\right)$, or a sodium-poor Na-Ca amphibole richterite and a sodium-rich tremolite, cannot be distinguished based on a qualitative determination of their chemical composition alone. However, for most minerals of concern, including amphiboles that make up asbestos in widespread commercial use, identification is often possible, especially if the mineralogy of the aerosol source is known. The International Mineralogical Association recommends that the name of the suspected amphibole be qualified by using terms such as "tremolitic" instead of tremolite or "anthophyllitic" instead of anthophyllite, etc., when the chemical analysis is qualitative and information about the source is lacking, although this convention is rarely followed by commercial laboratories.

Scanning electron microscopy

Scanning electron microscopes have the capacity for very high magnification and resolution. They are able to provide chemical information and morphology. They lack the ability to determine crystallographic information easily during routine analysis (excluding the still research-based scanning tunneling microscopy and analytical scanning transmission electron microscopy, or STEM-inSEM.) (Holm and Mansfield, 2024).

The SEM has the advantage over TEM of being able to see the entire length of fibers that are hundreds of micrometers in length, and a larger number of particles are available for observation. Larger particles may exhibit habit characteristics, such as the fibrillar structure of asbestos, that are not normally observed or recorded by TEM. Also, because a single preparation for observation contains many times the amount of material on a TEM grid, the sensitivity to detect low-abundance minerals is higher. For these reasons, lengths and widths generated by TEM and SEM from the same material are not usually comparable, especially for chrysotile but also for amphibole. In general, the narrowest and shortest fibers are reported as more abundant in a TEM analysis than in one done by SEM.

TABLE 2.4
Proportions of amphibole asbestos by width and method of analysis

Width range (μm)	Fraction by SEM	Fraction by TEM
Amosite		
< 0.125	0.014	0.035
0.125–0.275	0.089	0.094
0.275– 0.375	0.175	0.074
> 0.375	0.72	0.80
Crocidolite		
< 0.125	0.042	0.13
0.125–0.275	0.42	0.27
0.275– 0.375	0.37	0.26
> 0.375	0.17	0.34

In comparison to the measurement of length by optical microscopy, SEM reports a higher number of shorter particles (Wylie, 1993), but in comparison to TEM, SEM includes longer fibers because of the larger field of view.

In addition to differences in the range of length observed by scanning electron microscopy, there are differences in the measurement of length among the data sets in our database. Many of the SEM measurements were made many years ago, and modern SEMs, including FESEMs (Field Emission Scanning Electron Microscopes), may have much improved sensitivity for narrow fibers.

Table 2.4 shows the fraction of four width categories for EMPs longer than 5 μm of two materials: amosite from the Transvaal and crocidolite from South Africa. The number of fibers in each set shown below are amosite SEM n = 801, amosite TEM n = 202, crocidolite SEM n = 497, and crocidolite TEM n = 204. While the data demonstrate the capacity for the SEM to measure the narrowest widths, the method is not as sensitive in these narrow width ranges.

Chrysotile is a particular problem for many SEMs to visualize. Chrysotile fibrils can be as small as 10 nanometers. In our database, we have fibers longer than 5 μm that are only 13 nm in width. Such a small fibril is already 14% water, with an empty tube (or sometimes filled) providing very little mass to interact with the incident electron beam; however, they are readily visible by TEM. Dodson et al. (2008) compared asbestos concentrations from paraffin blocks of lung tissue determined by SEM and TEM. Analysis by SEM at 1000 magnification overlooked many uncoated chrysotile fibers.

Transmission electron microscopy

An aerosol prepared by direct transfer for TEM analysis, as described by ISO 10312 and ASTM D7201, provides the opportunity to measure with great precision the dimensions of elongate particles and to determine their identity from a qualitative chemical analysis and indexed zone axis electron diffraction patterns. For positive identification of an unknown, two indexable zone axis electron diffraction patterns are required in addition to chemical information.

Operating at about 20,000 magnification, the data could be recorded in 0.05 µm increments, although it may be reported in 0.1 µm increments. At higher magnification, much greater precision is possible. Given the recognition of the importance of width in carcinogenicity, it is recommended that for the measurement of narrow widths, a magnification of 40,000 or more should be used, such that the measurement bin is 0.025 µm. The difference in carcinogenicity between a fiber that is 100 nanometers in width and one that is 150 nanometers may be very significant (Lippmann, 2015), so precision that enables measurements of fibers in increments less than 20–30 nm may be important in evaluating their toxicity. Chrysotile fibrils and the smallest amphibole fibrils may be only 20 nm in width, and high magnification is necessary to measure them at all. For length, measurement intervals of 0.5 µm for fibers close to 5 µm in length and 1 µm for longer fibers are normally sufficient for hazard assessment.

Mineral fibers normally display parallel sides, and there is little variability in width. However, some particles of asbestiform material may be composite, with fibrils of different lengths, and fragments do not always break along continuous planes. Under these conditions, there may be a variation in width along the particle length. Often, an estimate of the average width is made, and if the material is a fiber bundle, that information is noted. Averages are most useful for determining mass. Alternatively, the largest dimension perpendicular to the length may be recorded as the width. If aerodynamic diameter is to be calculated from the measured length and width, the largest width rather than the average may be preferred. However, most elongate particles from aerosols of mineral fiber do not present this dilemma.

The formal methods for sample characterization described in Table 2.1 use differing criteria for including particles as fibers. As we will show in the rest of this chapter and in the book generally, not every one of these characterization methods would be satisfactory for sample characterization for toxicological purposes. First, all particles longer than 5 µm and with an aspect ratio of 3:1 and higher should be counted. These are the fibers that form the basis for epidemiological studies and risk assessment. When the data are restricted to 5:1, important data are lost because epidemiological data for asbestos-related cohorts included criteria of 3:1 for counting. Second, no lower limit of width should be applied. While there may be a lower limit of width for toxicity based on fiber rigidity (see Chapter 7), the narrowest rigid fibers are likely the most toxic. Furthermore, the lower limits of width imposed (0.25 or 0.2 µm) do not correspond to visibility limits in the membrane filter method in the first place. Finally, a lower limit of length of 0.5 µm is unnecessary. All evidence points to the body's treating short fibers as nuisance dust that is not carcinogenic, and the risk from short fibers has not been established, although some researchers believe that short fibers contribute to the toxicity of asbestos generally. If short fibers are to be counted, then a lower limit of length of 2 µm probably could be used. This level of 2 µm is the size of clay particles, a common exposure in every agricultural region in the world, and humans likely have evolved mechanisms to rid the body of such nuisance dust.

CHARACTERIZING THE DIMENSIONS OF MINERAL PARTICLE POPULATIONS

Because dimensions have been shown to be a primary determinant of EMP toxicity, their measurement may be particularly important in understanding and predicting diseases associated with inhalation exposure, particularly because the path of mineral fiber from inhalation to lung and mesothelial tissue is governed by particle dimensions. Frequency distributions of length and width reveal the habit of the source material, and if asbestiform, the size of fibrils. Frequency distributions of width for particles longer than 5 μm in length from the lung burden of asbestos-related disease cases provide a clear picture of the characteristics of mineral fiber carcinogens. QSAR analysis of epidemiological and dimensional data has produced robust models for mineral particle toxicity and risk analysis.

To understand mineral fiber carcinogenicity is to understand the origins of cancer generally, but to do so, we must first understand the carcinogen. Mineral fiber, such as asbestos, is highly inhomogeneous with respect to fiber dimensions, varying from location to location (Wylie, 2016; Korchevskiy & Wylie, 2025). The potency for mesothelioma also varies from location to location (Hodgson & Darnton, 2000; Darnton, 2023, 2024). Perhaps the key to explaining these observations lies in a common but variably abundant carcinogenic (lung cancer and mesothelioma) fiber that can be identified by its dimensions.

While the formal methods are described briefly at the beginning of the chapter, only a few are useful for understanding the toxicology of mineral fibers unless they are modified. PCM or modified TEM or SEM provide fiber concentrations, but only the TEM can be used to make dimensional measurements useful for toxicology, and those measurements should cover the full range of widths less than 3 μm. Some of the special conditions that asbestos presents in the measurement and characterization of its unusual dimensions are discussed below.

WIDTH

Many people assume that mineral fibers are microfibers, not nanofibers. In fact, most asbestos fibrils are nanofibers with widths that range from < 20 to > 100 nm. They form fibers from bundles of fibrils, and these bundles are microfibers. Elongate particles formed by comminution, on the other hand, are not nanofibers, and most rarely have widths less than 500 nm. Table 2.5 provides the range of widths of the 10 narrowest particles we have in our database for the common amphiboles by length and subdivided by method of measurement. It is clear that very narrow fibers can be found in all and that measurement protocols, including high magnification, should be developed with this range in mind.

It has become increasingly clear that differences in width on the order of tens of nanometers can have a profound impact on mineral particle carcinogenicity. Insights have come from experiments with carbon nanotubes, which can be produced with widths that range from a few nanometers to almost 200 nm. Zhu et al. (2016) showed that they could be too narrow (37 nm) because they lack rigidity below this width, and Nagai et al. (2011) suggested that carbon nanotubes (although perhaps not

TABLE 2.5
Dimensions of the smallest single fibrils by mineral and type of EM

Mineral type	EM	Length Range (μm)	Width Range (nm)
Tremolite	TEM	≤ 5	10–34
	TEM	5 ≤ 10	11–50
	TEM	10 ≤ 20	34–61
	TEM	> 20	60–90
Anthophyllite	TEM	≤ 5	69–100
	TEM	5 ≤ 10	96–103
	TEM	10 ≤ 20	50–240
	TEM	> 20	100–200
Amosite	TEM	≤ 5	20–40
	SEM	≤ 5	40–50
	TEM	5 ≤ 10	95
	SEM	5 ≤ 10	50–100
	TEM	10 ≤ 20	95
	SEM	10 ≤ 20	90–100
	TEM	> 20	50–95
	SEM	> 20	100–140
Crocidolite	TEM	≤ 5	50
	SEM	≤ 5	40–50
	TEM	5 ≤ 10	44
	TEM	10 ≤ 20	29–50
	SEM	10 ≤ 20	60
	TEM	> 20	50–80
	SEM	> 20	70
Chrysotile	TEM	≤ 5	10
	TEM	5 ≤ 10	13–17
	TEM	10 ≤ 20	13–20
	TEM	> 20	17–50

crocidolite) could be too wide (maybe > 145 nm) because wide fibers cannot break membranes or otherwise injure mesothelial cells. The potential for both upper and lower width thresholds for EMPs exists, as suggested by carbon nanotube studies, and must be tested, but it is clear that the measurement of width, in particular, should be made at high enough magnification that imprecision in the measurements does not affect the understanding of mineral fiber carcinogenicity.

Thickness of EMPs

To calculate surface area or volume for individual particles, direct measurements or assumptions of the thickness must be made. Thickness is also very important in determining the rigidity of EMPs, and rigidity is a necessary characteristic of carcinogenic mineral fiber.

Thickness can be measured directly by polarized light microscopy. Grains dispersed in a liquid can be rotated for visual estimates of width-to-thickness ratio. Alternatively, thickness can be determined from the interference colors produced by the two rays traversing the thickness in a birefringent mineral grain whose two indices of refraction are known. However, polarized light techniques are most effective for EMPs thicker than several micrometers and therefore may not be useful for most aerosol-sized mineral particles.

It is very common to see the width of a mineral fiber referred to as the diameter. Because diameter is the width of a circle, the use of the term implies a cylindrical shape. This assumption is technically only correct for rolled sheet silicates such as single chrysotile fibers or halloysite fibers and for carbon nanotubes, which are cylinders. Studies on amphibole fibrils have shown that they are irregular in cross-section, but that curved surfaces are not uncommon. Fragmented EMPs will have shapes that are determined primarily by cleavage and parting planes that follow well-known crystallographically controlled directions and are planar, not curved.

Only one study has measured the thickness of asbestos fibers directly. In 1987, Wylie et al. measured the thickness of crocidolite and amosite from South Africa by both TEM and SEM. From these two studies, a single equation relating width and thickness was derived:

$$\text{Log thickness} = 0.692 \log \text{width} - 0.493$$

We have used this equation for all asbestiform amphiboles.

Amphiboles have two directions of well-developed cleavage at 56-degree angles, and these cleavage planes bound the particles. These planes ideally form a rhombus shape perpendicular to elongation, resulting in an ideal width-to-thickness ratio of 1.88. This could be used for fragmented amphiboles with the assumption tested by examination by polarized light microscopy, where thickness can be directly estimated from known indices of refraction and interference colors.

Single-chain silicates such as pyroxenes have two well-developed directions at about 90 degrees, creating an ideal square cross-section. Other estimates we have used based on polarized light microscopy are erionite, 1:1; balangeroite, 1.1:1; and talc, 3:1. The latter estimate is based on studies of other sheet silicates (discussed in Wylie & Korchevskiy, 2025) as well as estimates from direct observation.

Because of the importance of rigidity in mineral carcinogenicity, the lack of direct measurement of thickness must be seen as a deficit in our knowledge. It is likely an important clue to understanding the potential carcinogenicity of all ribbon-shaped sheet silicate EMPs.

Frequency distributions of EMP width and length

Shape of frequency curves

It is often assumed that the frequency of width and length follows a log-normal distribution. In general, this is true for EMP mineral particle populations, but in detail, sometimes superimposed on the log-normal distributions are one or more modes of both length and width. During fragmentation in response to an applied force, width and length modes will reflect the spacing of planes of weakness in the mineral that are related to their atomic structures, to intergrowth relationships among minerals, and to planes of weakness related to strain developed in the rock from its geologic history. When mineral fibers form in nature, they can be very uniform and exhibit well-developed modes when the fibers are dispersed, especially in width. Crystals grown in the laboratory from supersaturated fluids are small and uniform in size. Asbestiform fibrils form in this same way, with several modes in either width or length likely reflecting changing conditions under which the single fiber crystals (fibrils) were forming (Wylie, 2016). Fibrils from the same mining district often exhibit remarkable uniformity, demonstrating regionally uniform physical and chemical factors at work during formation.

The choice of frequency bin intervals

Visualizing dimensional data in ways that are helpful in understanding mineral fiber carcinogenicity depends on the presentation of frequency diagrams that are based on clearly stated bin intervals, so frequency is a measure of number % in each bin. To make comparisons among and within populations possible, each bin should be the same size to the extent possible.

Frequency bin intervals themselves should be some multiple of the bin measurement interval. For example, measurements are recorded in mm, which is converted to μm and recorded. For most of the data in our database, the precision of the measurements and hence the bin measurement interval is determined by the magnification and the unit of measure on either the TEM screen when measurements are made directly or from photographs. Assuming a 1 mm minimum measurement interval, the minimum interval recommended in the TEM methods in Table 2.1 is 0.1 μm at 10,000x, 0.05 μm at 20,000, 0.025 μm at 40,000x, and 0.01 μm at 100,000. It is the intervals of the initial recording unit, the measurement interval that must be known to ensure that the frequencies depicted in a frequency diagram reflect the data collected, free from as many binning errors as possible. If possible, frequency bin intervals should be chosen that are multiples of the bin measurement interval, but offset slightly to prevent overlap of boundaries, especially if they are close in value. If the measurement interval is smaller than the frequency bin interval and the frequency interval is not a multiple of the measurement interval, some frequency intervals will include more measurement intervals than others, creating false modes. On the other hand, if the measurement interval is larger than the frequency bin interval, some bins would be empty. This happens with asbestos because the toxicological properties related to width can change on the scale of nanometers (e.g., rigidity and ability to penetrate a cell membrane under biological forces), so it is often the case that we are interested in measurements on the nanoscale where measurement bins and frequency bin intervals can be almost the same size. When each frequency bin interval contains many measurement intervals, the relationship between frequency bin boundaries and measurement boundaries becomes less important.

Frequency of particle number/unit sample mass

When Merle Stanton was using asbestos to implant on the pleura of animals, he devised a method to talk about both dimension and dose by first measuring the length and width from photographs of 1000 particles dispersed on TEM grids by weight. In this way, he could derive a measure of potency based on fiber number per microgram in specific length/width categories. In 1987, Stanton crocidolite samples were remeasured at the U.S. Bureau of Mines. They found that because the number of particles of particular sizes varied significantly among the materials, especially materials with fibers, they used the log #f/ug, which varied over many orders of magnitude. For this reason, experimental error suggested by the recount would likely make no more than 0.5 log units' uncertainty in the calculation of log #f/microgram. Given that the range is over six log units, an error of this size is relatively small.

Some general observations

There are many factors, from sampling to sample preparation to sample examination and recording, that influence the frequencies of length and width that are counted and reported as representative of an inhalable aerosol. In particular, discussions have centered around processes that increase fiber numbers and decrease fiber size, and some have asked if measurement can be relied on to describe carcinogenic mineral fibers. The variables are most evident in data collected by TEM because it is the frequencies of small fibers that are most affected.

Disaggregation may be a problem for regulatory purposes when a permissible exposure limit (PEL) has been established based on a particular sample collection and a method of analysis, and alternate protocols are used to measure it in practice. However, disaggregation is a property of a mineral carcinogen. In a sense, it is what makes it a carcinogen, and it means that dose may increase over time. Cleavage fragments do not disaggregate during sample collection or preparation.

The discussion of lung burden in Chapter 7 shows that, in those exposed to asbestos, lung burden is dominated by single fibrils, and those that are bundles are likely to disaggregate over time. As we will show, despite all of the variability in protocols, dimensions identify asbestiform mineral populations. Furthermore, we will also show that it is the presence of durable, rigid EMPs, which are derived from asbestiform minerals, that are of a particular size and occur in statistically significant amounts that signifies the presence of carcinogenic mineral fibers.

THE DATABASE

As long as certain elongated mineral particles are defined as carcinogens based on their dimensions, it is important that raw data from studies of mineral dimensions be retained. Over the last five years, we have assembled raw data for length and width of minerals from many locations. These data were gathered from many sources, including the University of Maryland, the U.S. Bureau of Mines, the U.S. EPA, NIOSH, and other public sources. The database benefited significantly from important contributions from Dr. Eric Chatfield and Drew Van Orden (R.J. Lee), Cook et al. (2016), and others identified in Table 2.6, and we are very grateful that they were willing to share their data. Where data were lacking, additional samples were measured and added to the database, enhancing the breadth of characterized minerals or mineral locations. With financial support from the National Stone Sand and Gravel Association, the database was established and organized by Chemistry & Industrial Hygiene, Inc. (C&IH). It has been the source of the data that we present in this book.

The database contains data on three mineral groups: amphibole, serpentine, and erionite. It includes measurements from air samples as well as from aerosol-sized, dispersed bulk samples. Most were measured by TEM, although a few used the SEM.

In assembling the database, the highest priority was measurements of mineral dusts associated with excess mesothelioma following animal or human exposure (see Chapter 1). In addition, many samples of asbestos from other locations are also included, as well as samples of fragmented minerals.

Table 2.6 contains the list of datasets in the database used in this book, as well as our previous publications on the toxicology of elongate mineral particles and epidemiology of asbestos-related disease. Where habit is listed as unknown, samples were air samples taken during construction or mining. Later analysis would show in many cases which habit likely dominated the aerosol.

TABLE 2.6
Datasets from the database included in the analysis

Mineral type Habit	Source, method of analysis, sample type	Source of the dataset	Number of particles
Actinolite Non-asbestiform	Marbridge Mine, La Motte, Quebec, Canada, TEM, bulk	Eric Chatfield (personal communication, 2021)	207
Actinolite Likely mixed	Boulder City Bypass construction, Nevada, TEM, airborne	EMSL, Nevada Department of Transportation	384
Actinolite Non-asbestiform	Shadwell Quarry, Virginia, MSHA filter SEM, airborne	Wylie, Virta, et al. (2015)	427
Actinolite Non-asbestiform	San Bernardino County, California, TEM, bulk	NIOSH communication, analysis by RTI	300
Actinolite Non-asbestiform	San Bernardino County, California, PCM, bulk	NIOSH communication, analysis by RTI	300
Actinolite Non-asbestiform	Grace Mine, Enoree, South Carolina, TEM, bulk	MRI report.Atkinson et al. (1981)	145
Actinolite Likely mixed	Rock Hill Quarry, East Rock Hill Township, Pennsylvania, TEM, bulk	Drew Van Orden (RJ Lee) (personal communication)	235
Actinolite Likely asbestiform	Rock Hill Quarry, East Rock Hill Township, Pennsylvania, TEM, bulk	Bradley Erskine (personal communication)	128
Actinolite Asbestiform	NIST SRM, TEM, bulk	Eric Chatfield (personal communication)	212

(Continued)

TABLE 2.6 *(Continued)*
Datasets from the database included in the analysis

Mineral type Habit	Source, method of analysis, sample type	Source of the dataset	Number of particles
Actinolite Asbestiform	HSE SRM, TEM, bulk	Eric Chatfield (personal communication)	222
Actinolite Asbestiform	ROM SRM, TEM, bulk	Eric Chatfield (personal communication)	200
Actinolite Asbestiform	HSE, TEM, bulk	Drew Van Orden (RJ Lee) (personal communication)	1622
Actinolite Non-asbestiform	San Bernardino, California, TEM, bulk	Drew Van Orden (RJ Lee) (personal communication)	1404
Actinolite Asbestiform	ROM SRM (Mean AD < 10 μm), TEM, bulk	Eric Chatfield (personal communication)	210
Actinolite Non-asbestiform	Vermont, TEM, bulk	Drew Van Orden (RJ Lee) (personal communication)	15
Actinolite Non-asbestiform	Italy, TEM, bulk	Drew Van Orden (RJ Lee) (personal communication)	113
Actinolite Unknown	Boulder City Bypass construction, Nevada, TEM, bulk	Bradley Erskine (personal communication)	56
Actinolite and other amphiboles Unknown	Boulder City Bypass construction, Nevada, TEM, airborne	Drew Van Orden (RJ Lee) (personal communication)	384
Actinolite, chrysotile Mixed	El Dorado Hills, California, TEM, bulk	Drew Van Orden (RJ Lee) (personal communication)	6871
Actinolite, other amphiboles Mixed	Boulder City Bypass construction, Nevada, TEM, airborne	Drew Van Orden (RJ Lee) (personal communication)	226
Actinolite, other amphiboles Mixed	Boulder City Bypass construction, Nevada, TEM, bulk, soil	Mark Bailey (personal communication)	456
Ferro-actinolite Asbestiform (Mountain Leather)	Transvaal, South Africa, SEM, bulk	Wylie and Virta (2016a)	562
Al2Oc-HC Laboratory sample	Stanton Alumina 1, unleached S, TEM, bulk	Cook et al. (2016)	311
Al2O3 GTC #3 Laboratory sample	Stanton Alumina 2, unleached S, TEM, bulk	Cook et al. (2016)	213
Al2O3 GTC #2 Laboratory sample	Stanton Alumina 5, unleached S, TEM, bulk	Cook et al. (2016)	296

TABLE 2.6 (Continued)
Datasets from the database included in the analysis

Mineral type Habit	Source, method of analysis, sample type	Source of the dataset	Number of particles
Al2O3 GTC #4 Laboratory sample	Stanton Alumina 6, unleached S, TEM, bulk	Cook et al. (2016)	111
Al2O3 HC Laboratory sample	Stanton Alumina 1, leached S, TEM, bulk	Cook et al. (2016)	311
Al2O3 GTC #3 Laboratory sample	Stanton Alumina 2, leached S, TEM, bulk	Cook et al. (2016)	213
Al2O53 GTC #2 Synthetic	Stanton Alumina 5, leached S, TEM, bulk	Cook et al. (2016)	296
Al2O3 GTC #4 Synthetic	Stanton Alumina 6, leached S, TEM, bulk	Cook et al. (2016)	111
Grunerite (Amosite) Asbestiform	Electric Company OSHA filters, SEM, airborne	Wylie, Virta, et al. (2015)	374
Grunerite (Amosite) Asbestiform	Shipyard OSHA filters, SEM, airborne	Wylie, Virta, et al. (2015)	839
Grunerite (Amosite) Asbestiform	South Africa Mine, TEM, air	Monte Carlo Simulation (MCS) from Pooley and Clark (1980)	1993
Grunerite (Amosite) Asbestiform	South Africa Mine, TEM, air	MCS from Gibbs and Hwang (1980)	2000
Grunerite (Amosite) Asbestiform	NIST Standard, TEM, bulk	Eric Chatfield (personal communication)	203
Grunerite (Amosite) Asbestiform	Penge, South Africa, TEM, bulk	Drew Van Orden (RJ Lee) (personal communication)	3433
Grunerite (Amosite) Asbestiform	South Africa Production, TEM, bulk	Drew Van Orden (RJ Lee) (personal communication)	726
Grunerite (Amosite), Asbestiform	South Africa UICC unleached U, TEM, bulk	Cook et al. (2016)	1197
Grunerite (Amosite) Asbestiform	South Africa UICC leached U, TEM, bulk	Cook et al. (2016)	338
Grunerite (Amosite) Asbestiform	South Africa Pooley, TEM, airborne	MCS from Pooley and Clark (1980)	1991
Grunerite (Amosite) Asbestiform	South Africa, TEM, lung burden	MCS from Pooley and Clark (1980)	1991
Grunerite (Amosite) Asbestiform	Pipe insulation finishing, TEM, airborne	MCS from Dement and Harris (1979)	183
Grunerite (Amosite) Asbestiform	Pipe insulation, TEM, airborne	MCS from Dement and Harris (1979)	212
Grunerite (Amosite) Asbestiform	Pipe insulation mixing, TEM, airborne	MCS from Dement and Harris (1979)	183

(Continued)

TABLE 2.6 *(Continued)*
Datasets from the database included in the analysis

Mineral type Habit	Source, method of analysis, sample type	Source of the dataset	Number of particles
Grunerite (Amosite), Asbestiform	South Africa UICC-Davis sample, SEM, bulk	MCS from Davis et al. (1986)	8303
Grunerite (Amosite) Asbestiform	Transvaal South Africa NIEHS, SEM, bulk	Wylie and Virta (2015)	1022
Amphiboles and chrysotile Mixed	El Dorado, California, TEM, air	Drew Van Orden (RJ Lee) (personal communication)	6871
Anthophyllite Asbestiform	HSE SRM Paakkila Karelia, Finland, TEM, bulk	Eric Chatfield (personal communication)	207
Anthophyllite Non-asbestiform	Montauban mine, Quebec, Canada, TEM, bulk	Eric Chatfield (personal communication)	205
Anthophyllite Asbestiform	NIST SRM Udaipur Rakabedo Mines, India, TEM, bulk	Eric Chatfield (personal communication)	202
Anthophyllite Asbestiform	Sal Mountain Mine, Georgia, TEM, bulk	Eric Chatfield (personal communication)	206
Anthophyllite Asbestiform	UICC SRM Pargas, Finland, TEM, bulk	Eric Chatfield (personal communication)	207
Anthophyllite Asbestiform	Western Moravia, Věžná, Czechoslovakia, TEM, bulk	Eric Chatfield (personal communication)	214
Anthophyllite Non-asbestiform	JAWE 431 Afghanistan, TEM, bulk	Eric Chatfield (personal communication)	208
Anthophyllite Asbestiform	UICC unleached U, TEM, bulk	Cook et al. (2016)	256
Anthophyllite Asbestiform	UICC leached U, TEM, bulk	Cook et al. (2016)	271
Anthophyllite Asbestiform	Finland UICC, TEM, bulk	Bureau Veritas, A. Segrave, analyst	205
Anthophyllite Asbestiform	Russia, TEM, bulk	RJ Lee, M. Sanchez, analyst	50
Balangeroite Asbestiform	Balangero, Italy (from F. Turci), TEM, bulk	EMSL, analysis for C&IH	148
Chrysotile Asbestiform	Calidria Mine, California, NIEHS Short Fiber, TEM, bulk	Wylie and Virta (2015)	1047

TABLE 2.6 *(Continued)*
Datasets from the database included in the analysis

Mineral type Habit	Source, method of analysis, sample type	Source of the dataset	Number of particles
Chrysotile Asbestiform	Canada, NIEHS long Fiber, TEM, bulk	Bureau Veritas, A. Segrave, analyst for C&IH	319
Chrysotile Asbestiform	Quebec, Canada, airborne	MCS from Gibbs and Hwang (1980)	2000
Chrysotile Asbestiform	Asbestos textile, South Carolina, TEM, airborne	MCS from Dement et al. (2011)	2000
Chrysotile Asbestiform	Balangero, Italy (from F. Turci), TEM, bulk	EMSL, analysis for C&IH	53
Chrysotile Asbestiform	Jeffrey Mine, Canada, grade 6, TEM, bulk	EMSL, measurements for C&IH	201
Chrysotile Asbestiform	Thetford Mine, Canada, TEM, bulk	EMSL, measurements for C&IH	201
Chrysotile Asbestiform	Europe textile, TEM, airborne	MCS from Rood and Streeter (1984)	500
Chrysotile Asbestiform	North Carolina textile, TEM, airborne	Simulation from Loomis et al. (2009)	500
Chrysotile Asbestiform	Armley, Leeds, England, TEM, bulk	EMSL, measurements for C&IH	201
Chrysotile Asbestiform	Cement pipe mixing, TEM, airborne	MCS from Dement and Harris (1979)	2172
Chrysotile Asbestiform	Cement pipe product finishing, TEM, airborne	MCS from Dement and Harris (1979)	4738
Chrysotile Asbestiform	Cement pipe product forming, TEM, airborne	MCS from Dement and Harris (1979)	2444
Chrysotile Asbestiform	Friction products mixing, TEM, airborne	MCS from Dement and Harris (1979)	5776
Chrysotile Asbestiform	Friction products finishing, TEM, airborne	MCS from Dement and Harris (1979)	3571
Chrysotile Asbestiform	Friction products forming, TEM, airborne	MCS from Dement and Harris (1979)	3570
Chrysotile Asbestiform	Quebec, Canada, Sample UICC, SEM, bulk	MCS from Davis et al. (1986)	55852
Chrysotile Asbestiform	Swift Creek, Sumas Mountain, Washington, TEM, bulk	Cyphert et al. (2012)	502
Riebeckite (Crocidolite) Asbestiform	Cape South Africa, TEM, air	MCS from Gibbs and Hwang (1980)	2000

(Continued)

TABLE 2.6 *(Continued)*
Datasets from the database included in the analysis

Mineral type Habit	Source, method of analysis, sample type	Source of the dataset	Number of particles
Riebeckite (Crocidolite) Asbestiform	South Africa, TEM, air	MCS from Pooley and Clark (1980)	1999
Riebeckite (Crocidolite) Asbestiform	South Africa, TEM, bulk	MCS from Shedd (1985)	4000
Riebeckite (Crocidolite) Asbestiform	Australia, TEM, bulk	MCS from Shedd (1985)	4000
Riebeckite (Crocidolite) Asbestiform	Australia amended, TEM, bulk	MCS from Shedd (1985)	4000
Riebeckite (Crocidolite) Asbestiform	South Africa amended	MCS from Shedd (1985)	4000
Riebeckite (Crocidolite) Asbestiform	UICC sample, TEM, bulk	NIOSH communication, analysis by RTI	768
Riebeckite (Crocidolite) Asbestiform	UICC U, unleached, TEM, bulk	Cook et al. (2016)	940
Riebeckite (Crocidolite) Asbestiform	UICC L3 unleached, TEM, bulk	Cook et al. (2016)	670
Riebeckite (Crocidolite) Asbestiform	Cape South Africa (SA), Stanton 2 Cook 21 unleached, TEM, bulk	Cook et al. (2016)	303
Riebeckite (Crocidolite) Asbestiform	Cape SA, Stanton 3 Cook 22 unleached, TEM, bulk	Cook et al. (2016)	284
Riebeckite (Crocidolite) Asbestiform	Cape SA, Stanton 4 Cook 23 unleached, TEM, bulk	Cook et al. (2016)	848
Riebeckite (Crocidolite) Asbestiform	Cape SA, Stanton 6 Cook 24 unleached, TEM, bulk	Cook et al. (2016)	437
Riebeckite (Crocidolite) Asbestiform	Cape SA, Stanton 7 Cook 25 unleached, TEM, bulk	Cook et al. (2016)	224
Riebeckite (Crocidolite) Asbestiform	Cape SA, Stanton 19 Cook 26 unleached, TEM, bulk	Cook et al. (2016)	229

TABLE 2.6 *(Continued)*
Datasets from the database included in the analysis

Mineral type Habit	Source, method of analysis, sample type	Source of the dataset	Number of particles
Riebeckite (Crocidolite) Asbestiform	Cape SA, Stanton 13 Cook 27 unleached, TEM, bulk	Cook et al. (2016)	182
Riebeckite (Crocidolite) Asbestiform	UICC Cook U leached, TEM, bulk	Cook et al. (2016)	559
Riebeckite (Crocidolite) Asbestiform	UICC Cook L3 leached, TEM, bulk	Cook et al. (2016)	670
Riebeckite (Crocidolite) Asbestiform	Cape SA, Stanton 2 Cook 21, TEM, bulk	Cook et al. (2016)	448
Riebeckite (Crocidolite) Asbestiform	Cape SA, Stanton 3 Cook 22 leached, TEM, bulk	Cook et al. (2016)	442
Riebeckite (Crocidolite) Asbestiform	Cape SA, Stanton 4 Cook 23 leached, TEM, bulk	Cook et al. (2016)	580
Riebeckite (Crocidolite) Asbestiform	Cape SA, Stanton 6 Cook 24 leached 6, TEM, bulk	Cook et al. (2016)	364
Riebeckite (Crocidolite) Asbestiform	Cape SA, Stanton 7 Cook 25 leached S, TEM, bulk	Cook et al. (2016)	340
Riebeckite (Crocidolite) Asbestiform	Cape SA, Stanton 10 Cook 26, leached, TEM, bulk	Cook et al. (2016)	466
Riebeckite (Crocidolite) Asbestiform	Cape SA, Stanton 13 Cook 27 leached, TEM, bulk	Cook et al. (2016)	182
Riebeckite (Crocidolite) Asbestiform	South Africa, TEM, airborne	MCS from Pooley and Clark (1980)	1991
Riebeckite (Crocidolite) Asbestiform	South Africa, TEM, Lung burden	MCS from Pooley and Clark (1980)	1991
Riebeckite (Crocidolite) Asbestiform	UICC, TEM, airborne	MCS from Wagner et al. (1985)	1996
Riebeckite (Crocidolite) Asbestiform	South Africa, Davis sample UICC, SEM, bulk	MCS from Davis et al. (1986)	21474

(Continued)

TABLE 2.6 *(Continued)*
Datasets from the database included in the analysis

Mineral type Habit	Source, method of analysis, sample type	Source of the dataset	Number of particles
Riebeckite (Crocidolite) Asbestiform	Cape South Africa, TEM, bulk	NIOSH communication, analysis by RTI	300
Riebeckite (Crocidolite) Asbestiform	Kuruman Hills, South Africa, NIEHS SEM, bulk	Wylie and Virta (2015)	1030
Grunerite Non-asbestiform	Homestake, South Dakota MSHA filters SEM, airborne	Wylie, Virta, et al. (2015)	578
Grunerite Non-asbestiform	Homestake, South Dakota, TEM, bulk	Eric Chatfield (personal communication)	210
Grunerite Non-asbestiform	Labrador 1, TEM, bulk	Eric Chatfield (personal communication)	195
Grunerite Non-asbestiform	Finland, TEM, bulk	Drew Van Orden (RJ Lee) (personal communication)	62858
Cumming-tonite-Grunerite Non-asbestiform	Homestake Mine, South Dakota, TEM, bulk	Drew Van Orden (RJ Lee) (personal communication)	57199
Dawsonite Synthetic	Stanton Sample 1 unleached, TEM, bulk	Cook et al. (2016)	318
Dawsonite Synthetic	Stanton Sample 3, unleached, TEM, bulk	Cook et al. (2016)	434
Dawsonite Unknown	Stanton Sample 4, Olduvai Gorge, Tanzania, unleached TEM, bulk	Cook et al. (2016)	348
Dawsonite Synthetic	Stanton Sample 5, unleached, TEM, bulk	Cook et al. (2016)	336
Dawsonite Synthetic	Stanton Sample 6, unleached S, TEM, bulk	Cook et al. (2016)	355
Dawsonite Synthetic	Stanton Sample 7, unleached S, TEM, bulk	Cook et al. (2016)	307
Dawsonite Synthetic	Stanton Sample 1, leached S TEM, bulk	Cook et al. (2016)	865
Dawsonite Synthetic	Stanton Sample 3, leached, TEM, bulk	Cook et al. (2016)	720
Dawsonite Unknown	Stanton Sample 4, Olduvai Gorge, Tanzania, leached S, TEM, bulk	Cook et al. (2016)	829
Dawsonite Synthetic	Stanton Sample 5, leached S, TEM, bulk	Cook et al. (2016)	1383

TABLE 2.6 *(Continued)*
Datasets from the database included in the analysis

Mineral type Habit	Source, method of analysis, sample type	Source of the dataset	Number of particles
Dawsonite Synthetic	Stanton Sample 6, leached S, TEM, bulk	Cook et al. (2016)	564
Dawsonite Synthetic	Stanton Sample 7, leached S, TEM, bulk	Cook et al. (2016)	506
Erionite Asbestiform	Oregon, North Dakota, TEM, bulk	NIOSH communication, analysis by RTI	658
Erionite Asbestiform	Oregon, North Dakota, TEM, bulk	EMSL, analysis for C&IH	203
Erionite Unknown	Karain, TEM, bulk	Simulation from Wagner et al. (1985)	2000
Erionite Asbestiform (wooly)	Oregon, TEM, airborne	Simulation from Wagner et al. (1985)	2000
Erionite Asbestiform (wooly)	Oregon, TEM, bulk	Simulation from Wagner et al. (1985)	2000
Erionite Asbestiform (wooly)	Oregon, SEM, bulk	Simulation from Davis et al. (1991)	7849
Ferroactinolite Asbestiform	EPA sample (Coffin et al., 1983), unleached, TEM, bulk	Cook et al. (2016)	1205
Ferroactinolite Asbestiform	EPA sample (Coffin et al., 1983), leached, TEM, bulk	Cook et al. (2016)	437
Ferroactinolite Non-asbestiform	Ontario PM2.5, TEM, bulk	Cyphert et al. (2012)	516
Fibrous talc Mixed	Gouverneur, New York, fibrous talc concentrate, TEM, bulk	EMSL, analysis for C&IH	200
Fluoro-edenite, Non-asbestiform	Sicily, Italy Set 1, TEM, bulk	Bureau Veritas, A. Segrave, analyst for C&IH	209
Fluoro-edenite Non-asbestiform	Sicily, Italy Set 2, TEM, bulk	Bureau Veritas, A. Segrave, analyst for C&IH	224
Fluoro-edenite Asbestiform	Biancavilla, Sicily, Italy, TEM, air	Compiled by Wylie from Paoletti and Bruni (2009)	110
Fluoro-edenite Mixed	Biancavilla, Sicily, Italy, biological	Compiled by Wylie from Paoletti and Bruni (2009)	197

(Continued)

TABLE 2.6 *(Continued)*
Datasets from the database included in the analysis

Mineral type Habit	Source, method of analysis, sample type	Source of the dataset	Number of particles
Fluoro-edenite Mixed	Basilicata, Sicily, Italy, TEM, biological	Compiled by Wylie from Paoletti and Bruni (2009)	296
Fybex Synthetic	Stanton Fybex, unleached S fybex 10, TEM, bulk	Cook et al. (2016)	382
Fybex Synthetic	Stanton Fybex, leached S fybex 10, TEM, bulk	Cook et al. (2016)	371
Grunerite Non-asbestiform	Canada, Labrador, TEM, bulk	Eric Chatfield (personal communication)	208
Grunerite Non-asbestiform	Unknown location, elutriated AD < 10 µm fraction	Eric Chatfield (personal communication)	210
Amosite Asbestiform	Stanton, non-leached, TEM, bulk	Cook et al. (2016)	495
Grunerite Non-fibrous	Stanton, leached, TEM, bulk	Cook et al. (2016)	288
Grunerite actinolite Non-asbestiform	Taconite mine, MN, MSHA filters, SEM, airborne	Wylie, Virta, et al. (2015)	119
Hornblende Group Asbestiform	Goonyella Mine, Australia, from Keeley, TEM, bulk	Bureau Veritas, A. Segrave, analyst for C&IH	209
Glaucophane Mixed	Calaveras Dam, California, TEM, environmental airborne	Bradley Erskine (personal communication)	27650
NaCa amphiboles winchite and richterite Asbestiform and fibrous	Libby, Montana (MT), TEM, airborne	RJ Lee, personal communication	1254
NaCa amphiboles winchite and richterite Asbestiform and fibrous	Libby, MT, exfoliation, TEM, bulk	MRI report.Atkinson et al. (1981)	568
NaCa amphiboles winchite and richterite Asbestiform and fibrous	Libby, MT, ore and mine, TEM, bulk	MRI report.Atkinson et al. (1981)	427
NaCa amphiboles winchite and richterite Asbestiform and fibrous	Libby, MT, EPA, TEM, airborne	EPA data from RJ Lee (personal communication)	3509

TABLE 2.6 *(Continued)*
Datasets from the database included in the analysis

Mineral type Habit	Source, method of analysis, sample type	Source of the dataset	Number of particles
Na-Ca amphiboles winchite and richterite Asbestiform and fibrous	Libby, MT, PM2.5, TEM, bulk	Cyphert et al. (2015)	532
Na-clinojimthomp-sonite Asbestiform and fibrous	Lab samples from Dr. David Jenkins, TEM, bulk	EMSL, analysis for C&IH, Ams and Jenkins (2011)	222
Richterite and Winchite Mixed	Libby, MT, TEM, bulk	Eric Chatfield (personal communication)	211
Riebeckite Non-asbestiform	St. Peter's Dome, Colorado, PCM, bulk	NIOSH communication, analysis by RTI	300
Riebeckite (Crocidolite) Asbestiform	NIST SRM, TEM, bulk	Eric Chatfield (personal communication)	203
Riebeckite Non-asbestiform	Australia, TEM, bulk	Drew Van Orden (RJ Lee) (personal communication)	3994
Riebeckite (Crocidolite) Asbestiform	HSE SRM Kuruman, South Africa, TEM, bulk	Eric Chatfield (personal communication)	208
Riebeckite (Crocidolite) Asbestiform	Pomfret, South Africa, TEM, bulk	Eric Chatfield (personal communication)	209
Riebeckite (Crocidolite) Asbestiform	Wittenoom, Australia, TEM, bulk	Eric Chatfield (personal communication)	215
Riebeckite Non-asbestiform	St. Peter's Dome, Colorado, TEM, bulk	Eric Chatfield (personal communication)	212
Riebeckite Asbestiform	Filadelfia Mine, Bolivia, TEM, bulk	Drew Van Orden (RJ Lee) (personal communication)	5592
Riebeckite Non-asbestiform	Location unknown, Air Elutriated AD < 10 μm, TEM, bulk,	Eric Chatfield (personal communication)	205
Riebeckite Non-asbestiform	Pikes Peak, Colorado, NIOSH, TEM, bulk	NIOSH communication, analysis by RTI	829
Riebeckite Non-asbestiform	Long Valley Creek Quarry, California, SEM, bulk	Wylie, Schweitzer, Siegrist (2015)	969

(Continued)

TABLE 2.6 *(Continued)*
Datasets from the database included in the analysis

Mineral type Habit	Source, method of analysis, sample type	Source of the dataset	Number of particles
Riebeckite Non-asbestiform	Location unknown, Riebeckite 1, TEM, bulk	Eric Chatfield (personal communication)	201
Riebeckite Non-asbestiform	Australia, FESEM, bulk	Drew Van Orden (RJ Lee) (personal communication)	30506
Riebeckite (Crocidolite) Asbestiform	UICC, TEM, bulk	Eric Chatfield (personal communication)	208
Riebeckite (Crocidolite) Asbestiform	Prieska, South Africa, TEM, bulk	Eric Chatfield (personal communication)	206
Riebeckite (Crocidolite) Asbestiform	Transvaal Kromdraai, South Africa, TEM, bulk	Eric Chatfield (personal communication)	212
Riebeckite (Crocidolite) Asbestiform	Cochabamba, Bolivia, TEM, bulk	Eric Chatfield (personal communication)	218
Riebeckite (Crocidolite) Asbestiform	NIST 2, TEM, bulk	Eric Chatfield (personal communication)	207
Silicon Carbide Manufactured product	Stanton sample, unleached S, TEM, bulk	Cook et al. (2016)	401
Silicon Carbide Manufactured product	Stanton sample, leached S, TEM, bulk	Cook et al. (2016)	401
Tremolite Non-asbestiform	Balmat, New York, NIEHS SEM, bulk	Wylie and Virta (2015)	481
Tremolite Asbestiform	Addison Davis sample, Korea, TEM, bulk	Verkouteren and Wylie (personal communication)	1443
Tremolite Asbestiform	Lone Pine, California, TEM, bulk	Bureau Veritas, A. Segrave, analyst for C&IH	102
Tremolite Asbestiform	Barstow, California, NIST SRM, TEM, bulk	NIOSH communication, analysis by RTI	300
Tremolite Non-asbestiform	Balmat, New York, NIEHS, TEM, bulk	NIOSH communication, analysis by RTI	300
Tremolite Asbestiform	Metsovo, Greece, TEM, bulk	Bureau Veritas, A. Segrave, analyst for C&IH	210

TABLE 2.6 *(Continued)*
Datasets from the database included in the analysis

Mineral type Habit	Source, method of analysis, sample type	Source of the dataset	Number of particles
Tremolite Asbestiform	Barstow, California, NIST SRM, PCM, bulk	NIOSH communication, analysis by RTI	300
Tremolite Non-asbestiform	Balmat, New York, NIEHS PCM, bulk	NIOSH communication, analysis by RTI	300
Tremolite Non-asbestiform	Ala di Stura, Italy, TEM, bulk	Eric Chatfield (personal communication)	193
Tremolite Asbestiform	NIST SRM, TEM, bulk	Eric Chatfield (personal communication)	205
Tremolite Asbestiform	Location unknown, HSE 1, TEM, bulk	Eric Chatfield (personal communication)	212
Tremolite Asbestiform	Location unknown, HSE 2, TEM, bulk	Eric Chatfield (personal communication)	206
Tremolite Asbestiform	Jamestown, California, TEM, bulk	Eric Chatfield (personal communication)	219
Tremolite Asbestiform	Korea, TEM, bulk	Eric Chatfield (personal communication)	197
Tremolite Asbestiform	Lone Pine, California, TEM, bulk	Eric Chatfield (personal communication)	210
Tremolite Asbestiform	Lone Pine, California (Selected), TEM, bulk	Eric Chatfield (personal communication)	208
Tremolite Unknown	Saltworks Mine, California 1, TEM, bulk	Eric Chatfield (personal communication)	226
Tremolite Unknown	Saltworks Mine, California 2, TEM, bulk	Eric Chatfield (personal communication)	205
Tremolite Non-asbestiform	Swansea, Wales-Davis Sample, TEM, bulk	Eric Chatfield (personal communication)	216
Tremolite Non-asbestiform but fibrous	Brazil 1, TEM, bulk	Eric Chatfield (personal communication)	219
Tremolite Non-asbestiform	Dornie, Scotland-Davis Sample, TEM, bulk	Eric Chatfield (personal communication)	195
Tremolite Non-asbestiform	Shinness, Scotland-Davis Sample, TEM, bulk	Eric Chatfield (personal communication)	193
Tremolite Non-asbestiform	Sparta, New Jersey, TEM, bulk	Eric Chatfield (personal communication)	202
Tremolite Asbestiform	HSE standard, TEM, bulk	Drew Van Orden (RJ Lee) (personal communication)	1954
Tremolite Non-asbestiform	Madagascar, FESEM, bulk	Drew Van Orden (RJ Lee) (personal communication)	30889

(Continued)

TABLE 2.6 *(Continued)*
Datasets from the database included in the analysis

Mineral type Habit	Source, method of analysis, sample type	Source of the dataset	Number of particles
Tremolite Asbestiform	Yamaga Mine, Japan, JAWE 531, TEM, bulk	Eric Chatfield (personal communication)	209
Tremolite Non-asbestiform	Massape, Brazil, TEM, bulk	Eric Chatfield (personal communication)	204
Tremolite Non-asbestiform	Shinness, Scotland-Davis sample, TEM, bulk	Eric Chatfield (personal communication)	208
Tremolite Unclassified	Brazil-Chatfield sample, elutriated AD<10 μm, bulk	Eric Chatfield (personal communication)	209
Tremolite Non-asbestiform	Shinness, Scotland-Chatfield sample, elutriated AD<10 μm, bulk	Eric Chatfield (personal communication)	207
Tremolite Non-asbestiform	Shinness, Scotland-Chatfield sample, TEM, bulk, combined size fractions	Eric Chatfield (personal communication)	19497
Tremolite Non-asbestiform	Dornie, Scotland-Chatfield sample, TEM, bulk, combined size fractions	Eric Chatfield (personal communication)	16675
Tremolite Non-asbestiform	Ala di Stura Italy-Davis Sample, TEM, bulk, combined size fractions	Eric Chatfield (personal communication)	7435
Tremolite Non-asbestiform	Swansea Lab Wales-Davis sample, TEM, bulk, combined size fractions	Eric Chatfield (personal communication)	7016
Tremolite Asbestiform	Jamestown, California, elutriated combined, TEM, bulk, combined size fraction	Eric Chatfield (personal communication)	11613
Tremolite Asbestiform	Korea, TEM, bulk, combined size fraction	Eric Chatfield (personal communication)	1631
Tremolite Non-asbestiform	NIOSH, TEM, bulk	NIOSH communication, analysis by RTI	704
Tremolite Asbestiform	Stanton sample, unleached, TEM, bulk	Cook et al. (2016)	1073
Tremolite Asbestiform	Stanton sample, leached, TEM, bulk	Cook et al. (2016)	667
Tremolite Non-asbestiform	Falls Village, CT, TEM, bulk	EMSL, analysis for C&IH	221
Tremolite Asbestiform	Eastern NY, TEM, bulk	EMSL, analysis for C&IH	211
Tremolite Habit	Quebec, TEM, bulk	EMSL, analysis for C&IH	209
Tremolite Fibrous	Udaipur, India, SEM, bulk	Wylie and Virta (2016b)	466

TABLE 2.6 *(Continued)*
Datasets from the database included in the analysis

Mineral type Habit	Source, method of analysis, sample type	Source of the dataset	Number of particles
Tremolite Non-asbestiform	Miners Bay, Canada, TEM, bulk	Bureau Veritas, A. Segrave, analyst	106
Tremolite Non-asbestiform	El Dorado Hills, California, TEM, bulk PM 2.5	Cyphert et al. (2015)	507
Tremolite, actinolite, hornblende, Unknown	El Dorado Hills, California, TEM, airborne	RL Lee, analysis by LabCorp (personal communication)	3219
Wollastonite, Non asbestiform	NYCO Processed Minerals, TEM, bulk	NIOSH communication, analysis by RTI	537

Toxicological requirements for measuring fiber dimensions

Generally, the analysis of toxic effects for elongate mineral particles should always include dimensional characteristics of the population based on measurements of length and width of individual particles. Preferably, dimensions should be reported as a length-to-width matrix. For example, Table 2.7 contains a dimensional matrix for non-asbestiform tremolite from Falls Village, Connecticut. The size categories can vary based on the analytical procedures and judgment of scientists.

It is very beneficial to use individual measurements of length and width for each of the particles gathered in any TEM mineral fiber analysis so they can be used in toxicological studies. To be most useful, and to understand mineral carcinogens better, measurements of widths should be made on a TEM at magnifications of about 50,000x so that the error in width is no greater than +−0.01 μm, as indicated in Table 2.7. This level of precision reflects the fact that 10 or 20 nanometers in width can make the difference between a rigid mesotheliomagenic fiber and a nonrigid fiber with no known mesotheliomagenic potential. This precision means that the width bins shown in Table 2.7 can fluctuate with individual samples. The error in length has not emerged as critical, and +−0.5 μm seems adequate.

For risk assessment and regulatory purposes, it seems to be beneficial to measure only elongate particles with length > 5 μm, while for scientific studies and potency determination, all ranges of length could be useful, especially those longer than 2 μm. However, all spectrums of widths should always be used in the range from about 0.02 μm to 3 μm.

Exposure concentrations and risk assessments are based on counting elongated particles with a length-to-width ratio of at least 3:1. However, many of the methods listed in Table 2.1 use 5:1 as a minimum aspect ratio for inclusion in an analysis. To be useful for risk assessment that can be used to protect worker health, concentrations of mineral fiber should apply to particles defined by the 3:1 standard for minimum aspect ratio.

TABLE 2.7
Example of a length/width matrix for non-asbestiform tremolite

	Width (µm) (+/–0.01)				
Length (µm)		≤0.15	0.15–0.25	0.25–0.38	>0.38
(+/–0.05)	< 1	3	3	0	0
	1–2	13	48	21	6
	2–3	7	13	11	26
	3–4	0	6	2	24
	4–5	0	2	1	10
	5–8	0	1	0	14
	8–10	0	1	0	4
	> 10	0	0	0	2

Surface area and specific surface area of elongate particles should be reported. It is expected that future laboratory methods will be able to evaluate 3D characteristics of fibers, including thickness. The dose should be expressed in terms of fiber number and surface area per exposed biological material or per unit of breathing air or per weight of instilled minerals in animals. The weight of fibers alone and concentrations by weight can be used as a supplement, but never as the only dose metric.

NOTE

1 At the time of this writing, ASTM is considering a revision to reduce the minimum width in conformity to NIOSH 7400 visibility determinations of 0.15 µm for chrysotile and 0.05 µm for amphibole.

REFERENCE LIST

American Society for Testing and Materials (ASTM). (2019). *Standard test method for wipe sampling of surfaces, indirect preparation, and analysis for asbestos structure number surface loading by transmission electron microscopy* (ASTM D6480-19). https://store.astm.org/d6480-19.html

American Society for Testing and Materials (ASTM). (2020). *Standard practice for sampling and counting airborne fibers, including asbestos fibers, in the workplace, by phase contrast microscopy (with an option of transmission electron microscopy)* (ASTM D7201-06). https://store.astm.org/d7201-06.html

American Society for Testing and Materials (ASTM). (2022). *Standard test method for determination of asbestos in soil* (ASTM D7521-22). https://store.astm.org/d7521-22.html

American Society for Testing and Materials (ASTM). (2023a). *Standard test method for airborne asbestos concentration in ambient and indoor atmospheres as determined by transmission electron microscopy direct transfer (TEM)* (ASTM D6281-23). https://store.astm.org/d6281-23.html

American Society for Testing and Materials (ASTM). (2023b). *Standard test method for analytical procedure using transmission electron microscopy for the determination of the concentration of carbon nanotubes and carbon nanotube-containing particles in ambient atmospheres* (ASTM D8526-23). https://store.astm.org/d8526-23.html

Ams, B. E., & Jenkins, D. M. (2011). Formation conditions for triple-chain silicates. *American Mineralogist, 96*(5–6), 814–819. https://doi.org/10.2138/am.2011.3568

Atkinson, G. R., Rose, D., Thomas, K., Jones, D., Chatfield, E., & Going, J. (1981). *Collection, analysis, and characterization of vermiculite samples for fibre content and asbestos contamination* (USEPA Contract No 68-01-5915 Report from MRI). USEPA.

Berry, D., Januch, J., Woodbury, L., & Kent, D. (2020). Detection of erionite and other zeolite fibers in soil by the fluidized bed preparation method. *Microscopy, 67*(4), 147–158. PMID: 32704189.

Burdett, G. (2024). Asbestos exposure measurements: principles of current and historical data interpretation. In A. Korchevskiy, J. Rasmuson, & E. Rasmuson (Eds.), *Health risk assessment for asbestos and other fibrous minerals*. John Wiley & Sons. ISBN: 978-1-119-43843-4. https://doi.org//10.1002/9781119438397

Chatfield, E. J. (1999). A rapid procedure for preparation of transmission electron microscopy specimens from polycarbonate filters. In M. E. Beard & H. L. Rook (Eds.), *Advances in environmental measurement methods for asbestos* (STP1342-EB). ASTM International. https://doi.org/10.1520/STP42341S

Chatfield, E. J. (2021). *Studies on the equivalence of air and water elutriation of amphibole elongate mineral particles* (STP 1632/2021). www.astm.org/https://doi.org/10.1520/STP163220200064

Chesson, J., Rench, J. D., Schultz, B. D., & Milne, K. L. (1990). Interpretation of airborne asbestos measurements. *Risk Analysis, 10*(3), 449–458. https://doi.org/10.1111/j.1539-6924.1990.tb00527.x

Coffin, D. L., Palekar, L. D., & Cook, P. M. (1983). Correlation of in vitro and in vivo methods by means of mass dose and fiber distribution for amosite and fibrous ferroactinolite. *Environmental Health Perspectives, 51*, 49–53. https://doi.org/10.1289/ehp.835149

Cook, P. M., Swintek, J., Dawson, T. D., Chapman, D., Etterson, M. A., & Hoff, D. (2016). Quantitative structure-mesothelioma potency model optimization for complex mixtures of elongated particles in rat pleura: A retrospective study. *Journal of Toxicology and Environmental Health, Part B, 19*(5–6), 266–288. https://doi.org/10.1080/10937404.2016.1195326

Cyphert, J. M., Carlin, D. J., Nyska, A., Schladweiler, M. C., Ledbetter, A. D., Shannahan, J. H., et al. (2015). Comparative long-term toxicity of Libby amphibole and amosite asbestos in rats after single or multiple intratracheal exposures. *Journal of Toxicological and Environmental Health A, 78*, 151–165. https://doi.org/10.1080/15287394.2014.947455

Cyphert, J. M., Nyska, A., Mahoney, R. K., Schladweiler, M. C., Kodavanti, U. P., & Gavett, S. H. (2012). Sumas mountain chrysotile induces greater lung fibrosis in Fischer 344 rats than Libby amphibole, El Dorado tremolite, and Ontario ferroactinolite. *Toxicological Sciences, 130*(2), 405–415. https://doi.org/10.1093/toxsci/kfs249

Darnton, L. (2023). Quantitative assessment of mesothelioma and lung cancer risk based on phase contrast microscopy (PCM) estimates of fibre exposure: An update of 2000 asbestos cohort data. *Environmental Research, 230*, 114753. https://doi.org/10.1016/j.envres.2022.114753

Darnton, L. (2024). The Hodgson and Darnton approach to quantifying the risks of mesothelioma and lung cancer in relation to asbestos exposure. In A. Korchevskiy, J. Rasmuson, & E. Rasmuson (Eds.), *Health risk assessment for asbestos and other fibrous minerals* (pp. 233–269). John Wiley & Sons, Inc. https://doi.org/10.1002/9781119438397

Davis, J. M., Addison, J., Bolton, R. E., Donaldson, K., Jones, A. D., & Smith, T. (1986). The pathogenicity of long versus short fibre samples of amosite asbestos administered to rats by inhalation and intraperitoneal injection. *British Journal of Experimental Pathology, 67*(3), 415–430.

Davis, J. M., Bolton, R. E., Miller, B. G., & Niven, K. (1991). Mesothelioma dose response following intraperitoneal injection of mineral fibres. *International Journal of Experimental Pathology, 72*(3), 263–274.

Dement, J. M., & Harris, R. L. (1979). *Estimates of pulmonary and gastrointestinal deposition for occupational fiber exposure* (NTIS PB80-149644, U.S. HEW Contract #78-2438). US EPA.

Dement, J. M., Loomis, D., Richardson, D., Wolf, S. H., & Kuempel, E. D. (2011). Estimates of historical exposures by phase contrast and transmission electron microscopy for pooled exposure – response analyses of North Carolina and South Carolina, USA asbestos textile cohorts. *Occupational and Environmental Medicine*, *68*(8), 593–598. https://doi.org/10.1136/oem.2010.059972

Dodgson, J. (1963). Use of interference microscopy for the mineralogical analysis of samples of airborne dust obtained with the thermal precipitator. *Nature*, *199*, 245–247. https://doi.org/10.1038/199245a0

Dodson, R. F., Hammar, S. P., & Poye, L. W. (2008). A technical comparison of evaluating asbestos concentration by phase-contrast microscopy (PCM), scanning electron microscopy (SEM), and analytical transmission electron microscopy (ATEM) as illustrated from data generated from a case report. *Inhalation Toxicology*, *20*(7), 723–732. https://doi.org/10.1080/08958370701883250

Gibbs, G. W., & Hwang, C. Y. (1980). Dimensions of airborne asbestos fibres. In J. C. Wagner (Ed.), *Biological effects of mineral fibres* (IARC Scientific Publication No. 30, pp. 69–78). IARC Scientific Publications, Lynn. PMID: 7239672.

Hodgson, J. T., & Darnton, A. (2000). The quantitative risks of mesothelioma and lung cancer in relation to asbestos exposure. *Annals of Occupational Hygiene, 44*(8), 565–601. https://doi.org/10.1093/annhyg/44.8.565

Holm, J.D. and Mansfield, E. (2024). Transmission electron imaging and diffraction of asbestos fibers in a scanning electron microscope. Analytical Methods, 16, 4570–4581. https://doi.org/10.1039/D4AY00555D

International Standards Organization (ISO). (2012). *Air quality – bulk materials. Part 1: Sampling and qualitative determination of asbestos in commercial bulk materials* (ISO 22262-1:2012). https://www.iso.org/standard/40834.html

International Standards Organization (ISO). (2014a). *Air quality – determination of the number concentration of airborne inorganic fibers by phase contrast optical microscopy – membrane filter method* (ISO 8672:2014(E)). https://cdn.standards.iteh.ai/samples/53413/f387df25c68f450d9da8d22b0c3c2ee3/ISO-8672-2014.pdf

International Standards Organization (ISO). (2014b). *Indoor air – part 27: Determination of settled fibrous dust on surfaces by SEM (scanning electron microscopy) (direct method)* (DIN ISO 16000-27:2014). https://www.iso.org/standard/50104.html

International Standards Organization (ISO). (2019a). *Ambient air – determination of asbestos fibres – direct transfer transmission electron microscopy method* (ISO 10312:2019(en)). https://www.iso.org/obp/ui/#iso:std:iso:10312:ed-2:v1:en

International Standards Organization (ISO). (2019b). *Ambient air – determination of asbestos fibers – indirect-transfer transmission electron microscopy method* (2nd ed., ISO 13794-2019). https://www.iso.org/standard/75576.html

International Standards Organization (ISO). (2019c). *Ambient air – determination of numerical concentration of inorganic fibrous particles – scanning electron microscopy (SEM) method* (ISO 14966-2019). https://www.iso.org/standard/75583.html

Korchevskiy, A. A., & Wylie, A. G. (2025). Habit of elongate amphibole particles as a predictor of mesothelial carcinogenicity. *Toxicology Reports*, *14*, 101908. https://doi.org/10.1016/j.toxrep.2025.101908

Lee, R. J., Dagenhart, T. V., Dunmyre, G. H., Stewart, I. M., & Van Orden, D. R. (1995). Effect of indirect sample preparation procedures on the apparent concentration of asbestos in settled dust. *Environmental Science and Technology, 29*(7), 1728–1736. https://doi.org/10.1021/es00007a006

Lippmann, M. (2015). Correction to: Lippmann, toxicological and epidemiological studies on effects of airborne fibers: Coherence and public health implications. *Critical Reviews in Toxicology*, *45*, 92. https://doi.org/10.3109/10408444.2014.964036

Longhurst, R. S. (1957). *Geometrical and physical optics*. Longmans.

Loomis, D., Dement, J., Richardson, D., & Wolf, S. (2009). Asbestos fibre dimensions and lung cancer mortality among workers exposed to chrysotile. *Occupational & Environmental Medicine*, *67*(9), 580–584. https://doi.org/10.1136/oem.2009.050120

Malinconico, S., Paglietti, F., Serranti, S., Bonifazi, G., & Lonigro, I. (2022). Asbestos in soil and water: A review of analytical techniques and methods. *Journal of Hazardous Materials*, *436*, 129083. https://doi.org/10.1016/j.jhazmat.2022.129083

Nagai, H., Okazaki, Y., Chew, S. H., Misawa, N., Yamashita, Y., Akatsuka, S., Ishihara, T., Yamashita, K., Yoshikawa, Y., Yasui, H., Jiang, L., Ohara, H., Takahashi, T., Ishihara, G., Kostarelos, K., Miyata, Y., Shinohara, H., & Toyokuni, S. (2011). Diameter and rigidity of multiwalled carbon nanotubes are critical factors in mesothelial injury and carcinogenesis. *Proceedings of the National Academies of Science*, *108*(49), E1330–E1338. https://doi.org/10.1073/pnas.1110013108

National Institute for Occupational Safety and Health (NIOSH). (1994, August 15). *Asbestos and other fibers by PCM: Method 7400, issue 2* (4th ed.). NIOSH Manual of Analytical Methods (NMAM). https://www.cdc.gov/niosh/docs/2003-154/pdfs/7400.pdf

National Institute for Occupational Safety and Health (NIOSH). (2019, June 14). *Asbestos and other fibers by PCM: Method 7400, issue 3* (5th ed.). NIOSH Manual of Analytical Methods (NMAM). https://www.cdc.gov/niosh/nmam/pdf/7400.pdf

National Institute for Occupational Safety and Health (NIOSH). (2022, August 1). *Asbestos by TEM. Method: 7402, issue 3* https://www.cdc.gov/niosh/nmam/pdf/7402.pdf

Occupational Safety and Health Administration (OSHA). (1997, July). *Method ID-160 (1988/1997): Asbestos in air. Branch of physical measurements and analysis* (T-ID160-FV-01–9707-PM). OSHA Salt Lake Technical Center. Revised July 1988. https://www.osha.gov/sites/default/files/methods/osha-id160.pdf

Paoletti, L., & Bruni, B. M. (2009). Caratterizzazione dimensionale di fibre anfiboliche nel polmone e nella pleura di casi di mesothelioma da esposizione ambientale. *Medicina del Lavoro*, *100*(1), 11–20.

Perkins, R. L., & Harvey, B. W. (1993). *Method for the determination of asbestos in bulk building materials* (EPA/600/R-93/116). U.S. Environmental Protection Agency. https://www.nist.gov/system/files/documents/nvlap/EPA-600-R-93-116.pdf

Pooley, F. D., & Clark, N. J. (1980). A comparison of fibre dimensions in chrysotile, crocidolite and amosite particles from samples of airborne dust and from post-mortem lung tissue specimens. *IARC Scientific Publications*, *30*, 79–86.

Pott, F. (1980). Animal experiments on biological effects of mineral fibres. *IARC Scientific Publications*, *30*, 261–272.

Rood, A. P., & Streeter, R. R. (1984). Size distributions of occupational airborne asbestos textile fibres as determined by transmission electron microscopy. *Annals of Occupational Hygiene*, *28*(3), 333–339. https://doi.org/10.1093/annhyg/28.3.333

Shedd, K. B. (1985). *Fiber dimensions of crocidolites from Western Australia, Bolivia, and the Cape and Transvaal Provinces of South Africa* (RI8998). U.S. Department of the Interior, Bureau of Mines Report of Investigations.

Stanton, M. F., Layard, M., Tegeris, A., Miller, E., May, M., Morgan, E., & Smith, A. (1981). Relation of particle dimension to carcinogenicity in amphibole asbestoses and other fibrous minerals. *Journal of the National Cancer Institute*, *67*(5), 965–975.

Turcotte, D. L. (1986). Fractals and fragmentation. *Journal of Geophysical Research, 91*(B2), 1921–1926. https://doi.org/10.1029/JB091iB02p01921

U.S. Environmental Protection Agency (U.S. EPA). (1993, July). *Test method: Method for the determination of asbestos in bulk building materials* (EPA 600 R-93/116). https://www.nist.gov/system/files/documents/nvlap/EPA-600-R-93-116.pdf

Verkouteren, J., & Wylie, A. (2002). Anomalous optical properties of fibrous tremolite, actinolite, and ferro-actinolite. *American Mineralogist, 87*(8–9), 1090–1095. https://doi.org/10.2138/am-2002-8-905

Wagner, J. C., Skidmore, J. W., Hill, R. J., & Griffiths, D. M. (1985). Erionite exposure and mesotheliomas in rats. *British Journal of Cancer*, *51*(5), 727–730. https://doi/10.1038/bjc.1985.108

Wylie, A. G. (1993). Modeling asbestos populations: A fractal approach. *Canadian Mineralogist, 30*, 437–446. https://doi.org/10.3749/1499-1276-31.2.437

Wylie, A. G. (2016). Amphibole dusts: Fibers, fragments, and mesothelioma. *The Canadian Mineralogist*, *54*(6), 1403–1435. https://doi.org/10.3749/canmin.1500109

Wylie, A. G., & Korchevskiy, A. A. (2023). Dimensions of elongate mineral particles and cancer: A review. *Environmental Research, 230*, 114688. https://doi.org/10.1016/j.envres.2022.114688

Wylie, A. G., & Korchevskiy, A. A. (2025). Critical values for dimensional parameters of mesotheliomagenic mineral fibers: Evidence from the dimensions and rigidity of MWCNT. *Frontiers in Toxicology, 7*, 1568513. https://doi.org/10.3389/ftox.2025.1568513

Wylie, A. G., Schweitzer, P., & Siegrist, H. G. (2015). *Size and shape characteristics of amphibole cleavage fragments from milled riebeckite*. Digital Repository at the University of Maryland. http://dx.doi.org/10.13016/M2S98X

Wylie, A. G., & Virta, R. L. (2015). *Size distribution measurements of amosite, crocidolite, chrysotile, and nonfibrous tremolite*. Digital Repository at the University of Maryland. http://dx.doi.org/10.13016/M2798Z

Wylie, A. G., & Virta, R. L. (2016a). *Size and shape characteristics of mountain-leather actinolite*. Digital Repository at the University of Maryland. http://dx.doi.org/10.13016/M2WT68

Wylie, A. G., & Virta, R. L. (2016b). *Size and shape characteristics of Indian tremolite asbestos*. Digital Repository at the University of Maryland. http://dx.doi.org/10.13016/M21H7S

Wylie, A. G., Virta, R., & Segretti, J. (1987). Characterization of mineral populations by index particle: Implications for the Stanton hypothesis. *Environmental Research, 43*, 427–439. https://doi.org/10.1016/S0013-9351(87)80043-9

Wylie, A. G., Virta, R. L., Shedd, K. B., & Snyder, J. G. (2015). *Size and shape characteristics of airborne amphibole asbestos and amphibole cleavage fragments*. Digital Repository at the University of Maryland. http://dx.doi.org/10.13016/M2HP87

Zhu, W., von dem Bussche, A., Yi, X., Qiu, Y., Wang, Z., Weston, P., Hurt, R. H., Kane, A. B., & Gao, H. (2016). Nanomechanical mechanism for lipid bilayer damage induced by carbon nanotubes confined in intracellular vesicles. *Proceedings of the National Academies of Science*, *113*(44), 12374–12379. https://doi.org/10.1073/pnas.1605030113

3 Fractional characteristics of elongate mineral particles and their relationships with cancer potency factors

A. Korchevskiy & A. Wylie

Elongate mineral particles (EMPs) in general, and asbestiform fibers in particular, are different from spherical particulates and/or nuisance dust by their properties and effects. From the earliest studies on asbestos toxicology, it was clear that the elongation of fibers plays an important role in the toxic response and makes fibrous minerals different from other types of respirable dust.

In the first paper on lung fibrosis caused by inhalation of asbestos dust, Cooke (1924) noted various sizes and shapes of asbestos particles in the lung sections of exposed workers. King et al. (1946) first reported that the effect of asbestos in laboratory animals depends on fiber length. In particular, the authors suggested that the fibers with low length were expected to be fully removed from the lungs, while longer fibers remain and cause the fibrotic reaction. Wagner et al. (1960) in their pioneering paper on the asbestos-related etiology of mesothelioma emphasized that the suspected agent was the "fibrous" form. Timbrell (1965) explored the deposition of asbestos fibers in the lungs and discussed the reasons why longer fibers can be found in the human alveoli vs. spherical particles. Based on experiments on animals, Pott (1978) published estimates that the most biologically active fibers were those with L>10 µm, W≤0.25 µm. Tilkes and Beck (1980) demonstrated by *in vitro* and *in vivo* tests that the toxicity of asbestos and man-made mineral particles increased with increasing length. At the same time, Bertrand and Pezerat (1980) argued that the predictor of fiber carcinogenicity is actually an aspect ratio, and it is "not possible to separate the effects of the two variables, length and diameter." Bonneau et al. (1986) also named aspect ratio, along with the "nature of the mineral" as two parameters defining the carcinogenic potency of a solid particle.

Stanton et al. (1977) demonstrated that fibers less than or equal to 1.5 µm in diameter and greater than 8 µm in length yielded the highest probability of pleural sarcomas, and probability trends suggested that pleural sarcoma incidence increased with increasing lengths of fibers. Later, Stanton et al. (1981) performed an experiment

DOI: 10.1201/9781003424277-4

with pleural implantation of amphibole asbestos and other materials in rats, concluding that short fibers and large-diameter fibers were inactivated by phagocytosis, but negligible phagocytosis of long, thin fibers occurred. Stanton concluded that the category of fibers with L>8 μm and W≤0.25 μm was most closely associated with tumor probability.

Bernstein and Hoskins (2006), in their comprehensive study on chrysotile, stated that fibers less than 5 μm in length are effectively not different from non-fibrous particles and are cleared with similar kinetics and mechanisms as isomorphous particles, presenting very little or no risk to human health. Roggli (2015) concluded that there is no convincing evidence for a pathogenic effect for fibers that are 5 μm or less in length. The length of 5 μm can be considered a type of "dimensional threshold" indicating the level of a parameter that conditionally subdivides all fibers into the "carcinogenic" and "non-carcinogenic" categories, in line with recent findings on a threshold-based dose-response in various agents, as in Golden et al. (2019). Wylie and Korchevskiy (2023) reviewed literature sources and performed quantitative structure-activity relationship (QSAR) modeling confirming that elongate particles shorter than 5 μm do not contribute to mesothelioma risk.

Korchevskiy et al. (2019) attempted to develop an empirical model that would reconstruct mesothelioma potency factors for various types of fiber based on their chemical composition and dimensionality. Typical chemical composition and dimensionality metrics (aspect ratios) were obtained and combined with mesothelioma potency factors estimated by the Hodgson and Darnton method for Quebec chrysotile, South African amosite, South African and Australian crocidolite, Russian anthophyllite, Libby amphibole, and Turkey erionite. The forward stepwise log-log regression method was utilized to determine the best combination of input parameters. Mesothelioma potency factors (R_M) for selected cohorts were effectively reconstructed utilizing the median aspect ratio of fibers and equivalent fractions of SiO_2, total Fe oxides or total equivalent Fe^{3+}as Fe_2O_3, and MgO. Modeled potency factors increase as the aspect ratio, SiO_2, and total Fe oxide (or Fe_2O_3) content grow, and as the MgO content diminishes. Correlation coefficients up to 0.999, $p < 0.01$, were achieved. The models also yield reasonable estimates of mesothelioma potencies for other fiber types, including Bolivian crocidolite, Russian chrysotile, fluoro-edenite, and others. It was concluded that the proposed models provide a starting point for targeted studies of mesothelioma mechanisms by elucidating significant contributing physicochemical factors. The models have an exploratory and preliminary character but can potentially be useful to introduce quantitative structure-activity relationship approaches for the toxicology of fibrous minerals. In 2024, the model by Korchevskiy, Rasmuson, and Rasmuson was further adjusted to the updated published information and expanded to predict potency factors for lung cancer along with mesothelioma (Korchevskiy et al., 2024).

In 2020, Wylie et al. modeled mesothelioma potency factors for amphibole fibers based on so-called fractional dimensional parameters. The purposes of the study by the authors were: a) to define relevant dimension subsets of *Total EMP* found in aerosols, allowing the characterization of mesothelioma potency for specific types of amphibole fibers, b) to test these sets as possible mesothelioma potency indicators by evaluating their abundances in relationship to R_M, the mortality from mesothelioma per f/cc-yr derived from well-studied epidemiology meta-analyses, and c) to apply these models as predictors of mesothelioma potency (modeled R_M) to amphibole aerosols from occurrences where epidemiological data for a quantitative assessment of R_M are lacking, but excess mesothelioma has been linked to exposure.

It was noted by the authors that transmission electron microscopy (TEM) studies of crocidolite from the Cape Province of South Africa (asbestiform riebeckite) by Gibbs and Hwang (1980) and Pooley and Clark (1980) describe mineral fiber that is uncommonly narrow (≤ 0.15 μm) dominating in the mine aerosol and lung burden. Aerosol-sized particles generated from Hamersley, Australia crocidolite are very similar in length and width to those from the Cape (Shedd, 1985). Occupational exposures to these two sources of asbestos have resulted in the highest known mesothelioma potency (Hodgson & Darnton, 2000; Garabrant & Pastula, 2018). The authors emphasized that in his extensive review of the issue of dimensions and disease, Lippmann (2014) suggested fibers with widths ≤ 0.15 μm as the main category producing elevated mesothelioma rates. For these reasons, the first set that the authors correlated to mesothelioma mortality was % Total EMP (longer than 5 μm) with width (W) ≤ 0.15 μm (EMPA). It should be mentioned that, given the visibility limits of phase contrast microscopy (PCM), chrysotile fibers with width (W) ≤ 0.15 μm would probably not have been counted during occupational exposure monitoring, although other types of asbestos have fibrils visible to W = 0.05 μm.

It is also widely recognized that the translation of fibers from lung to pleura (or other translocations) favors fibers of very narrow width specified as < 0.4 μm (Lentz et al., 2003), < 0.3 μm (Carbone et al., 2012), and < 0.2 μm (Pooley, 2018) and < 0.15 μm (Lippmann, 2014). To include more of these narrow fibers, a second set, EMPB, was defined as % Total EMP with width ≤ 0.25 μm. Many particles in this set would be visible by PCM although they were for a long time *excluded* from a full fiber count and from transmission electron microscopy (TEM) PCM-equivalent (PCME) that until recent times only included fibers with width >0.25 μm (NIOSH, 1989). EMPA is a subset of EMPB.

Table 3.1 contains EMPA and EMPB values derived by Wylie et al. (2020), for several types of mineral fiber, and corresponding mesothelioma potency factors (R_M, %), as initially published by Hodgson and Darnton (2000) and updated by Darnton (2023). The lung carcinoma potency factors (R_L, %) from the same sources are also included in Table 3.1. The data for crocidolite from South Africa came from mine and mill aerosols (Gibbs & Hwang, 1980; Pooley & Clark, 1980) and from bulk samples (Shedd, 1985); the data for Australian crocidolite came entirely from bulk samples of the ore (Shedd, 1985). The raw data were available from all sources except Gibbs and Hwang (1980), Pooley and Clark (1980), and Shedd (1985). These data sets were tabulated in enough detail to be useful for determining the abundances of the selected toxicity indices. For amosite, two data sources were air data from occupational monitoring (Wylie & Candela, 2015) and three were aerosols from the mine and mill (Gibbs & Hwang, 1980; Pooley & Clark, 1980). Four data sets were used for amphibole-asbestos from Libby: two represent aerosols from the town of Libby (U.S. EPA, 2014; Lee et al., 2009), and two were from fiber extracted from raw and exfoliated vermiculite (Atkinson et al., 1981).

We have treated these data sets as random samples of their respective populations and calculated standard deviations based on counting statistics (SD = $\sqrt{\#}$ counts).

TABLE 3.1
The data used for the modeling of mesothelioma potency based on fractional dimensionality parameters

Principal mineral and habit	Source	R_M, % per total expected mortality, per PCME f/cc-years, age-adjusted, average (95% CI)	R_L, % per baseline lung cancer mortality, per PCME f/cc-years, age-adjusted, average (95% CI)	EMPA, %, average (standard deviation)	EMPB, % average (standard deviation)
Asbestiform riebeckite (crocidolite)	Cape, South Africa	0.59 (0.36, 0.91)	5.2 (0.74, 12)	51.6 (3.4)	79.5 (7.8)
	Hamersley, Australia	0.51 (0.45, 0.57)	4.6 (3.6, 5.7)	46 8 (3.9)	71.1 (9.4)
Asbestiform Grunerite (Amosite)	Transvaal, South Africa	0.06 (0.016, 0.15)	1.9 (−0.44, 5.1)	8.0 (0.8)	25.3 (2.0)
Asbestiform Na-Ca amphibole	Libby, Montana, U.S.A.	0.03 (0.017, 0.050)	0.82 (0.43, 1.3)	2.1 (0.3)	18.4 (0.6)

For the data from Gibbs and Hwang (1980) and Pooley and Clark (1980), which are expressed in percentages, a standard deviation of 20% was assigned to reflect uncertainty introduced by interpolation of the data provided in tabular form. Some of the tabulated data from Pooley and Clark (1980) lacked the detail necessary to extract estimates of the abundances of EMPA and were therefore not included in calculations.

Following the methodology from Wylie et al. (2020), we can perform modeling of mesothelioma and lung cancer potency factors based on the EMPA and EMPB parameters.

The following regression equations can be derived from the data:

For mesothelioma,

$$R_M = -0.012 + 0.011 \text{ EMPA } \left(R = 0.998,\ R^2 = 0.996,\ F(1,2) = 520.88,\ p < 0.0019\right),$$

$$R_M = -0.159 + 0.0094 \text{ EMPB } \left(R = 0.999,\ R^2 = 0.998,\ F(1,2) = 839.77,\ p < 0.0012\right),$$

$$\text{Log}_{10}\left(R_M\right) = -1.929 + 0.966 \text{ LOG}_{10}\left(\text{EMPA}\right)\ (R = 0.984,\ R^2 = 0.969,$$

$$F(1,2) = 63.891,\ p < 0.015), \text{ and}$$

$$\text{Log}_{10}\left(R_M\right) = -4.109 + 2.05 \text{ LOG}_{10}\left(\text{EMPB}\right)\ (R = 0.999,\ R^2 = 0.999,$$

$$F(1,2) = 3182.6,\ p < 0.00031).$$

For lung cancer,

$$R_L = 0.923 + 0.081\ \text{EMPA}\ \left(R = 0.992,\ R^2 = 0.985,\ F(1,2) = 129.28,\ p < 0.00765\right),$$

$$R_L = -0.126 + 0.067\ \text{EMPB}\ \left(R = 0.993,\ R^2 = 0.985,\ F(1,2) = 135.66,\ p < 0.00729\right),$$

$$\text{Log}_{10}(R_L) = -0.252 + 0.56\ \text{LOG}_{10}(\text{EMPA})\ (R = 0.998,\ R^2 = 0.997,\ F(1,2) = 633.17,\ p < 0.0158), \text{ and}$$

$$\text{Log}_{10}(R_L) = -1.44 + 1.14\ \text{LOG}_{10}(\text{EMPB})\ (R = 0.973,\ R^2 = 0.947,\ F(1,2) = 35.981,\ p < 0.027).$$

The results of the modeling are demonstrated in Figure 3.1.

The model developed in 2020 can be expanded to include other types of mineral fibers. For example, Table 3.2 contains additional information: EMPA and EMPB for chrysotile (data from the dimensional database, described in Chapter 2) and Turkish erionite (data from Wagner et al., 1985). Also, Table 3.2 includes the data on the *in vitro* acellular dissolution of mineral fibers included in our study (based on Gualtieri et al., 2018).

Using the biopersistence data from Table 3.2, we can develop models to reconstruct R_M and R_L.

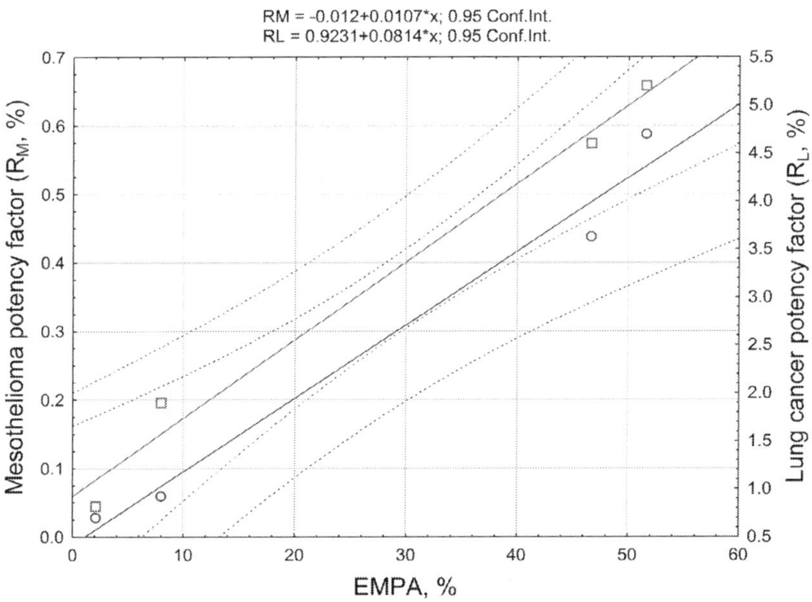

FIGURE 3.1 Relationship between mesothelioma and lung cancer potency factors and EMPA and EMPB parameters. Blue circles denote mesothelioma potency values, red squares denote lung cancer potency values, and the dotted lines denote the 95% confidence interval.

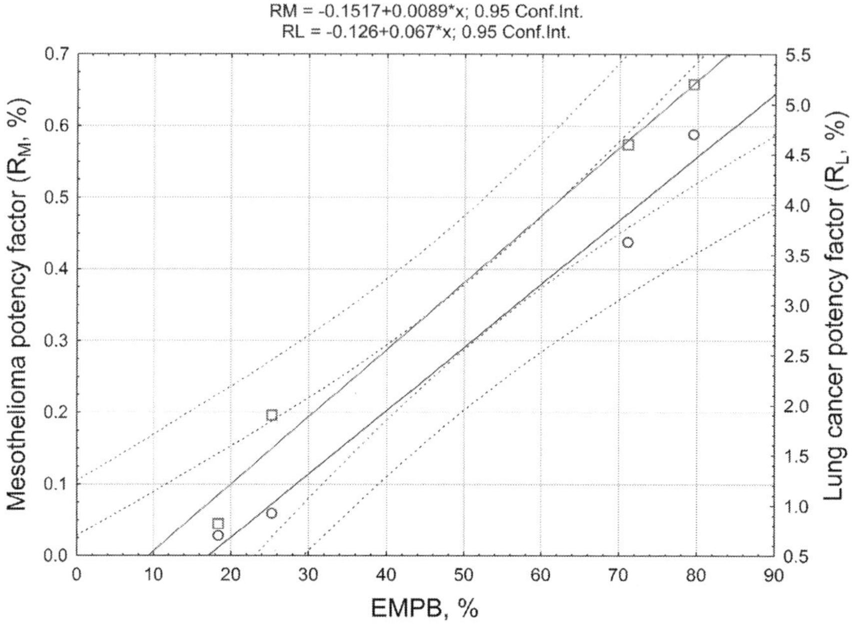

FIGURE 3.1 (Continued)

For mesothelioma,

$$\text{Log}_{10}\left(\text{R}_\text{M}\right) = -4.06 + 1.01\ \text{LOG}_{10}\left(\text{EMPA}\right) + 1.21\log_{10}\left(\text{BIOPER}\right)\ (\text{R} = 0.983,$$
$$\text{R}^2 = 0.967,\ \text{F}\left(2,3\right) = 44.186,\ \text{p} < 0.00595),\ \text{and}$$
$$\text{Log}_{10}\left(\text{R}_\text{M}\right) = -6.23 + 2.13\ \text{LOG}_{10}\left(\text{EMPB}\right) + 1.20\log_{10}\left(\text{BIOPER}\right)$$
$$\left(\text{R} = 0.973,\ \text{R}^2 = 0.946,\ \text{F}\left(2,3\right) = 26.365,\ \text{p} < 0.012\right).$$

For lung cancer,

$$\text{Log}_{10}\left(\text{R}_\text{L}\right) = -1.42 + 0.39\ \text{LOG}_{10}\left(\text{EMPA}\right) + 0.71\log_{10}\left(\text{BIOPER}\right)\ (\text{R} = 0.972,$$
$$\text{R}^2 = 0.944,\ \text{F}\left(2,3\right) = 25.7,\ \text{p} < 0.0129),\ \text{and}$$
$$\text{Log}_{10}\left(\text{R}_\text{L}\right) = -2.53 + 0.976\ \text{LOG}_{10}\left(\text{EMPB}\right) + 0.71\log_{10}\left(\text{BIOPER}\right)\ (\text{R} = 0.985,$$
$$\text{R}^2 = 0.971,\ \text{F}\left(2,3\right) = 49.648,\ \text{p} < 0.005).$$

The equations show that the values for R_M and R_L can be corrected for different types of mineral fibers to exclude the impact of the relative biopersistence of EMPs. For example, for chrysotile and mesothelioma, the correction factor between chrysotile and amphiboles would be estimated as about 203; recently, we estimated this factor empirically as 139 (Wylie & Korchevskiy, 2023). For lung cancer, the chrysotile correction factor as compared to amphiboles will be about 30.

TABLE 3.2
Expanded information for modeling

Principal Mineral and Habit	Source	R_M, % per total expected mortality, per PCME f/cc-years, age-adjusted, average (95% CI)	R_L, % per baseline lung cancer mortality, per PCME f/cc-years, age-adjusted, average (95% CI)	EMPA, %, average (standard deviation)	EMPB, % average (standard deviation)	Estimated fiber lifetime (years)
Asbestiform riebeckite (crocidolite)	Cape, South Africa	0.59 (0.36, 0.91)	5.2 (0.74, 12)	51.6 (3.4)	79.5 (7.8)	66
	Hamersley, Australia	0.51 (0.45, 0.57)	4.6 (3.6, 5.7)	46.8 (3.9)	71.1 (9.4)	66
Asbestiform grunerite (amosite)	Transvaal, South Africa	0.06 (0.016, 0.15)	1.9 (−0.44, 5.1)	8.0 (0.8)	25.3 (2.0)	74
Asbestiform Na-Ca amphibole	Libby, Montana, U.S.A.	0.03 (0.017, 0.050)	0.82 (0.43, 1.3)	2.1 (0.3)	18.4 (0.6)	49*
Chrysotile	Quebec, Canada	0.0009 (0.0006, 0.0013)	0.060 (0.042, 0.079)	30.4 (46.0)	50.5 (50.0)	0.36**
Erionite	Karain, Turkey	4.5 (1.83, 7.5)	3.3 (N/A)	43.7 (49.8)	50.4 (50.2)	181

* As for tremolite

** Average between several varieties

We can also determine if the proposed width criteria (0.15 μm for EMPA and 0.25 μm for EMPB) are good choices for the prediction of carcinogenic potency.

The performed modeling can be expanded by using the whole dimensional database developed in 2024. Table 3.3 shows the updated values, including the integrated values of the mineral types for various datasets included in the study.

It should be noted that the biopersistence derived from Gualtieri et al. (2018) can be related to other estimates of the toxicokinetics of fibers. For example, for tremolite, crocidolite, amosite, and chrysotile, the biopersistence by Gualtieri correlates well with the central tendency estimations of half-life for corresponding types of fibers as derived by Korchevskiy and Wylie (2022). The log-transformed biopersistence by Gualtieri et al. and by Korchevskiy and Wylie correlates with R=0.99, R^2=0.98,

TABLE 3.3
Integrated information for modeling based on combined database information

Principal mineral and habit	R_M, % per total expected mortality, per PCME f/cc-years, age-adjusted, average (95% CI)	R_L, % per baseline lung cancer mortality, per PCME f/cc-years, age-adjusted, average (95% CI)	EMPA, %, average (standard deviation)	EMPB, % average (standard deviation)	Estimated fiber lifetime (years)
Asbestiform riebeckite (crocidolite)	0.52 (0.47, 0.6)	4.8 (3.8, 5.9)	33.8 (47.3)	56.9 (49.5)	66
Asbestiform grunerite (amosite)	0.11 (0.070, 0.15)	4.0 (3.3, 4.9)	8.9 (28.6)	27.2 (44.5)	74
Asbestiform Na-Ca amphibole	0.03 (0.017, 0.050)	0.82 (0.43, 1.3)	2.6 (16.0)	18.9 (39.1)	49*
Anthophyllite	0.056 (N/A)	1.8 (N/A)	2.5 (15.6)	7.2 (25.7)	245
Fluoro-edenite	0.12 (N/A)	2.34 (N/A)	1.9 (13.7)	18.8 (39.1)	N/A
Glaucophane	0.0085 (N/A)	0.08 (N/A)	2.3 (15.1)	14.1 (34.7)	N/A
Balangeroite	0.04 (0.0058, 0.16)	1.28 (0.75, 1.77)	5.4 (22.7)	8.9 (28.7)	N/A
Chrysotile, Quebec	0.0009 (0.0006, 0.0013)	0.060 (0.042, 0.079)	30.4 (46.0)	50.5 (50.0)	0.36**
Erionite, Karain	4.5 (1.83, 7.5)	3.3 (N/A)	43.7 (49.8)	50.4 (50.2)	181

*As for tremolite

**Average between several varieties

p <0.0096. Using the relationship between two estimations of biopersistence, we can evaluate the estimated fiber lifetime of balangeroite for Table 3.3 as 61 years.

For the updated and combined information, we can derive the relationships for amphiboles and single-chain silicates (balangeroite), similar to those determined in 2020.

In particular,

for mesothelioma,

$$R_M = 0.004 + 0.015\ \text{EMPA}\ \left(R = 0.969,\ R^2 = 0.939,\ F(1,5) = 76.52,\ p < 0.00032\right),$$
and

$$R_M = -0.099 + 0.0099\ \text{EMPB}\ \left(R = 0.943,\ R^2 = 0.889,\ F(1,5) = 40.214,\ p < 0.0014\right),$$
and

for lung cancer,

$$R_L = 1.22 + 0.114\ \text{EMPA}\ \left(R = 0.780,\ R^2 = 0.608,\ F(1,5) = 7.75,\ p < 0.038\right),\ \text{and}$$

$$R_L = 0.39 + 0.08\ \text{EMPB}\ \left(R = 0.802,\ R^2 = 0.644,\ F(1,5) = 9.05,\ p < 0.029\right),$$

Biopersistence can also be included in the modeling, if chrysotile and erionite are included as datapoints.

Using the biopersistence data from Table 3.2, we can develop models to reconstruct R_M and R_L.

For mesothelioma,

$$\text{Log}_{10}(R_M) = -3.78 + 1.45\ \text{LOG}_{10}(\text{EMPA}) + 0.90\log_{10}(\text{BIOPER})\ (R = 0.950,$$

$$R^2 = 0.904,\ F(2,3) = 14.19,\ p < 0.029),\ \text{and}$$

for lung cancer,

$$\text{Log}_{10}(R_L) = -1.53 + 0.723\ \text{LOG}_{10}(\text{EMPA}) + 0.51\ \log_{10}(\text{BIOPER})\ (R = 0.964,$$

$$R^2 = 0.929,\ F(2,3) = 19.69,\ p < 0.018),\ \text{and}$$

$$\text{Log}_{10}(R_L) = -2.26 + 0.85\ \text{LOG}_{10}(\text{EMPB}) + 0.73\log_{10}(\text{BIOPER})\ (R = 0.967,$$

$$R^2 = 0.936,\ F(2,3) = 21.89,\ p < 0.017).$$

It is noteworthy that the models above allow reconstruction of the biopersistence for various types of mineral fibers. For example, the estimated lifetime of glaucophane fibers would be 40 years, and that of balangeroite 55.6 years, close to the estimation we provided based on Korchevskiy and Wylie (2022). This calculation, however, demonstrates that fluoro-edenite and erionite are expected to have a very long lifespan.

Figure 3.2 demonstrates the relationship between cutpoint fiber width and Pearson's correlation between the fraction of fibers longer than 5 μm and thinner than the cutpoint, and mesothelioma potency (P values are demonstrated as well).

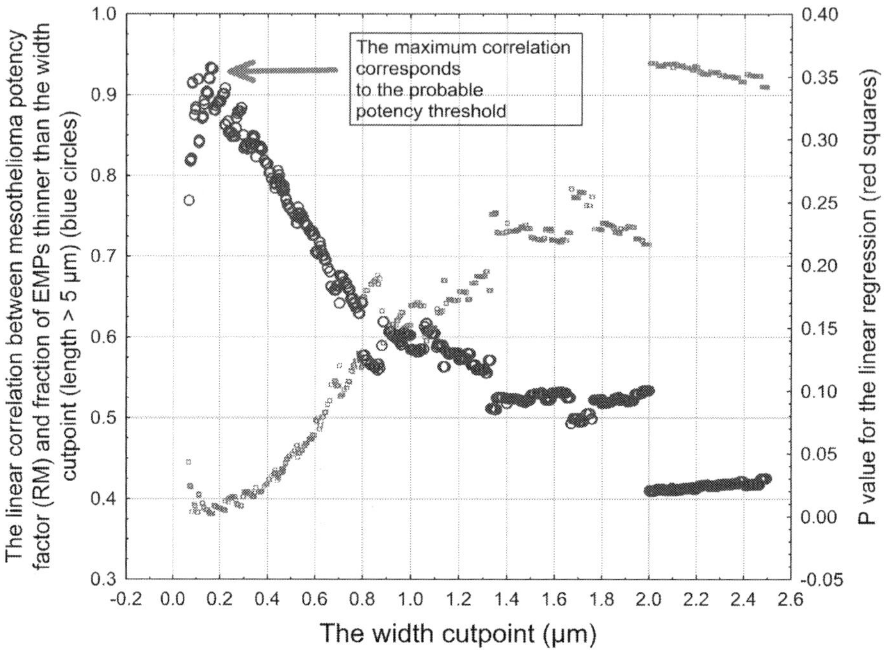

FIGURE 3.2 The results of Monte Carlo modeling for the correlation between RM and the fraction of the fibers limited by a cutpoint (threshold) width. Blue circles – correlation coefficients, red dots – P values.

It is noteworthy that the correlation curve increases up to a certain value and then decreases.

The following explanation can be given for the correlation between threshold width and mesothelioma potency. Let's assume f(w) to be a fraction of all fibers that are thinner than w, that w_0 is a threshold width, and that all fibers have a potency of 1 when the width is less than w_0 and 0 if it is greater than w_0. In this case, $f(w_0)$ provides us with full information about the potency of the fiber set.

However, if $w < w_0$, f(w) provides us with less information about the total potency of the fiber set than $f(w_0)$ would. Knowing f(w), we can only say that the potency is fluctuating somewhere between f(w) (if all potent fibers in reality are thinner than w) and $f(w_0)$ (if all fibers thicker than w would be thinner than w_0). The size of the interval from f(w) to 1 provides us with an estimation of the error for the potency estimation. The estimation of the maximum error in this case is

$$(f(w_0)-f(w))/f(w_0).$$

Now, if $w > w_0$, the information about the potency is limited again. If we know f(w), we can only conclude that the potency can be as low as 0 (if all fibers thinner than w will be at the same time thicker than w_0), or as high as f(w). The estimation of the error in this case is

$$f(w)/f(w_0).$$

A simple assumption would be that the function f is increasing with its argument w, changing from 0 when w = 0 and reaching 1 when w is at the maximum width value (e.g., it can be 3 μm).

With this assumption, we can say that the information error (1-f(w)) will decrease (and the corresponding correlation between the fraction f(w) and the potency factor will increase) while w is changing from 0 to w_0; then the correlation should reach its maximum (the error is 0 in this case), and then the error f(w) will increase (and the corresponding correlation will decrease) while w is changing from w_0 to the maximum width value.

We performed a statistical simulation to advance and check this explanation for the observed relationship between fractional characteristics of EMPs and the potency.

We conditionally assume that the potency is a random variable changing between 0.5 and 1 when the width is less than or equal to 0.15 μm, and equal to 0 otherwise (for widths between ≥0.05 μm and ≤3 μm). We assumed that the potency of any selection of fibers can be estimated as a sum of frequencies of each size group multiplied by the potency of each particle. Then, for each w in the range from 0.05 to 3 μm, we generated 100 random distributions of frequencies. We determined the linear correlation coefficient between the potency and the fraction of particles with width ≤w.

The correlations for each w are shown in Figure 3.3.

We can see that our simulation replicates well the observed trend of correlations between potency and fraction of particles, with the maximum reached at about the 0.15–0.17 μm cutpoint for width. In both cases, the correlations are lower at first but then reach the maximum at about the value separating datapoints with positive potency from datapoints with zero potency.

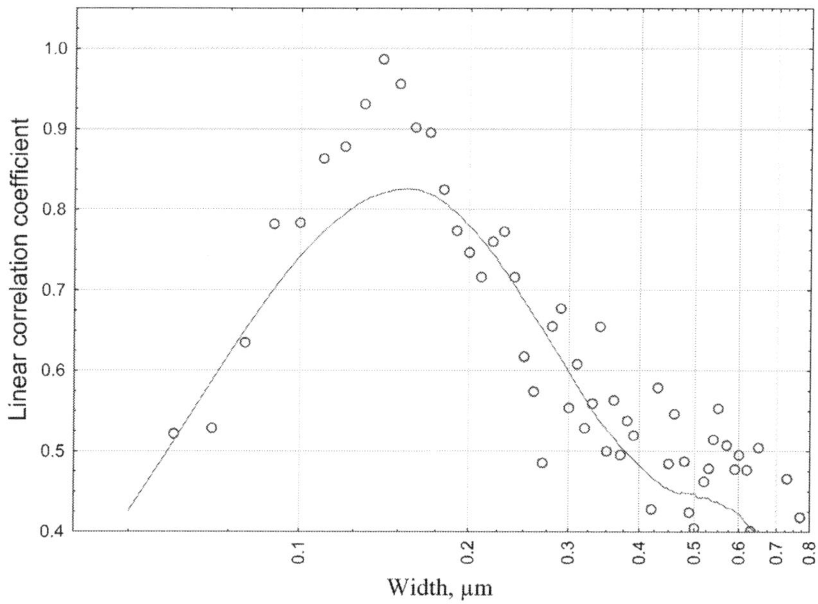

FIGURE 3.3 Correlation coefficient between the fraction of particles with width ≤w and accumulated potencies for the simulated selections of EMPs. Blue dots – datapoints. Red line – weighted-distance fitting curve.

In this sense, Figure 3.2 demonstrates that 0.17 μm can be considered a threshold for the mesothelioma potency in fibers longer than 5 μm. The fraction of fibers thinner than 0.17 μm is well approximated by the EMPA value. EMPB also serves as a good predictor of potency; most probably, it is another robust estimation of the fraction of very thin (and therefore mesotheliomagenic) asbestiform fibers.

We also performed a simulation study with both cutpoints for length and width tested to determine the highest correlation coefficients with mesothelioma potency. Only length values in the range from 5 to 30 μm were considered as cutpoints, along with width values in the range from 0.06 to 2.5 μm. Because some combinations of length and width cutpoints corresponded to a very small fraction of particles in the database, we included only combinations of length and width cutpoints that covered at least 5% of the fibers. The fraction of fibers in a specific length (greater than L_0) and width (not greater than W_0) group was determined as

$$\text{Fraction} = \frac{Number\ of\ particles\ longer\ than\ L_0\left(\mu m\right) and\ not\ thickers\ than\ W_0\left(\mu m\right)}{Number\ of\ particles\ longer\ than\ 5\left(\mu m\right).}$$

(denominator includes all particles longer than 5 μm to keep correspondence to the original definition of potency factor R_M, where it is related to the concentration of particles longer than 5 μm as well).

Figure 3.4 (a and b) shows the relationship between length and width cutpoint values with the correlation of the corresponding fraction of particles and potency factor as listed in Table 3.3 (only amphiboles and single-chain silicates included).

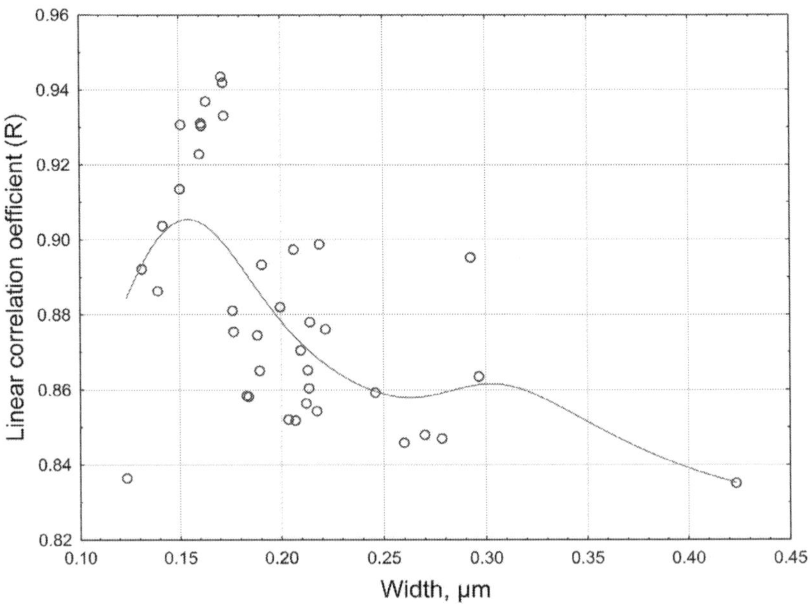

FIGURE 3.4 The results of Monte Carlo modeling for the correlation between R_M and cutpoints (threshold) for length and width. Only datapoints with P value <0.01 included. Red lines – fitting curves for the relationship between a parameter (width or length) and the correlation value.

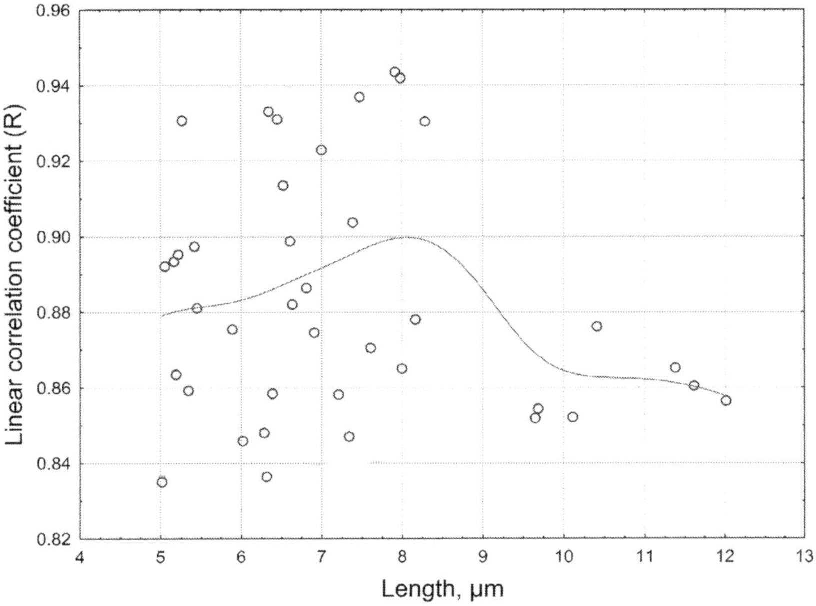

FIGURE 3.4 (Continued)

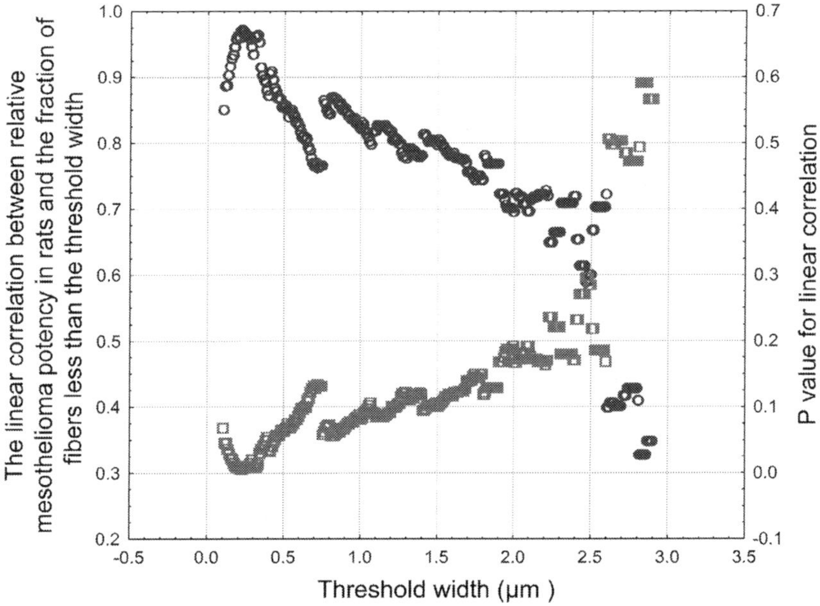

FIGURE 3.5 The results of Monte Carlo modeling for the correlation between R_M and the fraction of the fibers limited by a cutpoint (threshold) width. Blue circles – correlation coefficients. Red squares – P values.

The highest correlation was found for the dimensional fraction of particles with length >7.92 μm and width ≤0.17 μm ($R = 0.94$, $P \leq 0.0004$, fraction among all particles in the database with length >5 μm, length/width ≥3, width ≥0.06 μm, width ≤3 μm 6%).

Interestingly, the Cook et al. (2016) data on the potency of different types of fibers installed in rats intrapleurally can be modeled in a similar way, with the maximum potency associated with a slightly higher value, $w_0 = 0.21$ μm.

The results of the simulation are demonstrated in Figure 3.5.

In this case,

$$\text{MesoPotency} = 0.382 + 0.025 \text{ x } \text{EMP}_{0.21},$$

$$R = 0.969, R^2 = 0.939, p < 0.00637,$$

where MesoPotency is the published relative potency of various fibers with UICC amosite potency assumed equal to 1, and

$EMP_{0.21}$ is the fraction of fibers thinner than 0.21 μm among fibers longer than 5 μm. In our modeling, we took into account only asbestiform amphibole fibers (crocidolite, amosite, anthophyllite, tremolite, and ferro-actinolite) to make the results comparable with R_M modeling above.

The fraction of very thin fibers among the fibers longer than 5 μm demonstrates its predictive ability for mesothelioma and lung cancer potency in different settings and for various mineral fibers, if the potency is adjusted for biopersistence. It is reasonable to suggest that fibers longer than 5 μm and thicker than 0.25 μm are not demonstrated to produce mesothelioma in humans without the presence of thinner fibers. However, not all elongate mineral particles thinner than 0.15 μm are carcinogenic as well. With very small probability, cleavage fragments, or in general non-asbestiform elongate mineral particles that thin can be produced by mechanical forces, and not natural growth, although they are rare. These particles can accidentally be found in non-asbestiform datasets. However, being mechanically "carved" from the solid mineral, they are expected to lack the qualities typical for asbestos fibers and necessary to make them biologically active.

It is important to see that among 15,328 non-asbestiform EMPs longer than 5 μm, with AR ≥3 and width ≤3 μm, only 11 particles (0.07%) would adhere to EMPA criteria. This number is well within the error rate for the counting of elongate mineral particles in specific size categories.

We can therefore conclude that the criteria can be utilized for distinguishing between carcinogenic and non-carcinogenic EMP exposure in humans and predicting the potency of the EMPs, as demonstrated in Figure 3.6.

The idea of the statistical significance of the EMPA parameter as a predictor of carcinogenicity can also be illustrated by using the data from Cook et al. (2016).

We combined the data on the EMPA parameter and tumor incidence/potency of various types of amphibole fibers from the Cook study in Table 3.4.

As can be seen from Table 3.4, the only type of EMP not producing a statistically significant elevation in tumor incidence in rats, non-fibrous grunerite, was at the same time the only mineral type with EMPA not significantly different from 0.

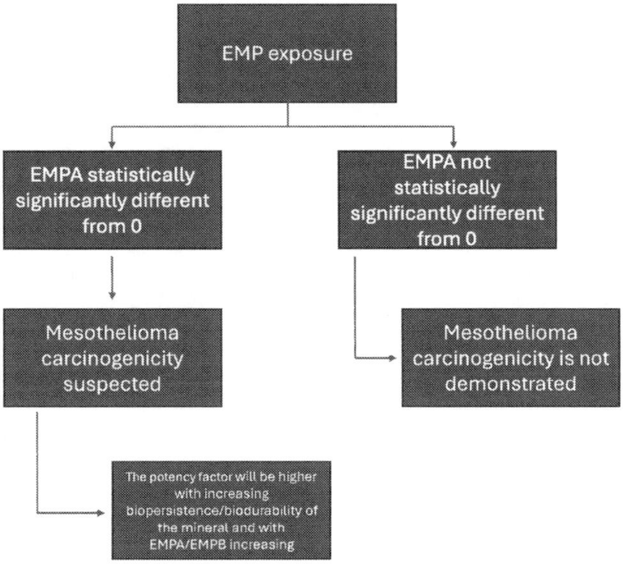

FIGURE 3.6 The suggested criteria for mesotheliomagencity of EMPs

TABLE 3.4
The integrated data from Cook et al. (2016) on mesothelioma in rats after intrapleural injection of EMPs

	EMPA (%)			Tumor incidence in 20 mg exposure group (%)			
Mineral type	**Average**	**95% CI lower bound**	**95% CI upper bound**	**Average**	**95% CI lower bound**	**95% CI upper bound**	**Relative potency factor for 20 mg exposure**
Crocidolite	15.34	13.38	17.30	57.47	47.08	67.86	1.37
Amosite	2.43	1.07	3.79	34.33	27.76	40.89	0.73
Anthophyllite*	3.88	1.62	6.14	34.38	22.74	46.01	0.47
Ferroactinolite	4.62	2.74	6.51	22.96	15.87	30.06	0.54
Tremolite	3.36	1.31	5.40	38.39	25.65	51.13	0.66
Non-fibrous grunerite	2.91	−0.33	6.16	2.22	−0.26	4.71	0.1

* Cook et al (2016) data reported anthophyllite UICC samples as having EMPA=0% and EMPB=1.75% (atypical for asbestiform anthophyllite). At the same time, the UICC anthophyllite sample used by Cook was analyzed repeatedly by different laboratories. The average value between various estimations of EMPA for anthophyllite from the dimensional database is reported here with the assumption that the original data from the Cook study was not fully reflective of the exposure material.

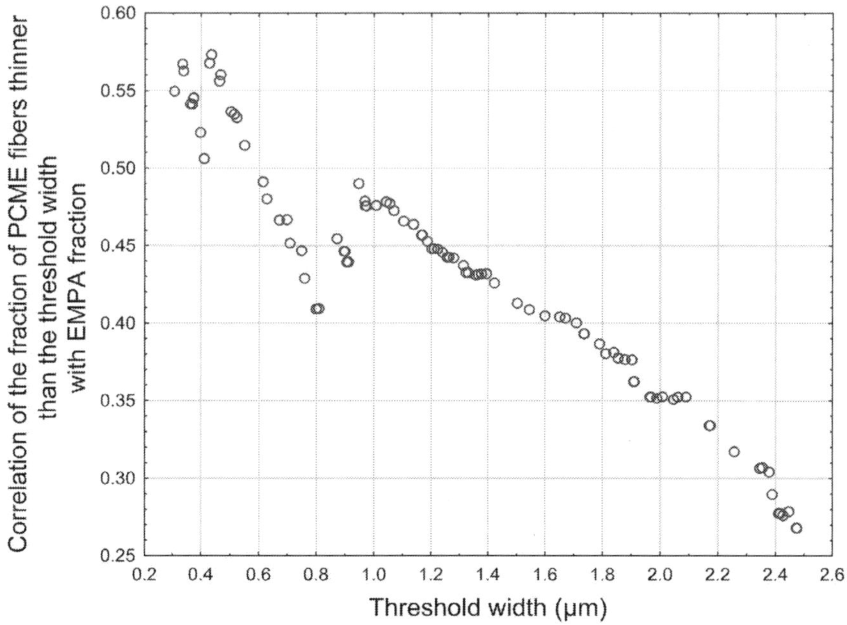

FIGURE 3.7 The results of Monte Carlo modeling for the correlation between EMPA and fractions of PCME fibers limited by a cutpoint (threshold) width.

It is also very important that artificially limiting the fiber counting criteria can significantly decrease the quality of toxicological analysis and modeling of potency. For example, Figure 3.7 demonstrates the correlation of various fractions of so-called PCME fibers (longer than 5 µm and thicker than 0.25 µm) with a certain width cutpoint and the EMPA fiber fraction. For the simulation, we used the separate estimations of EMPA and each of the other size of fractions for 240 cohorts included in the database. It can be seen that the correlations are pretty weak, though statistically significant, and the highest correlation is achieved for a width of 0.475 µm ($R = 0.573$, $R^2 = 0.33$, $p < 0.00001$). There is no fraction of PCME fibers that would be able to predict EMPA (and consequently the carcinogenic potency of fibers).

In general, the analysis of fractional characteristics of various datasets in our study shows that the hypothesis of very thin fibers longer than 5 µm being the exclusive mesotheliomagenic category is supported by the data. Also, the quantitative carcinogenicity of fibers depends on their biopersistence. We demonstrated an empirical approach where biopersistence is quantified in terms of the dissolution lifetime of various mineral types of fibers. In particular, for mesothelioma, the relative correction factor for biopersistence can be estimated as 1 for amphiboles, 0.0015 for chrysotile, and 1.8 for erionite.

REFERENCE LIST

Atkinson, G. R., Rose, D., Thomas, K., Jones, D., Chatfield, E., & Going, J. (1981). *Collection, analysis, and characterization of vermiculite samples for fibre content and asbestos contamination* (US EPA Contract No. 68-01-5915 report from MRI). US EPA.

Bernstein, D. M., & Hoskins, J. A. (2006). The health effects of chrysotile: Current perspective based upon recent data. *Regulatory Toxicology and Pharmacology, 45*(3), 252–264. https://doi.org/10.1016/j.yrtph.2006.04.008

Bertrand, R., & Pezerat, H. (1980). Fibrous glass: Carcinogenicity and dimensional characteristics. *IARC Scientific Publications, 30*, 901–911.

Bonneau, L., Malard, C., & Pezerat, H. (1986). Studies on surface properties of asbestos. II: Role of dimensional characteristics and surface properties of mineral fibers in the induction of pleural tumors. *Environmental Research, 41*(1), 268–275. https://doi.org/10.1016/s0013-9351(86)80188-8

Carbone, M., Ferris, L. K., Baumann, F., Napolitano, A., Lum, C. A., Flores, E. G., Gaudino, G., Powers, A., Bryant-Greenwood, P., Krausz, T., Hyjek, E., Tate, R., Friedberg, J., Weigel, T., Pass, H. I., & Yang, H. (2012). BAP1 cancer syndrome: Malignant mesothelioma, uveal and cutaneous melanoma, and MBAITs. *Journal of Translational Medicine, 10*, 179. https://doi.org/10.1186/1479-5876-10-179

Cook, P. M., Swintek, J., Dawson, T. D., Chapman, D., Etterson, M. A., & Hoff, D. (2016). Quantitative structure-mesothelioma potency model optimization for complex mixtures of elongated particles in rat pleura: A retrospective study. *Journal of Toxicology and Environmental Health, Part B, 19*(5–6), 266–288. https://doi.org/10.1080/10937404.2016.1195326

Cooke, W. E. (1924). Fibrosis of the lungs due to the inhalation of asbestos dust. *British Medical Journal, 2*(3317), 147. https://doi.org/10.1136/bmj.2.3317.147

Darnton, L. (2023). Quantitative assessment of mesothelioma and lung cancer risk based on phase contrast microscopy (PCM) estimates of fibre exposure: An update of 2000 asbestos cohort data. *Environmental Research, 230*, 114753. https://doi.org/10.1016/j.envres.2022.114753

Garabrant, D. H., & Pastula, S. T. (2018). A comparison of asbestos fiber potency and elongate mineral particle (EMP) potency for mesothelioma in humans. *Toxicology and Applied Pharmacology, 361*, 127–136. https://doi.org/10.1016/j.taap.2018.07.003

Gibbs, G. W., & Hwang, C. Y. (1980). Dimensions of airborne asbestos fibres. In J. C. Wagner (Ed.), *Biological effects of mineral fibres* (IARC Scientific Publications No. 30, pp. 69–78). IARC Scientific Publications, Lynn. PMID: 7239672.

Golden, R., Bus, J., & Calabrese, E. (2019). An examination of the linear no–threshold hypothesis of cancer risk assessment: Introduction to a series of reviews documenting the lack of biological plausibility of LNT. *Chemico Biological Interactions, 301*, 2–5. https://doi.org/10.1016/j.cbi.2019.01.038

Gualtieri, A. F., Pollastri, S., Gandolfi, N. B., & Gualtieri, M. L. (2018). In vitro acellular dissolution of mineral fibres: A comparative study. *Scientific Reports, 8*, 7071. https://doi.org/10.1038/s41598-018-25531-4

Hodgson, J., & Darnton, A. (2000). The quantitative risks of mesothelioma and lung cancer in relation to asbestos exposure. *The Annals of Occupational Hygiene, 44*, 565–601.

King, E. J., Clegg, J. W., & Rae, V. M. (1946). The effect of asbestos, and of asbestos and aluminum, on the lungs of rabbits. *Thorax, 1*(3), 188–197. https://doi.org/10.1136/thx.1.3.188

Korchevskiy, A. A., Rasmuson, J. O., & Rasmuson, E. J. (2019). Empirical model of mesothelioma potency factors for different mineral fibers based on their chemical composition and dimensionality. *Inhalation Toxicology, 31*(5), 180–191. https://doi.org/10.1080/08958378.2019.1640320

Korchevskiy, A. A., Rasmuson, J. O., & Rasmuson, E. J. (2024). Mathematical modeling of cancer potency for various fibrous minerals. In A. A. Korchevskiy, J. O. Rasmuson, & E. J. Rasmuson (Eds.), *Health risk assessment for asbestos and other fibrous minerals*. John Wiley & Sons, Inc.

Korchevskiy, A. A., & Wylie, A. (2022). Asbestos exposure, lung fiber burden, and mesothelioma rates: Mechanistic modelling for risk assessment. *Computational Toxicology, 24*, 100249. https://doi.org/10.1016/j.comtox.2022.100249

Lee, R. J., Van Orden, D. R., Allison, K. A., & Bunker, K. L. (2009). Characterization of airborne amphibole particles in Libby, MT. *Indoor Build Environment, 18*(6), 524–530.

Lentz, T. J., Rice, C. H., Succop, P. A., Lockey, J. E., Dement, J. M., & LeMasters, G. K. (2003). Pulmonary deposition modeling with airborne fiber exposure data: A study of workers manufacturing refractory ceramic fibers. *Applied Occupational and Environmental Hygiene, 18*(4), 278–288. https://doi.org/10.1080/10473220301404

Lippmann, M. (2014). Toxicological and epidemiological studies on effects of airborne fibers: Coherence and public [corrected] health implications. *Critical Reviews in Toxicology, 44*(8), 643–695. https://doi.org/10.3109/10408444.2014.928266

National Institute for Occupational Safety and Health (NIOSH). (1989). *Asbestos and other fibers by PCM: Method 7400, issue 1*. NIOSH.

Pooley, F. D. (2018). Characterization of lung burden EMPs. *Toxicology and Applied Pharmacology, 361*, 18–20. https://doi.org/10.1016/j.taap.2018.10.019

Pooley, F. D., & Clark, N. J. (1980). A comparison of fibre dimensions in chrysotile, crocidolite and amosite particles from samples of airborne dust and from Confirmed post-mortem lung tissue specimens. *IARC Scientific Publications, 30*, 79–86.

Pott, F. (1978). Some aspects on the dosimetry of the carcinogenic potency of asbestos and other fibrous dusts. *Staub-Reinhaltung der Luft, 38*(12), 486–490. WOS: A1978GC16500004.

Roggli, V. L. (2015). The so-called short-fiber controversy: Literature review and critical analysis. *Archives of Pathology and Laboratory Medicine, 139*(8), 1052–1057. https://doi.org/10.5858/arpa.2014-0466-RA

Shedd, K. B. (1985). *Fiber dimensions of crocidolites from Western Australia, Bolivia, and the Cape and Transvaal Provinces of South Africa* (8998). Report of Investigations (United States, Bureau of Mines). https://stacks.cdc.gov/view/cdc/10488

Stanton, M. F., Laynard, M., Tegeris, A., Miller, E., May, M., & Kent, E. (1977). Carcinogenicity of fibrous glass: Pleural response in the rat in relation to fiber dimension. *Journal of the National Cancer Institute, 58*(3), 587–603. https://doi.org/10.1093/jnci/58.3.587

Stanton, M. F., Layard, M., Tegeris, A., Miller, E., May, M., Morgan, E., & Smith, A. (1981). Relation of particle dimension to carcinogenicity in amphibole asbestos and other fibrous minerals. *Journal of the National Cancer Institute, 67*(5), 965–975. PMID: 6946253.

Tilkes, F., & Beck, E. G. (1980). Comparison of length-dependent cytotoxicity of inhalable asbestos and man-made mineral fibres. *IARC Scientific Publications, 30*, 475–483.

Timbrell, V. (1965, December). The inhalation of fibrous dusts. *Biological Effects of Asbestos: Annals of the New York Academy of Sciences, 132*(1), 255–273. https://doi.org/10.1111/j.1749-6632.1965.tb41107.x

U.S. EPA. (2014, December). *Toxicological review of Libby amphibole asbestos, in support of summary information on the integrated risk information system (IRIS)* (EPA/635/R-11/002F). U.S. EPA.

Wagner, J. C., Skidmore, J. W., Hill, R. J., & Griffiths, D. M. (1985). Erionite exposure and mesotheliomas in rats. *British Journal of Cancer, 51*(5), 727–730. https://doi.org/10.1038/bjc.1985.108

Wagner, J. C., Sleggs, C. A., & Marchand, P. (1960). Diffuse pleural mesothelioma and asbestos exposure in the North Western Cape province. *British Journal of Industrial Medicine, 17*, 260–271.

Wylie, A. G., & Candela, P. A. (2015). Methodologies for determining the sources, characteristics, distribution, and abundance of asbestiform and nonasbestiform amphibole and serpentine in ambient air and water. *Journal of Toxicology and Environmental Health, Part B, Critical Reviews, 18*, 1–42. https://doi.org/10.1080/10937404.2014.997945

Wylie, A. G., & Korchevskiy, A. A. (2023). Dimensions of elongate mineral particles and cancer: A review. *Environmental Research, 230*, 114688. https://doi.org/10.1016/j.envres.2022.114688

Wylie, A. G., Korchevskiy, A. A., Segrave, A. M., & Duane, A. (2020). Modeling mesothelioma risk factors from amphibole fiber dimensionality: Mineralogical and epidemiological perspective. *Journal of Applied Toxicology, 40*(4), 515–524. https://doi.org/10.1002/jat.3923

4 Mesothelial toxicity of elongate mineral particles

The mode of action and quantitative interpretation

A. Korchevskiy & A. Wylie

INTRODUCTION

This chapter attempts to provide a stage-by-stage quantitative exploration of the mesothelial toxicity of elongate mineral particles (EMPs) with the goal of understanding the reasons why different types of particles produce different levels of toxic response in similar environments. In particular, it is important to understand why non-elongate particles, at some point, change the biological response completely when one of their dimensions becomes significantly greater than another. This chapter provides a possible framework for toxicological studies rather than claiming to have the final answer for all possible questions. The approach here is to use various sources of information and utilize the quantitative structure-activity relationship (QSAR) model as a means to explore the validity of assumptions about the mode and mechanisms of action for EMPs in mesothelioma development. Undoubtedly, as knowledge progresses, new information will amend and potentially adjust this framework. However, we will demonstrate that our model is able to explain some of the key events in the mesothelial carcinogenicity of fibers and support a quantitative metric of risk fitting observed data and parameters.

DEPOSITION, RETENTION, AND ACCESS TO THE PLEURA

The toxicokinetics of elongate mineral particles is the critical element of their toxicity. To produce toxic effects in general, and carcinogenicity in particular, EMPs must gain access to the human respiratory system, penetrate deep enough, be deposited in the tissue, and withstand clearance long enough to produce a sustainable effect (for cancer, this effect could be responsible not just for one, but for several mutations). A detailed analysis of the available scientific information on the behavior of fibers in human lungs is provided in Chapter 6 of this book.

It should be noted that there are still many controversies around the issues of deposition, clearance, and biopersistence of elongate particles. In particular, existing models on the deposition of fibers in the lungs are limited by the insufficient amount of

 DOI: 10.1201/9781003424277-5

experimental data and an overreliance on mathematical modeling of the transfer of particles. The multi-path particle dosimetry (MPPD) model by the United States Environmental Protection Agency (U.S. EPA) apparently still requires additional validation when applied to different sizes and habits of elongate mineral particles (Jarabek, 2021; Asgharian et al., 2018). The recent publication by Mori et al. (2024) demonstrated the need for revision of the MPPD model as applied to complex composites of aerosols. Specifically for asbestos fibers, our calculations show that MPPD does not demonstrate significant differences in the deposition rates of elongate particles among dimensional groups known to vary from lung burden/aerosol comparisons and target health effects. For example, MPPD predicts similar deposition rates for long, thin and short, thick particles of several mineral types, counterintuitive to what is observed in the fibers derived from human lungs, where long, thin particles appear to prevail (see Chapter 6).

Available data and epidemiological observations allow us to conclude that elongate mineral particles differ from spherical ones in their deposition, clearance, and biopersistence in human lungs.

Particles enter the human respiratory tract through nasal or oral pathways, reach the tracheobronchial region, and enter the pulmonary or alveolar area. The particles in the upper respiratory tract are cleared by direct breathing out and also by ciliary cleaning, while there is no direct "way back" for the particles penetrating the alveolar area. Particles can be retained in or cleared from all parts of the respiratory system over prolonged time. Once deposited in the lung, bundles of mineral fibers may disaggregate, increasing the number of narrow fibers interacting independently with cells. Although the mechanism is not fully known, inhaled fibers appear to be translocated throughout the body. They can be found in the visceral and parietal pleural and peritoneal, the locations of mesothelioma related to asbestos exposure, and elsewhere. It is believed that fibers move through the human body either through the lymphatic system (probably the most important pathway) and/or by mechanical penetration through tissue.

During all stages of particle deposition, translocation, and clearance from the lung, in comparison to spherical particles, the dimensions of elongate particles, including length, width, thickness, and aspect ratio, significantly affect these processes, resulting in sorting by dimension at any moment in time. In particular, lengthier particles are more easily deposited by impaction; at the same time, small-diameter particles are expected to penetrate more easily through narrow lymphatic channels and through tissue itself. Small-diameter particles with the same length would go deeper into the lungs and potentially reach the pleura (Pooley & Clark, 1980; Miserocchi et al., 2008).

Korchevskiy and Wylie (2022) suggested the following way to estimate the lung burden of asbestos fibers in human lungs t years after the last exposure. They found that if the exposure to C f/cc with a duration of D years is treated as a time sequence consisting of D independent year-long events, the lung fiber burden can be conditionally approximated by the following mechanistic model:

$$\mathrm{B}_{\mathrm{wet}} = \sum_{i=1}^{D} \frac{C\,x1{,}000{,}000\,x\,BR\,x\,Rate_{dep}\,x\,DPY\,x\,e^{-\lambda(D+t-i)}}{LungWeight}$$

$$= \frac{C\,x1{,}000{,}000\,x\,BR\,x\,Rate_{dep}\,x\,DPY\,x\,e^{-\lambda(D+t-1)}(1-e^{\lambda D})}{LungWeight\,x\left(1-e^{\lambda}\right)},$$

$$\mathrm{B}_{\mathrm{dry}}=\mathrm{B}_{\mathrm{wet}}*\mathrm{DW},$$

where B_{wet} is the lung burden (fibers longer than 5 μm per 1 g of the lung wet weight),

B_{dry} is the lung burden (fibers longer than 5 μm per 1 g of the lung dry weight),

BR is the breathing rate of a worker (≈10 m^3/shift),

DPY is the working days per year (250 days),

LungWeight is the weight of human adult lungs (g),

t is the time since last exposure (years),

$Rate_{dep}$ is the initial alveolar deposition coefficient of fibers in lungs during exposure (unitless fraction),

λ is the elimination coefficient for a specific type of fibers ($years^{-1}$), and

DW is the coefficient between wet and dry weight of human lungs (unitless).

It should be noted that the initial alveolar deposition coefficient of fibers in the lungs is a function of various factors by itself. In our paper (Korchevskiy & Wylie, 2022), we used generalized published estimations of this parameter; however, various assumptions can be made on the deposition rate for fibers with different dimensions.

The authors estimated the following elimination coefficients for various types of mineral fibers. They concluded that the observed level in the lung tissue (as observed in a British case-control study, Gilham et al., 2016) would be achieved if the elimination coefficients were

- 0.169 (5th to 95th percentile range 0.14, 0.21) $years^{-1}$ for amosite,
- 0.0993 (5th to 95th percentile range 0.08, 0.12) $years^{-1}$ for crocidolite, and
- 6.45 (5th to 95th percentile range 5.34, 8.01) $years^{-1}$ for chrysotile.

The average elimination coefficients correspond to the values of 4.06 years half-life for amosite, 6.98 years for crocidolite, and 1.29 months for chrysotile.

The comparison of the modeled values of the elimination coefficient with selected previously published estimations is given in Table 4.1.

The reported elimination coefficients can be interpreted in several ways. They can be used along with Equation 4.1, to predict lung concentrations of fibers, assuming that the clearance process follows an exponential law. However, if the exponential elimination is limited by some other factors, the elimination can be slowed down. In this case, the elimination rate coefficients could be considered as relative values, allowing us to compare lung burden levels for various mineral types and sizes of fibers. This can be the case for chrysotile, which can still be found in the lungs even after an effective ban on chrysotile in Western countries. Potentially, low-level exposure to this type of fiber continues, despite the decrease in environmental and occupational exposure. Alternatively, we can also hypothesize that chrysotile has very limited access to the pleura, even if some fibers are still found in human lungs after cessation of exposure. It is quite possible that the transport of fibers from the pulmonary area to the pleura would be the last step of biological dissolution and elimination of fibers.

Remarkably, the elimination coefficient reported by Korchevskiy and Wylie (2022) is highly correlated with the log-transformed biopersistence of particles reported by Gualtieri et al. (2018) ($R = -0.998$, $R^2 = 0.996$, $P < 0.05$) (Table 4.2). At the same time (see Chapters 3 and 8 of this book), biopersistence (reversed biosolubility) by

TABLE 4.1
Comparison of the modeled and published estimations of elimination coefficients for various types of asbestiform mineral fibers (derived from Korchevskiy & Wylie, 2022)

Mineral type, source	Estimated elimination coefficient ($years^{-1}$) (5th to 95th percentile range)	Published elimination coefficients ($years^{-1}$)	The combined average published estimation ($years^{-1}$) (Range)
Amosite, South Africa	0.169 (0.14, 0.21)	0.28 (Hesterberg et al., 1998) 0.03 (Churg & Vedal, 1994) 0.46 (Rendall & Du Toit, 1994 in baboons)	0.19 (0.03–0.46)
Crocidolite, Australia and South Africa	0.099 (0.08, 0.12)	0.09 (de Klerk et al., 1996) 0.068 to 0.15 (Berry et al., 2012) 0.11 (Du Toit, 1991) 0.166 (Rendall & Du Toit, 1994 in baboons) 0.05 (Werner et al., 1995)	0.092 (0.01–0.166)
Chrysotile, Quebec, Canada	6.45 (5.35, 8.01)	15.76 (Bernstein & Hoskins, 2006) 3.92 – 25.3 (Searl, 1997) 2.18 (Coin et al., 1992) 1.18 (Jurinski & Rimstidt, 2001) 0.086–0.18 (Finkelstein & Dufresne, 1999)	6.36 (0.086 25.3)
Tremolite	0.14 (N/A)	0.17 (Oze & Solt, 2010)	0.17
Libby amphiboles	-	0.068 (U.S. EPA, 2014) 0.15 (U.S. EPA, 2014)	0.11

Gualtieri et al. (2018), along with the fraction of fibers longer than 5 μm and thinner than 0.15 μm (EMPA category), are some of the strongest predictors of mesothelioma potency of mineral fibers.

The following regression (Equation 4.1) can be found in this case:

$$\mathrm{Log}_{10}(\lambda) = 0.42 - 0.718\ \log_{10}\ (\text{Biopersistence}), \tag{4.1}$$

where λ is the elimination coefficient, $years^{-1}$, and

TABLE 4.2
The biopersistence (reversed biosolubility) and elimination rate for various types of asbestiform mineral fibers (λ)

Mineral type, source	Biopersistence (reversed biosolubility), per fiber of 0.25 μm (years to fully dissolve)	Elimination rate ($years^{-1}$)****
Chrysotile, Quebec, Canada	0.36*	6.243
Amosite, South Africa	74*	0.12
Crocidolite, South Africa	66*	0.13
Anthophyllite, Finland	245*	0.051
Glaucophane, California, U.S.A.	N/A	N/A
Libby amphiboles, Montana, U.S.A.	49**	0.161
Fluoro-edenite, Biancavilla, Italy	N/A	N/A
Erionite (Karain and Oregon, combined)	181*	0.063
Balangeroite, Italy	55.6***	0.147
Tremolite (different locations)	49*	0.161

* Gualtieri et al., 2018
** As for tremolite
*** Korchevskiy & Wylie, 2023
**** Equation (4.1)

Biopersistence is the fiber lifetime in the acellular dissolution process in terms of Gualtieri's acellular dissolution rate for a standard width of elongate particles ($R = 0.92$, $R^2 = 0.85$, $p < 0.00858$).

From this relationship, we can predict the fiber elimination rate for various types of mineral fibers (Table 4.2).

It should be noted that Table 4.2 reflects the overall biopersistence of elongate mineral particles in the lungs, not specifically in the pleura. We will further discuss the access of retained fibers to mesothelial tissue.

Also, we can estimate biopersistence for each fiber width, using data from Gualtieri et al. (2018) and Equation 4.2:

$$\text{Biopersistence for fibers with width of W (μm)} = W/0.25 \times \text{Biopersistence for fibers with width 0.25 μm} \tag{4.2}$$

Also, elongate particles must reach mesothelial tissue to produce an adverse toxic effect, such as the formation of pleural plaques or malignant mesothelioma. Some authors (e.g., Gualtieri, 2023) argue that toxic mechanisms of elongate particles should not be confined just to physical contact between fibers and tissue and can happen at a distance (by generating reactive oxygen species and other agents that can reach the pleura or peritoneum). While this "remote" mode of action cannot be excluded from consideration, it seems counterintuitive given the peculiar specificity of the mesothelial outcomes of exposure. If a fiber physically contacting the tissue is not needed to produce mesothelioma, it is unclear why it is not observed for many other agents that can initiate an inflammatory process in the lungs. Most probably, the mesothelium is protected from distant impacts but would inflame if the source of damage is immediate or very close.

The process of the lymphatic transport of fibers to the pleura is not satisfactorily described (Donaldson et al., 2010; Kane et al., 2018). Gualtieri (2023) noted that "[w]hile there seems to be no doubt that fibers do translocate to the pleural cavity (a process called 'primary translocation'), the overall mechanism is still obscure." There are no quantitative models available to describe the probability of a fiber translocating to the pleura.

However, our hypothesis is that the fraction of inhaled fibers reaching the pleura should be proportional to the ratio of length to width in the third power, as in Equation 4.3,

$$\text{Ratio} \propto \text{length/Width}^3 \tag{4.3}$$

This hypothesis needs to be further tested; however, the following support can be provided for it.

Based on the preliminary data from the Cardiff lung deposition database (Korchevskiy et al., 2025), we can estimate the ratio between the frequency of a specific width category of fibers in the lungs (including all compartments) for patients with mesothelioma, and in the airborne TEM data from the overall database we created. The following size categories were used:

Width <0.15 µm; 0.15 µm ≤Width <0.250 µm; 0.250 µm ≤Width <0.375 µm; 0.375 µm ≤Width.

Length <1 µm; 1 µm ≤Length <2 µm; 2 µm ≤Length <3 µm; 3 µm ≤Length <4 µm; 4 µm ≤Length <5 µm; 5 µm ≤Length <8 µm; 8 µm ≤Length <10 µm; 10 µm ≤Length.

The following regression (Equation 4.4) can be found for the ratio of crocidolite in a specific width category deposited in the lungs of persons with pleural mesothelioma, as compared to airborne samples, assuming length/width ≥3:1, width >=0.05 µm, width ≤3 µm):

$$\text{Ratio} = 0.42 + 0.0008\text{xlength/Width}^3 \tag{4.4}$$

$$\left(R = 0.957,\ R^2 = 0.916,\ p < 0.000001\right).$$

The data for the derivation of Equation 4.4 can be found in Table 4.3.

We can assume that the ratio of the fraction of fibers in the lungs to environmental sample size fraction is predictive of the access to the pleura for various sizes of fibers.

TABLE 4.3
Frequency distribution of width for crocidolite fibers in the lungs of pleural mesothelioma patients and in the airborne TEM samples

		Frequency (%)		
Average length in the range, μm	Average width in the range, μm	Lungs of patients with pleural mesothelioma	Airborne samples	Ratio
0.50	0.1	0.76	13.11	0.06
1.50	0.1	10.71	17.20	0.62
2.50	0.1	12.62	4.20	3.00
3.50	0.1	6.12	4.28	1.43
4.50	0.1	8.99	2.80	3.21
6.50	0.1	13.77	2.15	6.40
9.00	0.1	4.97	0.78	6.37
20.00	0.1	7.65	0.48	15.94
0.50	0.2	0.00	2.08	0.00
1.50	0.2	3.63	8.41	0.43
2.50	0.2	3.44	3.73	0.92
3.50	0.2	6.31	4.45	1.42
4.50	0.2	3.44	2.95	1.17
6.50	0.2	4.59	3.39	1.35
9.00	0.2	2.10	1.30	1.62
20.00	0.2	4.97	0.93	5.34
0.50	0.312	0.00	0.05	0.00
1.50	0.312	0.38	1.27	0.30
2.50	0.312	0.96	0.98	0.98
3.50	0.312	0.19	3.03	0.06
4.50	0.312	0.76	3.27	0.23
6.50	0.312	0.76	3.36	0.23
9.00	0.312	0.38	2.19	0.17
20.00	0.312	1.15	1.43	0.80
1.50	0.8	0.19	0.06	3.17
2.50	0.8	0.00	0.67	0.00
3.50	0.8	0.00	2.11	0.00
4.50	0.8	0.19	1.41	0.13
6.50	0.8	0.19	3.97	0.05
9.00	0.8	0.19	2.18	0.09
20.00	0.8	0.57	1.79	0.32

Combining Equations 4.2 and 4.3, we may have a hypothetical estimation of the lifetime probability for elongate mineral particles to be retained in the lungs and reach pleural space at some point in time:

$$LPP \propto \text{Biopersistence x Length x Width /Width}^3 = \text{Biopersistence x Length/Width}^2,$$

where LPP is the lifetime probability of pleural transfer.

Table 4.4 contains the values of the estimation of the ratio for various types of airborne mineral fibers, considering the distribution of particle sizes for each mineral type.

MACROPHAGE FRUSTRATION, DISTRACTION, AND MEMBRANE PIERCING

Macrophages are the agents playing an important role in the protection of the organism from elongate mineral particles. It was also discussed in the toxicological literature that macrophages participate in the overall carcinogenic process when their activities would be disrupted by particles of specific shapes and sizes. Elongate mineral particles are just another type of dust; however, their size and shape make them a difficult substance to remove from the body if they penetrate the respiratory system deeply enough.

Macrophages encounter elongate mineral particles while in the tracheobronchial and pulmonary levels and may transport them to the pleura and outside of the respiratory system through the lymph system; at the pleural level, free particles can also be picked up by macrophages. Macrophages are able to expand, if needed, and engulf

TABLE 4.4
The average predicted fraction of fibers reaching the pleura during the lifetime

Mineral type, source	The predicted probability of lifetime pleural transfer (with a conditional coefficient of 0.000001)
Chrysotile, Quebec	0.0008
Amosite, South Africa	0.13
Crocidolite, South Africa	0.21
Anthophyllite, Finland	0.18
Libby amphiboles, Montana, U.S.A.	0.022
Erionite, Karain and Oregon, combined	0.36
Balangeroite, Italy	0.023
Tremolite, different locations	0.04

the fibers. It would seem that macrophages should be able to efficiently phagocytize the particles with a surface area less than their own surface. With the diameter of macrophages being about 25 μm in humans, the majority of elongate mineral particles should fit the size of macrophage surface area to be removed from the body (about 2,000 μm^2).

It should be noted that several macrophages can fuse to produce a giant cell formation if a single macrophage is not be able to engulf the foreign object (Jay et al., 2010), encasing the fiber and preventing translocation. It is also important that phagocytosis of various types of particles leads to the creation of a special structure inside the macrophage, called phagosome (a vesicle derived from the plasma membrane), that surrounds the foreign structure. The phagosome has different stages of development, including early formation and maturation (Rosales & Uribe-Querol, 2017).

However, it appears that the shape of elongate particles significantly affects the ability of macrophages to engulf and eliminate them, even if the surface area of the particles does not exceed the average surface area of macrophages. It is usually assumed that the process of engulfment for elongate particles may lead to "frustration," or incomplete encapsulation, causing cell damage and possible inflammation. If the fiber is not fully engulfed, the leakage of internal cell content to the extracellular space is possible; the gradient of potassium and calcium would change between the macrophage and the environment. In particular, frustrated phagocytosis may lead to lysosomal destabilization and subsequent leakage of cathepsin B (or other lytic proteases) into the cytosol (Honarpisheh et al., 2017). Qi et al. (2024) suggested that frustrated phagocytosis caused by long nanofibers triggers an intense ROS/RNS leakage.

However, it was concluded that macrophages have difficulty removing not only very long fibers but also fibers between 5 and 20 μm if they are thin, and for this reason, the meaning of frustrated phagocytosis has been questioned (Murphy et al., 2021). The work of Murphy et al. emphasized the need for a better definition of frustrated phagocytosis, beyond incomplete encapsulation.

For the purposes of this discussion, we define frustrated phagocytosis as

> *a complex event involving elongate particles when the immune system is unable to eliminate the particles from tissues because of size and shape of the structures. Frustrated phagocytosis can be manifested as (a) incomplete engulfing of particles in macrophages, (b) abnormal reaction of actin filament, (c) secretion of various harmful agents to cellular environment, (d) unprogrammed death of macrophages, (e) cascading inflammatory reaction, (f) and other processes involving macrophages and elongate particles, leading to adverse toxicological reactions.*

The prerequisites for the ability of fibers to produce macrophage frustration are

- long length
- small width
- sufficient rigidity.

For example, as a rule, amphibole EMPs are rigid enough to pierce cell membranes and cause macrophage frustration. However, long chrysotile fibrils and talc fibers are not sufficiently rigid and would bend when engulfed by macrophages rather than cause significant frustration. Also, the wider particles, although being rigid enough, would not produce a piercing effect because of their larger cross-section.

At the same time, macrophage frustration is not expected to be a factor for short particles (L < 2 μm) that can be easily phagocytized even without stretching the macrophages. It appears that short and very narrow particles (< 30 nm) should also not be sufficiently active to produce a piercing effect (Wang, F. et al., 2019).

The propensity of long, thin fibers to damage cell membranes of macrophages and other cells in the tissue was partially explained by Baranov et al. (2021), who noted that needle-like particles cause inflammasome activation, with larger particles being more active. The authors name ROS production and cathepsin B as drivers of inflammation from large aspect ratio particles, with mechanisms related to macrophage frustration and related leakage of ROS and lytic enzymes into the extracellular environment. Also, Baranov et al. (2022) demonstrated the ability of elongate objects (protruding parts of hexapod-shaped particles) to cause membrane damage during phagocytosis.

Recently, Gu et al. (2023) suggested that one of the mechanisms of carcinogenicity of elongate mineral particles may be in attracting significant populations of macrophages, which otherwise would be able to scavenge and remove the cells with initial mutations leading to future mesothelial malignancies.

We hypothesize that the combined effect of macrophage frustration and distraction, along with membrane piercing of the frustrated macrophages, can be expressed as a function of length, rigidity, and width as

$$\text{Length}^{C} \text{x RI}^{D} / \text{Width}^{E},$$

where RI is the rigidity index of fibers (see Chapter 7).

Specific values for C, D, and E will be suggested later.

CHEMICAL COMPOSITION AND SURFACE CHARGE

Mineral fibers produce their toxic effects not only by their size and shape but also by chemical composition and atomic structure, which control dissolution and surface properties.

In particular, the biosolubility of fibers can be related to their chemical composition.

For example, the following regression has statistical significance for the fiber-forming silicate minerals:

$$\text{Log}_{10}(\text{Biosolubility}) = 2.31 - 0.04\text{MgO},$$

where Biosolubility is the biosolubility in terms of acellular dissolution lifetime of fibers (years),

MgO denotes magnesium oxide content (wt. %), and

$$\left(R = 0.615, R^2 = 0.378, p < 0.0439\right).$$

The chemical composition of fibers obviously may have not only a protective function, but it may also play a role in toxicity when the particle is interfering with cells and tissue. In particular, the iron content of fibers was demonstrated to correlate with mesothelioma potency factors (Korchevskiy et al., 2019).

Specifically, iron "overload" was suggested to play an important role in asbestos fiber toxicity (Quinlan et al., 1994). Iron (Fe^{+2}) and magnesium readily substitute for one another stoichiometrically because they have the same charge and are similarly sized. Iron is a common component in amphiboles such as crocidolite and amosite, while in chrysotile, it is usually very minimal (Schwarz & Winer, 1971; De Waele et al., 1984). It was suggested that asbestos fibers are able to adsorb iron from the cellular environment, creating an iron-containing coating around the fibers, sometimes leading to the formation of asbestos bodies. Some view the iron coating as a step in the mechanism of toxicity while others believe the coating is protective (Gilmour et al., 1997; Jaurand, 1997; Xu et al., 1999).

The role of the two chemical forms of iron, Fe^{3+} and Fe^{2+}, in asbestos cancer development is not completely clear. Fe^{3+} was demonstrated to have a more pronounced effect on the reduction of human enzyme activity than Fe^{2+} (Karami et al., 2010). Fisher et al. (1998) emphasized the role of Fe^{3+} in fiber toxicity. Ghio et al. (1992) determined that the generation of hydroxyl radical by crocidolite asbestos is proportional to surface Fe^{3+}. Toyokuni (1996) emphasized that different compounds of Fe^{3+} are carcinogenic in animals. For example, intraperitoneal injections of ferric saccharate followed by administration of nitrilotriacetate (NTA) caused a high incidence of malignant mesotheliomas. Intraperitoneal injections of Fe-NTA can induce peritoneal mesotheliomas in rats as well (Toyokuni, 1996; Okada et al., 1989).

Some authors hypothesized that the toxicity of fibers depends not on the iron content in the chemical composition or on the surface per se, but rather on the "deficiency" of iron that fibers may create in the cell, attracting iron ions from elsewhere. Ghio et al. (2008) suggested that differences between serpentine and amphibole fibers in oxidative stress and biological effects do not reflect the inclusion of iron in the crystal lattice, but rather larger numbers of surface functional groups (first, silanol) in amphiboles which can mobilize iron from the host. It is possible that either or both iron in fibers and extracellular iron may play a mechanistic role in the carcinogenicity process.

In the process of quantitative structure-activity relationship (QSAR) modeling, it was shown that the mesothelioma potency of elongate particles is proportional to a combination of the fractions for chemical constituents:

$$\mathrm{IC} = \frac{SiO2^{2.12}\, Fe^{0.24}}{MgO^{1.60}},$$

where

IC is the index of chemical composition,

SiO2 is the fraction of SiO2 in the chemical composition of a fiber (weight %),

MgO is the fraction of MgO in the chemical composition of a fiber (weight %), and

Fe is the fraction of iron oxides in the chemical composition of a fiber (weight %) (Korchevskiy et al., 2024).

Table 4.5 contains the typical values of IC for various types of mineral fibers (for sources of data, see Korchevskiy et al., 2019).

The chemical composition of the elongate mineral particles, atomic structure, and their size determine the surface charge, which in turn can also be a factor of damage to biological systems. According to the Agency for Toxic Substances Disease Registry (ATSDR, 2023) – "Because of their surface charge, asbestos fibers can adsorb to cellular macromolecules (proteins, DNA, RNA) and cell surface proteins. Binding of asbestos fibers to these cellular components is believed to induce changes in macromolecular conformation, thereby affecting macromolecule function."

One of the measurable parameters for characterizing the surface charge of mineral fibers is the zeta potential, the electric potential of the solid in the liquid phase environment (e.g., in distilled water) produced in close proximity to the surface compared to the surrounding layers of the liquid. The reported zeta potential values of the standard UICC asbestos at pH 7.4 are +40.5 to +52.5 mV for chrysotile, −50.5 mV for crocidolite, −58.5 mV for amosite, −54.0 mV for anthophyllite; erionite also has a negative zeta potential (Pollastri et al., 2014).

TABLE 4.5
Index of chemical composition for various types of mineral fibers

Mineral type	Source	IC
Chrysotile	Quebec	7.61
Amosite	Transvaal, South Africa	545.8
Crocidolite	Cape Province, South Africa	1810.5
	Bolivia	170.3
	Australia	1179.0
Na-Ca amphiboles	Libby, Montana, U.S.A.	67.0
Anthophyllite	Russia	47.1
Balangeroite	Italy	10.35
Minnesotaite	Minnesota, U.S.A.	283.6
Erionite*	Turkey	15408.4

* Iron content in erionite fibers is very small. Some sources suggest that iron is absent in the composition of erionite fibers or present only as an impurity (Gualtieri et al., 2016). However, even with a small content of iron (1.5%, as quoted in Korchevskiy et al., 2019), erionite apparently has the highest IC among the considered mineral fibers (because of high silica and low magnesium content).

Pollastri suggested that decreasing the surface potential is deemed to be a defensive chemical response of the macrophage cells to minimize hemolytic damage. Negatively charged surfaces favor the binding of collagen and redox-activated Fe-rich proteins to form the so-called asbestos bodies and prompt the formation of HO·via the reaction with peroxide $(H_2O_2 + e- \rightarrow HO + HO-)$. An additional mechanism accounting for higher carcinogenicity is possibly related to the Ca^{2+} sequestration by the fibers with surface negative potential, impairing the mitochondrial apoptotic pathway. It was also found that with a negative zeta potential, the attractive forces prevailed over repulsions and favored processes such as agglomeration responsible for tumorigenic chronic inflammation. It is unclear if the same logic can be applied to chrysotile (with positive surface charge) as compared to more biologically active amphiboles (with negative surface charge).

Fröhlich (2012) noted that cationic nanoparticles (NPs) cause more pronounced disruption of plasma membrane integrity, stronger mitochondrial and lysosomal damage, and a higher number of autophagosomes than anionic NPs. In general, non-phagocytic cells ingest cationic NPs to a higher extent, but charge density and hydrophobicity are equally important; phagocytic cells preferentially take up anionic NPs. Cells do not use different uptake routes for cationic and anionic NPs, but high uptake rates are usually linked to greater biological effects.

Nolan et al. (1991) noted that at a physiological pH of 7.4, six tremolite asbestos specimens had an average zeta potential of -44.9 ± 10.4 mV while the two non-asbestos tremolites averaged -13.4 ± 0.1 mV. Surface charge heterogeneity has also been reported between amphibole cleavage fragments and their asbestos analogues due to differences in shape, not differences in surfaces themselves (Schiller et al., 1980).

In general, chemical composition and surface charge affect the toxicological potency of elongate mineral particles. However, they also correlate with the dimensions and biosolubility of fibers. If chemical composition or surface charge are primarily variables, it is hard to explain why materials as different in composition and surface charge as carbon nanotubes (C), erionite $(Mg_2Al_4Si_{14}O_{36}.15H_2O)$, tremolite-asbestos $(Ca_2Mg_5Si_8O_{22}(OH)_2$, and crocidolite $(Na_2Fe^{+2}{}_3Fe^{+3}{}_2Si_8O_{22}(OH)_2$ all induce mesothelioma in animals. Furthermore, there is a very high correlation between dimensions and carcinogenicity, consistent with the Stanton Hypothesis that is independent of chemistry. Despite these uncertainties in the exact role of surface chemical activity, it is hard to imagine that surface-cell interaction does not play a role in carcinogenicity, and in the overall model of toxicity, chemical constituents and surface charge should be considered along with other parameters, or separately, to avoid intercorrelation issues.

INFLAMMATION AND CYTOTOXICITY

Elongate mineral particles retained in the lungs and specifically in the pleural area are able to produce chronic inflammation and cytotoxicity.

For example, Wright et al. (1986) demonstrated the cytotoxicity of 13 fibrous samples in P388D1 cells, with chrysotile proving to be more cytotoxic than amphiboles. Matsuzaki et al. (2018) explored cytotoxicity caused by crocidolite asbestos fibers and the acquisition of resistance by continuous exposure in human T cells (exhibiting a reduction of antitumor immunity with time). Cytotoxicity of short-fiber chrysotile for human alveolar macrophages was studied by Yeager, Jr., et al. (1983). Studies were performed to compare the cytotoxicity for human alveolar macrophages of a naturally occurring short-fiber chrysotile asbestos (RG 144) to that of a standard reference mixed-fiber (long and short) chrysotile asbestos (UICC chrysotile A, Rhodesian). Parallel studies were also performed with quartz (Min-U-Sil 15), a known macrophage toxin. On a mass basis, and after 24-hour incubation, RG 144 was more cytotoxic than the UICC standard reference fiber and less toxic than quartz (silica). The cytotoxic potential of RG 144 chrysotile was further enhanced after size reduction by milling.

Hesterberg et al. (1987) studied mechanisms of cytotoxicity of crocidolite and chrysotile asbestos fibers in rat tracheal epithelial cells. The authors concluded that this potentially important pathway of fiber toxicity involved binding, phagocytosis, nuclear damage, disruption of mitosis, inhibition of proliferation, and/or cell death. Fiber dimensions and surface charge were named as factors defining the degree of toxicity. Goodglick and Kane (1990) explored cytotoxicity of long and short crocidolite fibers *in vitro* and *in vivo*. Both long and short crocidolite asbestos fibers were toxic to elicited macrophages *in vitro*. Similar to native crocidolite asbestos, long and short fibers stimulated the release of reactive oxygen metabolites from elicited macrophages *in vitro*. They evaluated whether *in vitro* cytotoxicity was dependent on the production of reactive oxygen metabolites. In the presence of the reactive oxygen metabolite scavenging enzymes superoxide dismutase or catalase, the toxicity of long and short crocidolite fibers to macrophages was prevented. Furthermore, macrophages were not killed when either long or short fibers were soaked in the iron chelator deferoxamine. Native, long, and short crocidolite fibers also caused depolarization of the mitochondrial membrane potential prior to cell death. *In vivo*, a single intraperitoneal injection of long crocidolite fibers stimulated an intense inflammatory reaction, release of reactive oxygen metabolites near sites of fiber deposition, and cell death. In contrast, these events were minimal after a single injection of short fibers due to the rapid removal of fibers from the peritoneal cavity. However, fibers were present on the surface of the mesothelium and provoked an inflammatory response after five daily injections of short fibers. *In vivo*, short fibers were cytotoxic when the clearance of these fibers was prevented. It should be noted that the cytotoxicity of short fibers is not expected to correspond with mesothelial cancer development. To the contrary, we assume that if short fibers were to cause cytotoxic effects in vivo, it would eliminate cells with damaged genetic material, not elevate the probability of cancer.

The most efficient predictor of the inflammatory and cytotoxic potential for elongate mineral particles is their surface area (Duffin et al., 2002). The fibrosis response also depends on the accumulated surface area of inhaled particles (Bonner, 2007). Timbrell (1965) demonstrated that the rate of asbestosis among miners exposed to different forms of asbestos can best be understood by surface area/fiber rather than fiber number.

A good illustration of this fact can be found in Donaldson et al. (1989), where the inflammatory potential of "long" amosite fibers was higher than the UICC amosite sample, which in turn was higher than the potential for "short" amosite fibers. We estimated the values of the corresponding median surface area of fibers as 13.6 μm^2 (long) 4.95 μm^2 (UICC), and 2.89 μm^2 (short), respectively. The Pearson correlation between surface area and inflammatory markers on the second day after peritoneal instillation of fibers in Donaldson's experiment was 0.92 (P=0.06), and the Spearman rank correlation was 1.0.

Also, specific surface area (area per unit of volume and mass) was demonstrated to play a role in pulmonary fibrosis, in particular the case of crystalline silica (Byrne & Baugh, 2008). For asbestos, however, surface area per fiber and specific surface area (per volume or mass) are negatively correlated, though the correlation is weak (see Korchevskiy & Wylie, 2022).

Another confirmation of surface area being a predictor of inflammation and cytotoxicity can be found in Nolan et al. (1991). Table 4.6 contains the values of HC50 estimated by Nolan in mg/ml, indicating the weight of various types of mineral fibers that produce a hemolytic effect in 50% of the cell culture; we supplemented the data from Nolan including the estimation of HC50 in units of

TABLE 4.6
HC50 and surface area of fibers

Mineral type, source	Habit: asbestiform (A), non-asbestiform (NA), or mixed (M)	HC50, mg/ml (average)	HC50, fibers x10^9/ml (average)	Surface area, average/fiber (fibers with length >5 μm, length/width ≥3, width ≥0.05 μm, width ≤3 μm (μm^2)
Tremolite, Metsovo, Greece	A	3.06	1.700	7.61
Tremolite, Korea	A	1.38	0.509	11.93
Na-Ca amphiboles, Libby, Montana, U.S.A.	M	2.07	0.218	23.08
Tremolite, Swansea, Wales	A	2.53	0.091	38.08
Tremolite, Jamestown	A	1.14	0.174	17.13
Tremolite, India	A	2.81	0.414	18.15
Tremolite, Gouvernour, New York, U.S.A.	NA	5.21	0.118	44.92
Crocidolite, South Africa	A	4.05	1.007	15.03
Amosite, Transvaal	A	1.76	0.185	32.5
Anthophyllite, Finland	A	3.76	0.464	22.23
Chrysotile, Quebec, Canada	A	0.08	0.006	22.07

fibers x 10^9 per ml, using the average estimation of fiber weight from our database. The higher level of HC50 corresponds to a lower level of cytotoxicity per fiber. Table 4.6 contains an average level of surface area for each type of mineral fiber, also derived from our database.

Based on the data from Table 4.6, HC50 in fibers per ml negatively correlates with surface area divided by length:

$$\text{HC50}\left(\text{x } 10^9\text{fibers/ml}\right) = 1.11 - 0.03 \text{ SA}\left(\mu\text{m}^2\right),$$

$$R = 0.66, R^2 = 0.43, p < 0.027.$$

While the relationship is not very strong, it is statistically significant, with the slope factor being negative and statistically significantly different from 0.

This means that the inflammogenicity and cytotoxicity of the fibers increase with increased surface area per fiber.

Elongate mineral particles as inflammatory agents are strongly cytotoxic (Yang et al., 2006; Matsuzaki et al., 2018). However, it should be noted that the cytotoxicity of fibers competes with their carcinogenic potential because cells with possible mutations can be eliminated by cytotoxic agents.

Henzi et al. (2009) noted that SV40-induced expression of calretinin protects mesothelial cells from asbestos cytotoxicity, contributing to mesothelioma pathogenesis.

Carbone et al. (2023) stated,

> When added to human mesothelial cells in tissue culture, asbestos is cytotoxic and the entire cell population is wiped out in a matter of a few days. This is because mesothelial cells attempt to phagocytize asbestos fibers and die in the process . . . . In these tissue culture experiments, it is often possible to see asbestos fibers "perforating" mesothelial cells, sometimes perforating the nuclei of these cells. Some of these cells may attempt to divide while showing asbestos fibers going through their nuclei. This led to the hypothesis that asbestos could cause cancer by mechanically causing genetic damage . . . . However, we have never seen primary human mesothelial cells exposed to asbestos alone survive. Indeed, transformed cell lines were never derived from such experiments.

It should be noted that the relationship between cytotoxicity and carcinogenicity is complex. For example, repeated injury was suggested as one of the mechanisms of cancer promotion, in particular because of the increased proliferation of cells surrounding the injured tissue (Kuraishy et al., 2011). Liver and skin cancers were mentioned in the context of the tumor relationship with cell death. It is known that cancer cells can resist cytotoxicity using various mechanisms (Tuomela et al., 2022).

Still, the direction of cytotoxicity (carcinogenic or anti-cancer) obviously depends on the specific types of injury and types of tissue (regular proliferation of mesothelial tissue is very slow). For example, Korchevskiy et al. (2024) noted that the cytotoxicity of asbestos fibers by mineral type negatively correlates with mesothelioma potency factors.

DIRECT VS. INDIRECT GENOTOXICITY

There are several hypotheses about the carcinogenicity of elongate mineral particles and the role of genotoxicity in this process. Genotoxicity involves damage to DNA that transforms cells from a benign to malignant state. Normal repair mechanisms should return DNA to a normal state. Also, apoptosis (controlled death) removes abnormal cells if their DNA cannot be repaired. There are also mechanisms to prevent enhanced mitotic activity that promotes carcinogenesis. Failure of any of the repair processes can cause tumorigenesis.

Other (non-genotoxic) pathways of carcinogenicity also exist. They include promoters of mitosis and inhibitors of apoptosis (Klaassen & Watkins, 2010). Genotoxic carcinogens can be considered primary (direct or indirect) or secondary. The distinction between direct and indirect genotoxic agents is very important for the characterization of carcinogenicity for elongate mineral particles.

Barabadi et al. (2019) stated that

> [N]anogenotoxicity can be classified as primary or secondary. Primary NP [nanoparticles]-induced genotoxicity can be attributed to the direct or indirect interaction of NPs with genetic material. During direct primary genotoxicity, NPs directly interact with chromosomes during interphase and may bind with DNA molecules and prevent DNA replication or transcription. In addition, NPs could interact with chromosomes during mitosis, causing chromosomal breakage (clastogenic effect) or loss (aneugenic effect) mechanically or by chemical binding. During indirect primary genotoxicity, NP-mediated ROS generation and the release of toxic ions from soluble NPs are indirect interactions that can interfere with proteins essential for DNA replication, transcription, or repair as well as the mitotic spindle apparatus, centrioles or their associated proteins; these interactions can inactivate the proteins by structural modifications.

Moreover, the secondary genotoxicity mechanism of NPs is attributed to the excessive generation of ROS by activated phagocytes, including neutrophils and macrophages, through a chronic *in vivo* inflammatory response.

Given what is known today, it appears that elongate mineral particles are indirect primary or secondary genotoxic agents, and their genotoxicity is caused by intermediate reactions, like inflammation and the production of reactive oxygen species. For example, Xu et al. (2002) demonstrated evidence that the mutagenicity of asbestos is mediated by reactive oxygen species. The World Health Organization (WHO, 1986) concluded that the UICC reference samples of asbestos do not show mutagenic activities in bacterial assays. Shukla et al. (2003) showed that DNA damage by asbestos was preceded by oxidant stress.

We assume that the probability of indirect genotoxicity for elongate particles in mesothelioma depends on the length and width of particles:

$$GT \propto \text{Length}^{F}\text{Width}^{G},$$

where GT is the probability of indirect genotoxic event and

I, J are constants.

SUPPRESSION OF CELL DEATH AS A POSSIBLE KEY EVENT IN EMP CARCINOGENESIS

As noted previously, one key to understanding mesothelial carcinogenesis may be related to the prevention of cell death. Asbestos is a strong cytotoxic agent that brings in inflammatory processes and general activation of the immune system and apoptosis, the benign pathway for elimination of damaged cells, which may carry mutated genetic material. However, if elongate mineral particles are as cytotoxic to mesothelial cells as they are able to prevent cell death pathways, it might be consequential for carcinogenesis. The most dangerous EMPs, therefore, should be those that cause inflammation proportionally to cell immortalization.

One of the most important mutations tied to mesothelioma development is a deletion of BAP1; as a result of this mutation, cell death is significantly suppressed. According to Kuroda (2021), the following chain of events can be suggested, which can explain "the paradox of asbestos carcinogenicity." First, the phagocytosed asbestos in macrophages and mesothelial cells in the pleura may cause a mutagenic microenvironment due to frustrated phagocytosis reactions, enhancing mutations in mesothelial cells. Then, BAP1-mutated mesothelial cells may escape cell death and accumulate further DNA damage.

Recently, it was suggested that High Mobility Group Box 1 (HMGB-1) proteins are closely involved in mesothelioma development (Wang, Y. et al., 2019). The secretion of acetylated HMGB-1 from the nucleus to the intra- and extracellular environment was detected in patients with asbestos exposure, and also with pleural mesothelioma. The plasma level of HMGB-1 was found to be highly predictive in distinguishing between animals exposed to non-mesotheliomagenic particles vs. highly asbestiform fibers (Xue et al., 2020). Also, groups of mesothelioma patients, individuals exposed to amphibole asbestos (insulators), and general populations can be determined based on the level of acetylated HMGB-1 secretion (Napolitano et al., 2016). The short-term exposure of cells to amphibole asbestos caused HMGB-1 secretion, while only persistent chronic exposure could lead to this type of secretion of HMGB-1 by chrysotile asbestos (Qi et al., 2013). The sample of palygorskite fibers (with substantial iron content, but shorter than 5 μm) did not cause elevated HMGB-1 secretion, nor mesothelioma production in experimental animals (Larson et al., 2016). The secretion of HMGB-1 because of asbestos exposure was apparently noted in pleural macrophages and mesothelial cells as well (Suarez et al., 2023).

The mechanism of the induction of malignant mesothelioma in EMP exposure through elevated HMGB-1 can be explained by the fact that this protein group can promote so-called autophagy, or a process of immortalization for cells with mutations (Xue et al., 2020). In this case, inflammation caused by elongate particles creates a so-called field effect when initial mutations originate (Carbone et al., 2023).

Zolondick et al. (2021) reviewed HMGB-1 and stated,

> A recent study . . . identified a key mechanism by which HMGB1 favors mesothelioma development. It was found that asbestos induces HMGB1 translocation from the nucleus to the cytoplasm, which leads to the activation of autophagy in HM [human mesothelial cells]. It was also shown previously that asbestos exposure causes DNA

> damage, such as double-strand breaks . . ., which are associated with the loss of nuclear HMGB1. Therefore, following asbestos exposure, increased cytoplasmic HMGB1 induces autophagy, which allows the cells to escape cell death despite DNA damage . . . . In contrast, when HM were silenced for HMGB1, autophagy activation was reduced and HMGB1-silenced HM exhibited increased cell death by apoptosis and necrosis upon asbestos exposure.

While immortalization may not be a necessary step for carcinogenesis, it appears as one of the possible mechanisms to reduce the cytotoxicity of asbestos at a high level of chronic inflammation. We see "immortalization" as a general name for a wider class of processes where cytotoxicity is limited by the same factor that caused it. This process seems to be highly specific for elongate mineral particles and substantially different from other strongly inflammatory agents that apparently do not produce mesothelioma in humans.

Under normal conditions, mesothelial or immune cells with mutations would perish in significant fractions because of the direct cytotoxicity of the immediate cell environment and/or by macrophage intervention. However, HMGB-1 apparently changes the process by promoting cell immortalization and downregulating the immune response. This mechanism in mesothelial tissue appears to be specific to the combination of two factors: chronic inflammation and the HMGB-1-related autophagy process.

How EMP exposure causes a very specific type of HMGB-1 secretion from the nucleus is not fully clarified. However, it can be hypothesized that long, thin fibers, most involved in frustrated phagocytosis, can create a possible "bridge" between the intra- and extracellular environment, causing the nuclear membrane to be irritated, leading to acetylation and secretion of HMGB-1, which would then be transported out of the cell. It is also possible that the higher concentrations of HMGB-1 in the extracellular environment cause further stimulation of the cells to produce more of this type of protein before saturation is reached. It is also possible that this happens when fibers pierce the nuclear membrane.

While HMGB-1 secretion can be caused by numerous factors in various types of cells (in particular, silica exposure and viruses can be implicated as well) (Chen et al., 2022), elongate mineral particles seem to have an unusually high potential for stimulating this process in pleural macrophages. We can hypothesize that some evolutionary mechanisms could precede the model of action that we observe now. Just theoretically, some prehistorical biological objects could have an elongate shape resembling asbestos fibers. The induced secretion of HMGB-1 could exist as a factor of advantage rather than hazard, and it could have been historically caused by unknown elongate structures. The existence of this long, thin organic "proto asbestos" (the size of which would not be that different from bacterial flagella) can be imagined but needs to be further explored.

It is also known that asbestos stimulates other pathways of apoptosis inhibition and cell immortalization. Yang et al. (2006) demonstrated that treatment of human mesothelial (HM) cells with TNF-α significantly reduced asbestos cytotoxicity. TNF-α signaling, induced by asbestos exposure, increases the percentage of HM cells that survive asbestos exposure, thus increasing the pool of asbestos-damaged HM that are susceptible to malignant transformation.

It is important to note that asbestos is not only inflammogenic but also immunosuppressive. Based on Nishimura et al. (2020), asbestos exposure of cell cultures resulted in decreased natural and acquired cytotoxicity exerted by NK cells and CTLs, and reduced ability of Th1 cells to activate and support antitumor immunity. In contrast, asbestos exposure augmented Treg cell function and the generation of fibrogenic/suppressive macrophages. Mesothelioma patients also showed similar characteristics in certain alterations caused by asbestos exposure.

We hypothesize that the probability of a mutation, caused by inflammatory mechanisms, and consequent suppression of cytotoxicity caused by elongate mineral particles, can be size-dependent and approximated as being a function of the length and width of fibers:

$$IM \propto Length^I/Width^J,$$

where IM is the probability of immortalization and
I, J are constants.

Further studies are needed to understand the role of the immune system in the process of mesothelial carcinogenicity. Macrophages seem to be one of the drivers of chronic inflammation in pleural tissue. However, the direct impact of asbestos fibers on mesothelial cells can also be considered a stimulus for cytotoxicity and potential cancer, even if no specific macrophage-related events were involved. It seems that we deal with two possible processes (macrophage-involving vs. not-involving) that can manifest in mesothelioma. In both cases, we deal with cytotoxicity and malignant cell transformation that would be supplemented with counteraction of immune suppression necessary for abnormal cell proliferation. The future will show which of the processes can be determined as prevailing, and in what proportion.

GENERAL QUANTITATIVE MODEL OF MESOTHELIAL CARCINOGENESIS

While there can be various interpretations of a certain order of events in asbestos mesothelial carcinogenicity, it is reasonable to assume that they can be seen as shown in Figure 4.1.

Each of the stages of the carcinogenic process can be quantitatively assessed by assigning a level of probability as a function of various factors. We can empirically conclude that the following relationships may exist for the probabilities of each of the events (see the sections of this chapter above) in terms of measurable properties:

$$\text{Pulmonary deposition, retention, and pleural transfer} \sim \text{BiopersistencexLength/Width}^2,$$

$$\text{Macrophage frustration and/or mesothelial cell damage} \sim \text{Length}^C \text{ x } \text{RI}^D/\text{Width}^E,$$

$$\text{Induction of inflammation/cytotoxicity} \sim \text{Surface Area},$$

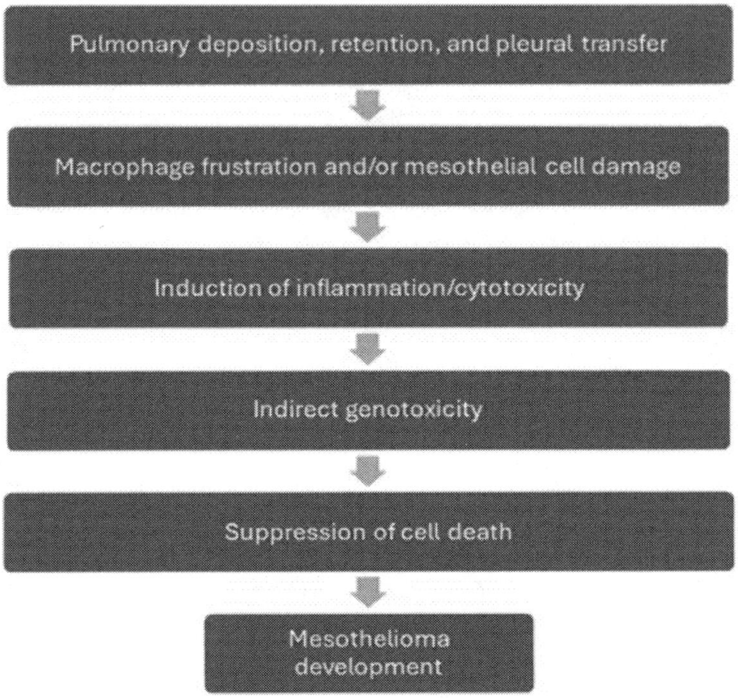

FIGURE 4.1 Mode of action of EMPs in mesothelioma development

$$\text{Indirect genotoxicity} \sim \text{Length}^{F}/\text{Width}^{G}, \text{ and}$$

$$\text{Suppression of cell death} \sim \text{Length}^{I}/\text{Width}^{J}.$$

In a wider mathematical interpretation, the relationships with width of fibers in these probability estimations are most probably more complex, as demonstrated in Table 4.7.

We can therefore propose a dimensionality-specific metric of mesothelial carcinogenicity for EMPs, proportional to the product of the probabilities of each of the stages of carcinogenesis, with some coefficients that can be found empirically to scale the values as a probability (from 0 to 1).

While the coefficients for the formulas in Table 4.7 are generally unknown, we can empirically suggest some combinations of the parameters to derive various empirical estimations of cancer risk and then check if the results are (a) reasonable from a toxicological perspective, b) confirmed by biological tests, and (c) in correlation with observed epidemiological data.

The probability of cancer caused by elongate particles can be expressed in this case as a product of the expressions in Table 4.7. We utilized the formula for the rigidity index as described in Chapter 7 of this book, considering that

$$\text{RI} \propto \frac{Width^{4}}{Length^{2}}.$$

TABLE 4.7
Stages of mesothelial carcinogenesis

Stage of the mesothelioma development	Probability proportion
Pulmonary deposition, retention, and pleural transfer	Biopersistence/Width^2
Induction of inflammation/cytotoxicity	Surface Area
Macrophage frustration and/or mesothelial cell damage	Length^C x RI^D/Width^E
Indirect genotoxicity	Length^F/Width^G
Suppression of cell death	Length^{I}Width^J

For example, if we assume the combination of parameters C=1/3, D=1, E=5/3, F=1/3, G=5/3, I=1/3, and J=5/3, the probability of a mesothelial cancer event can be considered to be proportional to

$$\frac{Length}{Width^3}\times BS\times Width\times SA\times\frac{Length^{1/3}}{Width^{5/3}}\times\frac{Width^4}{Length^2}\times\frac{Length^{1/3}}{Width^{5/3}}\times\frac{Length^{1/3}}{Width^{5/3}}=BS\times\frac{SA}{Width^3}.$$

This logic can serve as an explanation of the earlier proposed empirical metric for the dimensional component of mesothelial carcinogenicity of fibers. Korchevskiy and Wylie (2025a) demonstrated that the following formula can be used to estimate the potential of dimensional-based mesothelial carcinogenicity:

$$\text{DCC} = 1\text{-exp}\left(\text{-}0.11\text{*SA}/\left(1000\ \text{Width}^3+1\right)\right),$$

where DCC is the dimensional coefficient of mesothelial carcinogenicity.

As is seen from the formula, DCC is affected by two major factors that increase carcinogenic potential:

(a) fibers should have a significant surface area to promote chronic inflammation and create the "field effect" of cancer initiation, and
(b) fibers should have a low width and be transferred to the pleura to cause macrophage frustration and/or alteration of mesothelial cells, and to produce acetylated HMGB-1 proteins, promoting autophagy and immortalization of the cell (cancer promotion).

We demonstrated that DCC can serve as an empirical metric for the carcinogenicity of both elongate mineral particles and carbon nanotubes (Korchevskiy & Wylie, 2025a, 2025b). Figure 4.2 demonstrates the relationship between the proposed dimensional coefficient of carcinogenicity and the width of particles, including mineral fibers and carbon nanotubes.

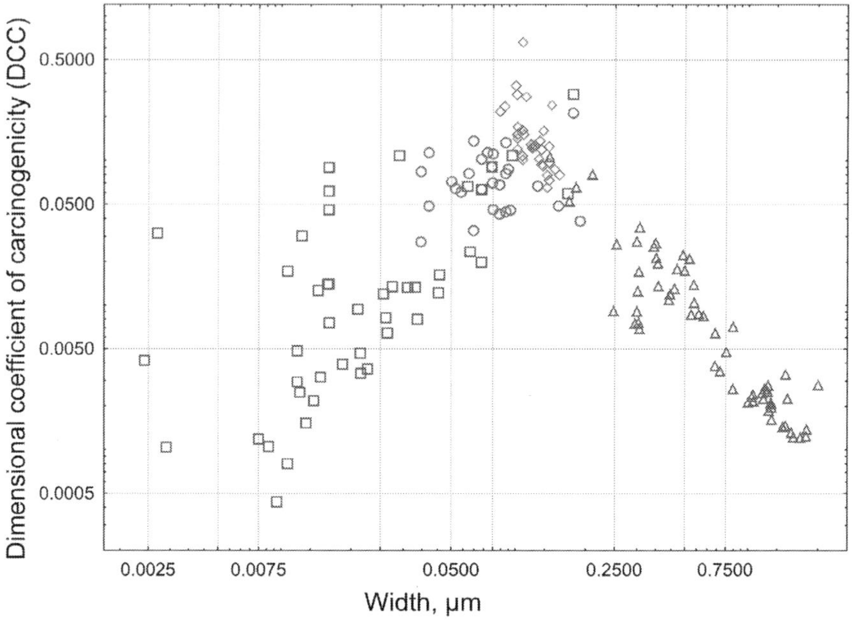

FIGURE 4.2 The relationship between the proposed dimensional coefficient of carcinogenicity and the width of EMPs, including mineral fibers and carbon nanotubes. Magenta circles denote mesotheliomagenic CNTs; blue squares denote CNTs with no reported mesothelioma, lung cancer, or fibrosis; red rhombuses denote mesotheliomagenic EMPs (EMPA)[1] (including EMPs longer than 5 μm and thinner than 0.15 μm); and green triangles denote non-mesotheliomagenic EMPs (including EMPs shorter than 5 μm, and EMPs longer than 5 μm and thicker than 0.15 μm).

As can be seen in Figure 4.2, despite all uncertainties, the probability of carcinogenicity increases with width up to a certain point (about 0.15 μm) and then decreases with increasing width. The majority of EMPs not belonging to the EMPA class and "no effect" CNTs have a probability of less than 0.05. It should be noted that the dimensional coefficient reflects only one aspect of carcinogenicity (dimensions), while leaving aside the biosolubility persistence that should be included in the consideration. More exactly, even if the DCC is lower than 0.05, a true mesotheliomagenic potential can still exist for these fibers because of biopersistence. However, it was suggested that no mesotheliomagenic particles are expected to have DCC <0.01 (Korchevskiy & Wylie, 2025a, 2025b).

Figure 4.3 shows the distribution of the dimensional coefficient of carcinogenicity in so-called criteria (asbestiform, as defined in Chapter 9) and "non-criteria" particles in the EMP database (length >5 μm, length/width ≥3:1, width ≥0.05 μm, width ≤3 μm), related to the aerodynamic diameter of EMPs. As can be seen, all non-criteria particles have DCC below the level of statistical significance.

Figure 4.4 shows the distribution of dimensional coefficient of carcinogenicity in short and long particles in our database (length/width ≥3:1, width ≥0.05 μm, width ≤3 μm) as related to the width of EMPs.

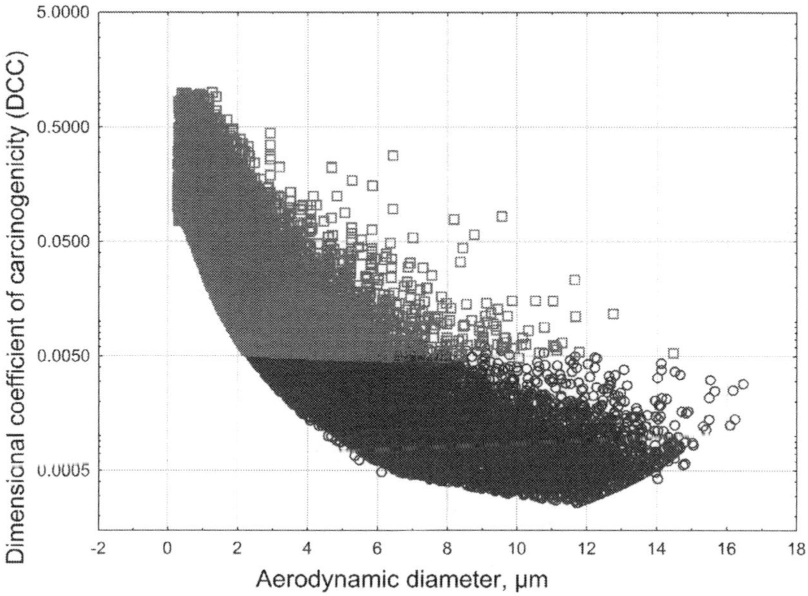

FIGURE 4.3 Relationship between the dimensional coefficient of carcinogenicity and aerodynamic diameter of particles. Blue circles denote non-asbestiform particles and red squares denote asbestiform particles.

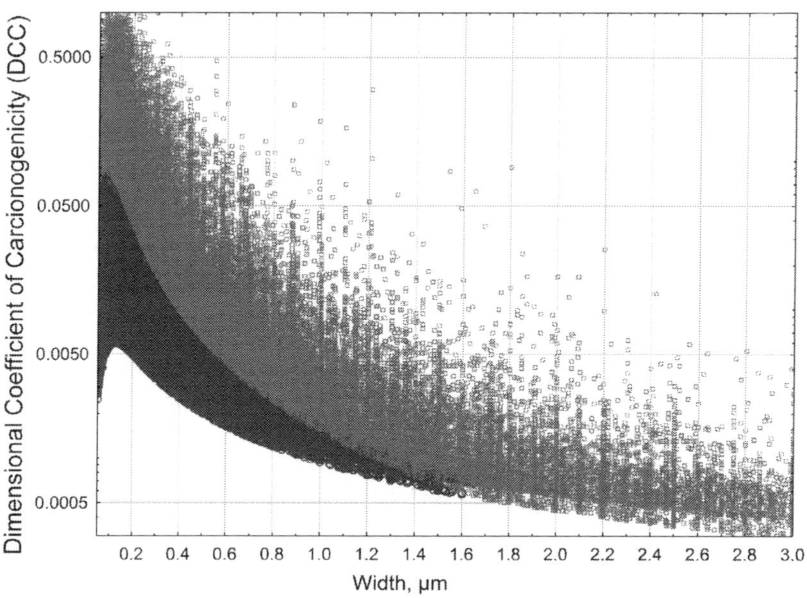

FIGURE 4.4 Relationship between the dimensional coefficient of carcinogenicity and width of particles. Blue circles – particles with length shorter than or equal to 5 µm, red dots – particles longer than 5 µm.

Only 2.3% of particles shorter than 5 μm have DCC higher than 0.05 (apparently within the margin of statistical error), while for particles longer than 5 μm, this fraction is 26.5%.

Table 4.8 contains estimations of biopersistence and DCC for various types of EMPs, along with their mesothelioma carcinogenic potency (R_M, %). Only particles longer than 5 μm were included in the calculations.

From here, the following regression equation can be found:

$$\text{Log}_{10}\left(R_M\right) = -0.13 + 2.03\ \text{Log}_{10}\left(\text{DCC}\right) + 1.11\text{Log}\left(\text{Biopersistence}\right),$$
$$\left(R = 0.94,\ R^2 = 0.89,\ p < 0.00137\right), \text{ and}$$

(length >5 μm, length/width ≥3:1, width ≥0.05 μm, width <3 μm).
Figure 4.5 demonstrates the relationship between predicted and published mesothelioma potency based on DCC and biopersistence.

This model would predict chrysotile mesothelioma potency of 0.0011% (published value 0.0014%), crocidolite potency of 0.79% (published value 0.52%), and fibrous talc potency of 0.00008% (most probably lower than the level of statistical significance). The estimation of erionite potency would be 1.2%, less than it was estimated earlier, but this could possibly be caused by other factors impacting the toxicity of erionite fibers from Turkey and other regions (Stevens et al., 2024). In particular,

TABLE 4.8
Biopersistence and dimensional coefficient of carcinogenicity (EMPs) for various types of fibers.

Mineral type	R_M, %	Average DCC (EMPs with length >5 μm, length/width ≥3:1, width ≥0.05 μm, width <3 μm)	Biopersistence (reversed biosolubility) (in terms of Gualtieri fiber dissolution lifetime, years)
Chrysotile	0.0014*	0.08	0.3
Amosite	0.11*	0.064	74
Crocidolite	0.52*	0.093	66
Anthophyllite	0.056**	0.02	245
Glaucophane	0.0085**	0.013	40
Libby amphiboles	0.03*	0.019	49
Fluoro-edenite	0.12**	0.034	140
Erionite	4.5**	0.065	181
Balangeroite	0.045***	0.03	55.6

* Darnton, 2024
** Korchevskiy et al., 2019
*** Korchevskiy & Wylie, 2023:

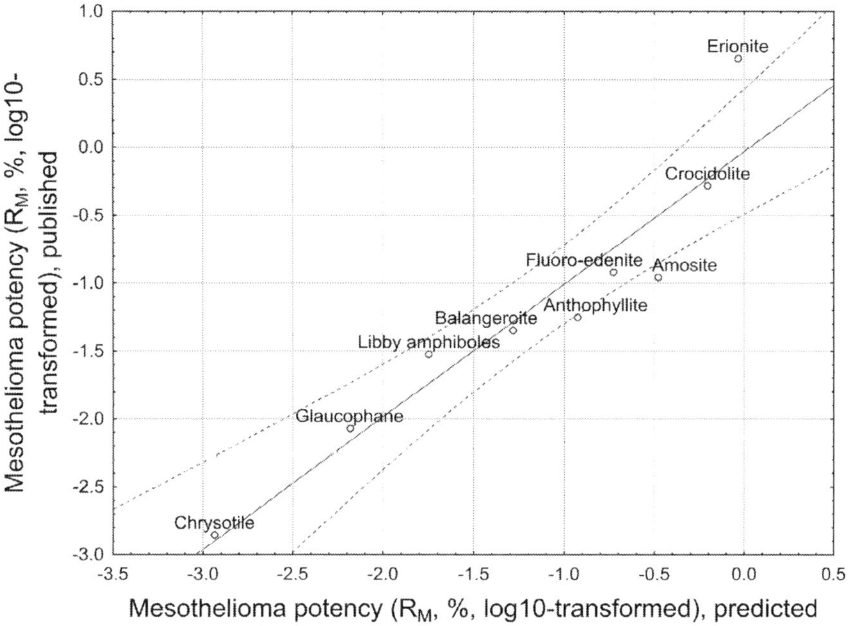

FIGURE 4.5 Published and predicted mesothelioma potency.

genetic factors were implicated in the toxicity of Turkey erionite (Carbone & Testa, 2001). It should be noted, however, that a hypothesis of increased genetic susceptibility in Turkish populations exposed to erionite was criticized as not supported by the data (Saracci & Simonato, 2001; Metintas et al., 2010).

Another model can be proposed that would include a parameter of Biopersistence x Width/0.25 as better accounting for slower biodissolution of thick particles:

$$\text{Log}_{10}\left(\text{R}_\text{M}\right) = -0.36 + 2.07\ \text{Log}_{10}\left(\text{DCC}\right) + 1.04\ \text{Log}_{10}\ (\text{Biopersistence x Width}/0.25),$$

$$\left(\text{R} = 0.93,\ \text{R}^2 = 0.85,\ \text{p} < 0.003\right),\ \text{and}$$

(length >5 μm, length/width ≥3:1, width ≥0.05 μm, width <3 μm).

In this case, the model fully characterizes the long-term persistence of fibers in mesothelial tissue as a function of biosolubility for fibers with width of 0.25 μm, and the actual width of fibers (the thicker fibers will dissolve more slowly).

We can also include the chemical composition index (IC), as described above, for modeling of the potency factor.

The following regression equation was determined:

$$\text{Log}_{10}\left(\text{R}_\text{M}\right) = -2.38 + 0.49\ \text{Log}_{10}\left(\text{IC}\right) + 0.75\ \text{Log}_{10}\left(\text{DCC}\right) + 0.64\,\text{Log}\left(\text{Biopersistence x Width}\right.$$

where IC is the index of chemical composition,
DCC is the dimensional coefficient of carcinogenicity,

Biopersistence (reversed biosolubility) denotes biopersistence by Gualtieri et al. (2018) method,

$$\left(R = 0.97, R^2 = 0.95, p < 0.0011\right), \text{ and}$$

(length >5 μm, length/width ≥3:1, width ≥0.05 μm, width <3 μm).

THRESHOLD LEVEL OF MAJOR CHARACTERISTICS

The proposed general model of carcinogenesis provides opportunities to estimate the limits of various parameters determining the carcinogenic potential of elongate mineral particles.

The following statements can be supported based on the studies reviewed and generalized in this chapter:

1. Particles with a rigidity index less than 0.05 are not mesothelial carcinogens.
2. Elongate mineral particles with a length less than 5 μm are not mesothelial carcinogens.
3. Elongate mineral particles with length >5 μm and width ≤0.15 μm are potential mesothelial carcinogens if they have low biosolubility and sufficient rigidity.

It should be noted that some scientists suggested earlier that not only long, thin fibers are responsible for mesothelioma development, but also short, thin ones. In particular, Suzuki et al. (2005) analyzed the pathology materials of 168 mesothelioma cases and determined that the majority of chrysotile fibers in the lung and mesothelial tissue were shorter than 5 μm. The authors concluded that short chrysotile fibers should be the major contributor to mesothelioma development. Similar reasoning was used by Suzuki and Yuen (2002). Schneider et al. (2023), based on the TEM analysis of lung pathology in 44 malignant mesothelioma cases, 28 cases of asbestosis, and 105 cases of lung cancer, confirmed that chrysotile has lower biopersistence than amphibole fibers; the authors also selected fibers longer than 5 μm, with a width diameter of less than 3 μm, and an aspect ratio not lower than 3:1 as "especially relevant for carcinogenicity and fibrogenicity."

Suzuki et al. correctly identified thin chrysotile fibers as being easily translocated to the pleura; chrysotile fibrils are one of the thinnest types of asbestos fibers. Based on the theory outlined in this chapter, the transfer of inhaled fibers to the pleura is determined by reciprocal width. However, the presence of a specific type of elongate particles in the pleura does not mean that the fibers will contribute to mesothelioma development. Chrysotile has a low biopersistence, which means that it will be efficiently cleared, and also that the clearance of short chrysotile is not expected to cause macrophage frustration (in a wider understanding of this term, as we used in this analysis) or mesothelial cell damage sufficient to produce a sufficient secretion of HMGB-1 proteins or other factors preventing tumor cell scavenging and death. Leinardi et al.

(2023) recently determined that short and long amosite fibers produce different signaling cascades in murine macrophages. The internalization of short fibers resulted in pyroptotic-related immunogenic cell death (ICD) characterized by the release of the pro-inflammatory damage signal (DAMP) IL-1α after inflammasome activation and gasdermin D (GSDMD)-pore formation. In contrast, macrophage responses to non-internalizable long fibers were associated with tumor necrosis factor alpha (TNF-α) release, caspase-3 and -7 activation, and apoptosis. The short fibers' effects exclusively resulted from Toll-like receptor 4 (TLR4), a pattern recognition receptor (PRR) recognized for its ability to sense particles, while the response to long fibers was elicited by a multifactorial ignition system involving the macrophage receptor with collagenous structure (SR-A6 or MARCO), reactive oxygen species (ROS) cascade, and TLR4. These results can be interpreted to mean that the tissue does not recognize short asbestos fibers in the same way as long ones; most probably, the reaction to short fibers is actually a reaction to dust, while longer fibers obviously belong to the EMP category with different risk mechanisms. In general, we believe that the scientific data provide an accurate assessment, with a length of 5 μm being an empirical threshold for mesothelioma-related fibers, along with a width cutpoint of about 0.15 μm.

Also, it is remarkable that DCC can be used to define the best fractional characteristic of the fiber's width that is reflective of mesothelial carcinogenesis.

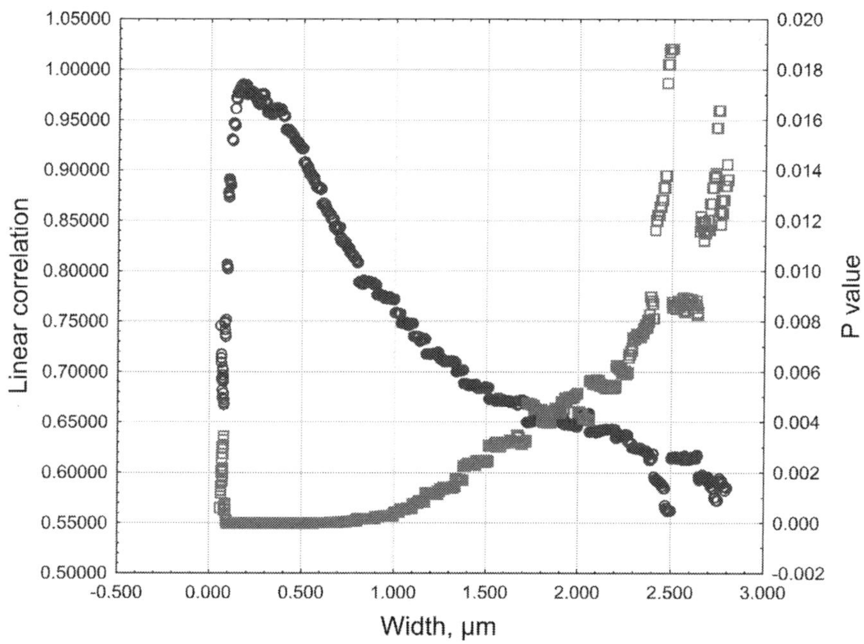

FIGURE 4.6 Correlation (blue circles) and P values (red squares) of the average DCC value and the fraction of fibers less than a specific width cut-off (the grouping is performed by mineral types, including chrysotile, asbestiform and non-asbestiform riebeckite, asbestiform and non-asbestiform cummingtonite-grunerite, asbestiform and non-asbestiform fluoro-edenite, Libby amphiboles, glaucophane, balangeroite, and erionite).

Figure 4.6 demonstrates the correlation between various fractional parameters (fraction of fibers longer than 5 μm that have width less than a specific cutpoint) with the DCC.

Also, for all cohorts in our database, the average DCC for fibers shorter than 5 μm is 0.013, and the minimum and maximum are 0.0019 and 0.035, respectively.

The average DCC value for non-EMPA particles longer than 5 μm is 0.019; minimum value is 0.0011 and the maximum 0.116; only 6% of non-EMPA datapoints have a DCC higher than 0.05.

METHODOLOGICAL NOTES

The surface area of each of the particles was estimated for non-serpentine particles as

$$\text{Surface Area} = 2LW + 2LT + 2WT,$$

where L denotes length, W denotes width, and T denotes thickness,

and for serpentine as

$$\text{Surface Area} = 0.5\pi W^2 + \pi WL.$$

The thickness of particles (T) was determined by the following empirical algorithm:

for erionite, $T = W$,

for balangeroite, $T = W/1.1$,

for fibrous talc $T = W/3$,

for asbestiform and mixed amphiboles, $\log_{10}(T) = 0.692\log_{10}(W) - 0.493$, and

for other non-serpentine EMPs, $T = W/1.9$.

The aerodynamic diameter (AD) of each particle was calculated by a formula derived by Timbrell (1965):

$$AD = 66W\ (AR/(2 + 4\ AR))^{2.2} \text{ x } (\rho p/\rho_0)^{0.5},$$

where AD denotes aerodynamic diameter, W denotes measured width of the EMP, AR denotes length/width, ρp is the density in gm/cm^3, and ρ0 is 1.0 gm/cm^3. The density of minerals is provided as basic information in descriptive mineral texts. The influence of small density variations (second decimal place) on AD is minor, so the use of literature values for mineral compositions is reasonable even if the exact composition can only be approximated from a qualitative chemical analysis or precise determination of the indices of refraction.

NOTE

1 EMPA (L > 5 μm W ≤ 0.015 μm) is referred to as mesotheliomagenic based on its ubiquity in exposures associated with elevated mesothelioma, and the fact that its abundance correlates significantly with the relative potency of the exposure as a whole (Wylie et al., 2020). For the purposes of this discussion, all other mineral particle populations are referred to as nonmesotheliomagenic, recognizing that neither length nor width at a single point is likely to separate carcinogenic from non-carcinogenic fibers.

REFERENCE LIST

Agency for Toxic Substances Disease Registry (ATSDR). (2023). *Asbestos toxicity: How does asbestos induce pathogenic changes?* Retrieved July 9, 2024, from www.atsdr.cdc.gov

Asgharian, B., Owen, T. P., Kuempel, E. D., & Jarabek, A. M. (2018). Dosimetry of inhaled elongate mineral particles in the respiratory tract: The impact of shape factor. *Toxicology and Applied Pharmacology*, *361*, 27–35. https://doi.org/10.1016/j.taap.2018.05.001

Barabadi, H., Najafi, M., Samadian, H., Azarnezhad, A., Vahidi, H., Mahjoub, M. A., Koohiyan, M., & Ahmadi, A. (2019). A systematic review of the genotoxicity and antigenotoxicity of biologically synthesized metallic nanomaterials: Are green nanoparticles safe enough for clinical marketing? *Medicina (Kaunas)*, *55*(8), 439. https://doi.org/10.3390/medicina55080439

Baranov, M. V., Ioannidis, M., Balahsioui, S., Boersma, A., de Boer, R., Kumar, M., Niwa, M., Hirayama, T., Zhou, Q., Hopkins, T. M., Grijpstra, P., Thutupalli, S., Sacanna, S., & van den Bogaart, G. (2022). Irregular particle morphology and membrane rupture facilitate ion gradients in the lumen of phagosomes. *Biophysical Reports, 2*(3), 100069. https://doi.org/10.1016/j.bpr.2022.100069

Baranov, M. V., Kumar, M., Sacanna, S., Thutupalli, S., & van den Bogaart, G. (2021). Modulation of immune responses by particle size and shape. *Frontiers in Immunology, 12*(1), 607945. https://doi.org/10.3389/fimmu.2020.607945

Bernstein, D. M., & Hoskins, J. A. (2006). The health effects of chrysotile: Current perspective based upon recent data. *Regulatory Toxicology and Pharmacology*, *45*, 252–264. https://doi.org/10.1016/j.yrtph.2006.04.008

Berry, G., Reid, A., Aboagye-Sarfo, P., de Klerk, N. H., Olsen, N. J., Merler, E., Franklin, P., & Musk, A. W. (2012). Malignant mesotheliomas in former miners and millers of crocidolite at Wittenoom (Western Australia) after more than 50 years follow-up. *British Journal of Cancer, 106*, 1016–1020. https://doi.org/10.1038/bjc.2012.23

Bonner, J. C. (2007). Lung fibrotic responses to particle exposure. *Toxicologic Pathology*, *35*(1), 148–153. https://doi.org/10.1080/01926230601060009

Byrne, J. D., & Baugh, J. A. (2008). The significance of nanoparticles in particle-induced pulmonary fibrosis. *McGill Journal of Medicine, 11*(1), 43–50. PMID: 18523535.

Carbone, M., Minaai, M., Takinishi, Y., Pagano, I., & Yang, H. (2023). Preventive and therapeutic opportunities: Targeting BAP1 and/or HMGB1 pathways to diminish the burden of mesothelioma. *Journal of Translational Medicine, 21*(1), 749. https://doi.org/10.1186/s12967-023-04614-5

Carbone, M., & Testa, J. R. (2001). Genetic susceptibility and familial malignant mesothelioma. *Lancet*, *357*, 1804. https://doi.org/10.1016/S0140-6736(00)04923-0

Chen, R., Kang, R., & Tang, D. (2022). The mechanism of HMGB1 secretion and release. *Experimental & Molecular Medicine*, *54*, 91–102. https://doi.org/10.1038/s12276-022-00736-w

Churg, A., & Vedal, S. (1994). Fiber burden and patterns of asbestos-related disease in workers with heavy mixed amosite and chrysotile exposure. *American Journal of Respiratory Critical Care Medicine, 150*, 663–669. https://doi.org/10.1164/ajrccm.150.3.8087335

Coin, P. G., Roggli, V. L., & Brody, A. R. (1992). Deposition, clearance, and translocation of chrysotile asbestos from peripheral and central regions of the rat lung. *Environmental Research, 58*, 97–116. https://doi.org/10.1016/S0013-9351(05)80207-5

Darnton, L. (2024). The Hodgson and Darnton approach to quantifying the risks of mesothelioma and lung cancer in relation to asbestos exposure. In A. Korchevskiy, J. Rasmuson, & E. Rasmuson (Eds.), *Health risk assessment for asbestos and other fibrous minerals* (pp. 233–269). John Wiley & Sons, Inc. https://doi.org/10.1002/9781119438397

de Klerk, N. H., Musk, A. W., Williams, V., Filion, P. R., Whitaker, D., & Shilkin, K. B. (1996). Comparison of measures of exposure to asbestos in former crocidolite workers from Wittenoom Gorge, W. Australia. *American Journal of Industrial Medicine, 30*, 579–587. https://doi.org/10.1002/(sici)1097-0274(199611)30:5%3C579::aid-ajim5%3E3.0.co;2-o

De Waele, J., Luys, M., Vansant, E., & Adams, F. (1984). Analysis of chrysotile asbestos by LAMMA and Mossbauer spectroscopy: A study of the distribution of iron. *Journal of Trace and Microprobe Techniques, 2*, 87–102.

Donaldson, K., Brown, G. M., Brown, D. M., Bolton, R. E., & Davis, J. M. (1989). Inflammation generating potential of long and short fibre amosite asbestos samples. *British Journal of Industrial Medicine, 46*(4), 271–276. https://doi.org/10.1136/oem.46.4.271

Donaldson, K., Murphy, F. A., Duffin, R., & Poland, C. A. (2010). Asbestos, carbon nanotubes and the pleural mesothelium: A review of the hypothesis regarding the role of long fibre retention in the parietal pleura, inflammation and mesothelioma. *Particle and Fibre Toxicology, 7*, 5. https://doi.org/10.1186/1743-8977-7-5

Duffin, R., Tran, C. L., Clouter, A., Brown, D. M., MacNee, W., Stone, V., & Donaldson, K. (2002). The importance of surface area and specific reactivity in the acute pulmonary inflammatory response to particles. *The Annals of Occupational Hygiene, 46*(Suppl 1), 242–245. https://doi.org/10.1093/annhyg/46.suppl_1.242

Du Toit, R. S. (1991). An estimate of the rate at which crocidolite asbestos fibres are cleared from the lung. *The Annals of Occupational Hygiene, 35*(4), 433–438. https://doi.org/10.1093/annhyg/35.4.433. PMID: 1750732.

Finkelstein, M. M., & Dufresne, A. (1999). Inferences on the kinetics of asbestos deposition and clearance among chrysotile miners and millers. *American Journal of Industrial Medicine, 35*, 401–412. https://doi.org/10.1002/(sici)1097-0274(199904)35:4%3C401::aid-ajim12%3E3.0.co;2-4

Fisher, C. E., Brown, D. M., Shaw, J., Beswick, P. H., & Donaldson, K. (1998). Respirable fibres: Surfactant coated fibres release more Fe3+ than native fibres at both pH 4.5 and 7.2. *The Annals of Occupational Hygiene, 42*(5), 337–345. https://doi.org/10.1093/annhyg/42.5.337

Fröhlich, E. (2012). The role of surface charge in cellular uptake and cytotoxicity of medical nanoparticles. *International Journal of Nanomedicine, 7*, 55775591. https://doi.org/10.2147/IJN.S36111

Ghio, A. J., Kennedy, T. P., Whorton, A. R., Crumbliss, A. L., Hatch, G. E., & Hoidal, J. R. (1992). Role of surface complexed iron in oxidant generation and lung inflammation induced by silicates. *The American Journal of Physiology, 263*(5 Pt 1), L511–L518. https://doi.org/10.1152/ajplung.1992.263.5.l511

Ghio, A. J., Stonehuerner, J. G., Richards, J. H., Crissman, K. M., Roggli, V. L., Piantadosi, C. A., & Carraway, M. S. (2008). Iron homeostasis and oxidative stress in idiopathic pulmonary alveolar proteinosis: A case-control study. *Respiratory Research, 9*. https://doi.org/10.1186/1465-9921-9-10

Gilham, C., Rake, C., Burdett, G., Nicholson, A. G., Davison, L., Franchini, A., Carpenter, J., Hodgson, J., Darnton, A., & Peto, J. (2016). Pleural mesothelioma and lung cancer risks in relation to occupational history and asbestos lung burden. *Occupational and Environmental Medicine, 73*(5), 290–299. https://doi.org/10.1136/oemed-2015-103074

Gilmour, P. S., Brown, D. M., Beswick, P. H., MacNee, W., Rahman, I., & Donaldson, K. (1997). Free radical activity of industrial fibers: Role of iron in oxidative stress and activation of transcription factors. *Environmental Health Perspectives, 105*(Suppl 5), 1313–1317. https://doi.org/10.1289/ehp.97105s51313

Goodglick, L. A., & Kane, A. B. (1990). Cytotoxicity of long and short crocidolite asbestos fibers in vitro and in vivo. *Cancer Research, 50*(16), 5153–5163.

Gu, S., Bull, A., Perry, J. K., Huang, A., Hourwitz, M. J., Abostate, M., Fourkas, J. T., Korchevskiy, A. A., Wylie, A. G., & Losert, W. (2023). Excitable systems: A new perspective on the cellular impact of elongate mineral particles. *Environmental Research, 230*, 115353. https://doi.org/10.1016/j.envres.2023.115353

Gualtieri, A. F. (2023). Journey to the centre of the lung. The perspective of a mineralogist on the carcinogenic effects of mineral fibres in the lungs. *Journal of Hazardous Materials, 442*, 130077. https://doi.org/10.1016/j.jhazmat.2022.130077

Gualtieri, A. F., Bursi Gandolfi, N., Pollastri, S., Pollok, K., & Langenhorst, F. (2016). Where is iron in erionite? A multidisciplinary study on fibrous erionite-Na from Jersey (Nevada, U.S.A.). *Scientific Reports, 6*, 37981. https://doi.org/10.1038/srep37981

Gualtieri, A. F., Pollastri, S., Gandolfi, N. B., & Gualtieri, M. L. (2018). In vitro acellular dissolution of mineral fibres: A comparative study. *Scientific Reports, 8*, 7071. https://doi.org/10.1038/s41598-018-25531-4

Henzi, T., Blum, W. V., Pfefferli, M., Kawecki, T. J., Salicio, V., & Schwaller, B. (2009). SV40-induced expression of calretinin protects mesothelial cells from asbestos cytotoxicity and may be a key factor contributing to mesothelioma pathogenesis. *American Journal of Pathology, 174*(6), 2324–2336. https://doi.org/10.2353/ajpath.2009.080352

Hesterberg, T. W., Hart, G. A., Chevalier, J., Miller, W. C., Hamilton, R. D., Bauer, J., & Thevenaz, P. (1998). The importance of fiber biopersistence and lung dose in determining the chronic inhalation effects of X607, RCF1, and chrysotile asbestos in rats. *Toxicology and Applied Pharmacology, 153*(1), 68–82. https://doi.org/10.1006/taap.1998.8522

Hesterberg, T. W., Ririe, D. G., Barrett, J. C., & Nettesheim, P. (1987). Mechanisms of cytotoxicity of asbestos fibres in rat tracheal epithelial cells in culture. *Toxicology In Vitro, 1*(2), 59–65. https://doi.org./10.1016/0887-2333(87)90001-4. PMID: 20647067.

Honarpisheh, M., Foresto-Neto, O., Desai, J., Steiger, S., Anguiano Gómez, L., Popper, B., Boor, P., Anders, H.-J., & Mulay, S. R. (2017). Phagocytosis of environmental or metabolic crystalline particles induces cytotoxicity by triggering necroptosis across a broad range of particle size and shape. *Scientific Reports, 7*, 15523. https://doi.org/10.1038/s41598-017-15804-9

Jarabek, A. (2021, May 4–10). *EPA background briefing: EPA multi-path particle dosimetry (MPPD) model 2021 (v. 1.01) technical support documentation & user's guide. external peer review of the EPA multi-path particle dosimetry (MPPD) model 2021 (v. 1.01)* Technical Support Documentation & User's Guide, NA.

Jaurand, M. C. (1997). Mechanisms of fiber-induced genotoxicity. *Environmental Health Perspectives, 105*(Suppl 5), 1073–1084. https://doi.org/10.1289/ehp.97105s51073

Jay, S. M., Skokos, E. A., Zeng, J., Knox, K., & Kyriakides, T. R. (2010). Macrophage fusion leading to foreign body giant cell formation persists under phagocytic stimulation by microspheres in vitro and in vivo in mouse models. *Journal of Biomedical Materials Research A*, *93*(1), 189–199. https://doi.org/10.1002/jbm.a.32513

Jurinski, J. B., & Rimstidt, J. (2001). Biodurability of talc. *American Mineralogist*, *86*(4), 392–399. https://doi.org/10.2138/am-2001-0402

Kane, A. B., Hurt, R. H., & Gao, H. (2018). The asbestos-carbon nanotube analogy: An update. *Toxicology and Applied Pharmacology*, *361*, 68–80. https://doi.org/10.1016/j.taap.2018.06.027

Karami, M., Ebrahimzadeh, M. A., Mahdavi, M. R., & Kazemi, A. (2010). Effect of Fe2+ and Fe3+ ions on human plasma cholinesterase activity. *European Review for Medical and Pharmacological Sciences*, *14*, 897–901.

Klaassen, C. D., & Watkins, J. B., III (Eds.). (2010). *Casarett & Doull's essentials of toxicology* (2nd ed., pp. 42–43). The McGraw-Hill Companies. https://accesspharmacy.mhmedical.com/content.aspx?bookid=449&sectionid=39910763

Korchevskiy, A., Attanoos, R., & Wylie, A. G. (2025). Size-dependent retention of elongate mineral particles in human lungs: Modeling and implications for risk assessment. *Frontiers in Public Health*, (2025), 13. https://doi.org/10.3389/fpubh.2025.1646016

Korchevskiy, A. A., Rasmuson, J. O., & Rasmuson, E. J. (2019). Empirical model of mesothelioma potency factors for different mineral fibers based on their chemical composition and dimensionality. *Inhalation Toxicology*, *31*(5), 180–191. https://doi.org/10.1080/08958378.2019.1640320

Korchevskiy, A. A., Rasmuson, J. O., & Rasmuson, E. J. (2024). Mathematical modeling of cancer potency for various fibrous minerals. In A. Korchevskiy, J. Rasmuson, & E. Rasmuson (Eds.), *Health risk assessment for asbestos and other fibrous minerals* (pp. 344–365). John Wiley & Sons. https://doi.org/10.1002/9781119438397

Korchevskiy, A. A., & Wylie, A. G. (2022). Asbestos exposure, lung fiber burden, and mesothelioma rates: Mechanistic modelling for risk assessment. *Computational Toxicology*, *24*, 100249. https://doi.org/10.1016/j.comtox.2022.100249

Korchevskiy, A. A., & Wylie, A. G. (2023). Toxicological and epidemiological approaches to carcinogenic potency modeling for mixed mineral fiber exposure: The case of fibrous balangeroite and chrysotile. *Inhalation Toxicology*, *35*(7–8), 185–200. https://doi.org/10.1080/08958378.2023.2213720

Korchevskiy, A. A., & Wylie, A. G. (2025a). Habit of elongate amphibole particles as a predictor of mesothelial carcinogenicity. *Toxicology Reports*, *14*, 101908. https://doi.org/10.1016/j.toxrep.2025.101908

Korchevskiy, A. A., & Wylie, A. G. (2025b, April 24). The empirical metric of mesothelial carcinogenicity for carbon nanotubes and elongate mineral particles. *Inhalation Toxicology* (online). https://doi.org/10.1080/08958378.2025.2486087

Kuraishy, A., Karin, M., & Grivennikov, S. I. (2011). Tumor promotion via injury-and death-induced inflammation. *Immunity*, *35*(4), 467–477. https://doi.org/10.1016/j.immuni.2011.09.006

Kuroda, A. (2021). Recent progress and perspectives on the mechanisms underlying asbestos toxicity. *Genes and Environment*, *43*(1), 46. https://doi.org/10.1186/s41021-021-00215-0

Larson, D., Powers, A., Ambrosi, J.-P., Tanji, M., Napolitano, A., Flores, E. G., Baumann, F., Pellegrini, L., Jennings, C. J., Buck, B. J., McLaurin, B. T., Merkler, D., Robinson, C., Morris, P., Dogan, M., Dogan, A. U., Pass, H. I., Pastorino, S., Carbone, M., & Yang, H. (2016). Investigating palygorskite role in the development of mesothelioma in southern Nevada: Insights into fiber-induced carcinogenicity. *Journal of Toxicology and Environmental Health, B Critical Reviews*, *19*(5–6), 213–230. https://doi.org/10.1080/10937404.2016.1195321

Leinardi, R., Petriglieri, J. R., Pochet, A., Yakoub, Y., Lelong, M., Lescoat, A., Turci, F., Lecureur, V., & Huaux, F. (2023). Distinct pro-inflammatory mechanisms elicited by short and long amosite asbestos fibers in macrophages. *International Journal of Molecular Sciences, 24*(20), 15145. https://doi.org/10.3390/ijms242015145

Matsuzaki, H., Lee, S., Kumagai-Takei, N., Min, Y., Sada, N., Yoshitome, K., Nishimura, Y., Maeda, M., & Otsuki, T. (2018). Cytotoxicity caused by asbestos fibers and acquisition of resistance by continuous exposure in human T cells. *Cytotoxicity InTech.* http://dx.doi.org/10.5772/intechopen.72064

Metintas, M., Hillerdal, G., Metintas, S., & Dumortier, P. (2010). Endemic malignant mesothelioma: Exposure to erionite is more important than genetic factors. *Archives of Environmental & Occupational Health, 65*(2), 86–93. https://doi.org/10.1080/19338240903390305

Miserocchi, G., Sancini, G., Mantegazza, F., & Chiappino, G. (2008). Translocation pathways for inhaled asbestos fibers. *Environmental Health, 7*, 4. https://link.springer.com/article/10.1186/1476-069x-7-4

Mori, A., Ito, S., & Sekine, T. (2024). A revision of the multiple-path particle dosimetry model focusing on tobacco product aerosol dynamics. *International Journal for Numerical Methods in Biomedical Engineering, 40*(3), e3796. https://doi.org/10.1002/cnm.3796

Murphy, F., Dekkers, S., Braakhuis, H., Ma-Hock, L., Johnston, H., Janer, G., di Cristo, L., Sabella, S., Jacobsen, N. R., Oomen, A. G., Haase, A., Fernandes, T., & Stone, V. (2021). An integrated approach to testing and assessment of high aspect ratio nanomaterials and its application for grouping based on a common mesothelioma hazard. *NanoImpact, 22*, 100314. https://doi.org/10.1016/j.impact.2021.100314

Napolitano, A., Antoine, D. J., Pellegrini, L., Baumann, F., Pagano, I., Pastorino, S., Goparaju, C. M., Prokrym, K., Canino, C., Pass, H. I., Carbone, M., & Yang, H. (2016). HMGB1 and its hyperacetylated isoform are sensitive and specific serum biomarkers to detect asbestos exposure and to identify mesothelioma patients. *Clinical Cancer Research, 22*(12), 3087–3096. https://doi.org/10.1158/1078-0432.ccr-15-1130

Nishimura, Y., Kumagai-Takei, N., Lee, S., Yoshitome, K., & Otsuki, T. (2020). Suppressed immune system caused by exposure to asbestos and malignant mesothelioma. In T. Otsuki (Ed.), *Asbestos-related diseases* (Chapter 1). IntechOpen. https://doi.org/10.5772/intechopen.90763

Nolan, R. P., Langer, A. M., Oechsle, G. W., Addison, J., & Colflesh, D. E. (1991). Association of tremolite habit with biological potential: Preliminary report. In R. C. Brown, J. A. Hoskins, & N. F. Johnson (Eds.), *Mechanisms in fibre carcinogenesis*. NATO ASI Series (Vol. 223). Springer. https://doi.org/10.1007/978-1-4684-1363-2_21

Okada, S., Hamazaki, S., Toyokuni, S., & Midorikawa, O. (1989). Induction of mesothelioma by intraperitoneal injections of ferric saccharate in male Wistar rats. *British Journal of Cancer, 60*(5), 708–711. https://doi.org/10.1038/bjc.1989.344

Oze, C., & Solt, K. L. (2010). Biodurability of chrysotile and tremolite asbestos in simulated lung and gastric fluids. *American Mineralogist, 95*(5–6), 825–831. https://doi.org/10.2138/am.2010.3265

Pollastri, S., Gualtieri, A. F., Lassinantti Gualtieri, M., Hanuskova, M., Cavallo, A., & Gaudino, G. (2014). The zeta potential of mineral fibres. *Journal of Hazardous Materials, 276*, 469–479. https://doi.org/10.1016/j.jhazmat.2014.05.060

Pooley, F. D., & Clark, N. J. (1980). A comparison of fibre dimensions in chrysotile, crocidolite and amosite particles from samples of airborne dust and from post-mortem lung tissue specimens. *IARC Scientific Publications, 30*, 79–86.

Qi, F., Okimoto, G., Jube, S., Napolitano, A., Pass, H. I., Laczko, R., DeMay, R. M., Khan, G., Tiirikainen, M., Rinaudo, C., Croce, A., Yang, H., Gaudino, G., & Carbone, M. (2013). Continuous exposure to chrysotile asbestos can cause transformation of human mesothelial cells via HMGB1 and TNF-α signaling. *The American Journal of Pathology, 183*(5), 1654–1666. https://doi.org/10.1016/j.ajpath.2013.07.029

Qi, Y.-T., Zhang, F.-L., Tian, S.-Y., Wu, H.-Q., Zhao, Y., Zhang, X.-W., Liu, Y.-L., Fu, P., Amatore, C., & Huang, W.-H. (2024). Nanosensor detection of reactive oxygen and nitrogen species leakage in frustrated phagocytosis of nanofibres. *Nature Nanotechnology, 19*, 524–533. https://doi.org/10.1038/s41565-023-01575-0

Quinlan, T. R., Marsh, J. P., Janssen, Y. M., Borm, P. A., & Mossman, B. T. (1994). Oxygen radicals and asbestos-mediated disease. *Environmental Health Perspectives*, *102*(Suppl 10), 107–110. https://doi.org/10.1289/ehp.94102s10107

Rendall, R. E. G., & Du Toit, R. S. J. (1994). The retention and clearance of glass fibre and different varieties of asbestos by the lung. *Annals of Occupational Hygiene, 38*(Suppl 1), 757–761. https://doi.org/10.1093/annhyg/38.inhaled_particles_VII.757

Rosales, C., & Uribe-Querol, E. (2017). Phagocytosis: A fundamental process in immunity. *Biomedical Research International,* 9042851. https://doi.org/10.1155/2017/9042851

Saracci, R., & Simonato, L. (2001). Familial malignant mesothelioma. *The Lancet*, *358*(9297), 1507. https://doi.org/10.1016/S0140-6736(01)06588-4

Schiller, J. E., Payne, S. L., & Khallafalla, S. E. (1980). Surface charge heterogenicity in amphibole cleavage fragments and asbestos fibers. *Science*, *204*(4464), 1530–1532. https://doi.org/10.1126/science.209.4464.1530

Schneider, J., Arhelger, R., Brückel, B., & Baur, X. (2023, March 27). Diagnostic limitations of lung fiber counts in asbestos-related diseases. *The Journal of Scientific Practice and Integrity* (online). https://doi.org/10.35122/001c.70352

Schwarz, E., & Winer, A. (1971). Magnetic properties of asbestos, with special reference to the determination of absolute magnetite contents. *CIM Bulletin*, *64*, 55–59. WOS: A1971L172100009.

Searl, A. (1997). A comparative study of the clearance of respirable para-aramid, chrysotile and glass fibres from rat lungs. *Annals of Occupational Hygiene*, *41*(2), 217–233. https://doi.org/10.1016/S0003-4878(96)00036-1. PMID: 9155241.

Shukla, A., Jung, M., Stern, M., Fukagawa, N. K., Taatjes, D. J., Sawyer, D., Van Houten, B., & Mossman, B. T. (2003). Asbestos induces mitochondrial DNA damage and dysfunction linked to the development of apoptosis. *American Journal of Physiology-Lung Cellular and Molecular Physiology, 285*(5), L1018–L1025. https://doi.org/10.1152/ajplung.00038.2003

Stevens, M. E., Paustenbach, D. J., Lockhart, N. J., Busboom, D. E., Deckard, B. M., & Brew, D. W. (2024). The presence of erionite in North American geologies and the estimated mesothelioma potency by region. *Inhalation Toxicology, 36*(3), 158–173. https://doi.org/10.1080/08958378.2024.2322496

Suarez, J. S., Novelli, F., Goto, K., Ehara, M., Steele, M., Kim, J.-H., Zolondick, A. A., Xue, J., Xu, R., Saito, M., Pastorino, S., Minaai, M., Takanishi, Y., Emi, M., Pagano, I., Wakeham, A., Berger, T., Pass, H. I., Gaudino, G., . . . Yang, H. (2023). HMGB-1 released by mesothelial cells drives the development of asbestos-induced mesothelioma. *Proceedings of the National Academy of Sciences, 120*(39), e2307999120. http://dx.doi.org/10.1073/pnas.2307999120

Suzuki, Y., & Yuen, S. R. (2002). Asbestos fibers contributing to the induction of human malignant mesothelioma. *Annals of the New York Academy of Sciences, 982*, 160–176. https://doi.org/10.1111/j.1749-6632.2002.tb04931.x. PMID: 12562635.

Suzuki, Y., Yuen, S. R., & Ashley, R. (2005). Short, thin asbestos fibers contribute to the development of human malignant mesothelioma: Pathological evidence.

International Journal of Hygiene and Environmental Health, 208(3), 201–210. https://doi.org/10.1016/j.ijheh.2005.01.015

Timbrell, V. (1965). The inhalation of fibrous dusts. *Biological Effects of Asbestos, Annals of the New York Academy of Sciences, 132*(1), 255–273. https://doi.org/10.1111/j.1749-6632.1965.tb41107.x

Toyokuni, S. (1996). Iron-induced carcinogenesis: The role of redox regulation. *Free Radical Biology and Medicine, 20*(4), 553–566. https://doi.org/10.1016/0891-5849(95)02111-6

Tuomela, K., Ambrose, A. R., & Davis, D. M. (2022). Escaping death: How cancer cells and infected cells resist cell-mediated cytotoxicity. *Frontiers in Immunology, 13*, 867098. https://doi.org/10.3389/fimmu.2022.867098

United States Environmental Protection Agency (U.S. EPA). (2014, July 25). *Risk assessment forum white paper: Probabilistic risk assessment methods and case studies* (EPA/100/R-14/004). https://www.epa.gov/sites/default/files/2014-12/documents/raf-pra-white-paper-final.pdf

Wang, F., Wang, Y., Yao, X., Ma, C., Yin, Y., & Song, M. (2019). Length and diameter-dependent phagocytosis and cytotoxicity of long silver nanowires in macrophages. *Chemosphere, 237*, 124565. https://doi.org/10.1016/j.chemosphere.2019.124565

Wang, Y., Jiang, Z., Yan, J., & Ying, S. (2019). HMGB1 as a potential biomarker and therapeutic target for malignant mesothelioma. *Disease Markers, 12*, 4183157. https://doi.org/10.1155/2019/4183157

Werner, A. J., Hochella, M. F., Guthrie, G. D., Hardy, J. A., Aust, A. E., & Rimstidt, J. D. (1995). Asbestiform riebeckite (crocidolite) dissolution in the presence of Fe chelators: Implications for mineral-induced disease. *American Mineralogist, 80*(11–12), 1093–1103. https://doi.org/10.2138/am-1995-11-1201

World Health Organization (WHO). (1986). *Asbestos and other natural mineral fibres: International programme on chemical safety*. Environmental Health Criteria 53. https://www.inchem.org/documents/ehc/ehc/ehc53.htm

Wright, A., Cowie, H., Gormley, I. P., & Davis, J. M. G. (1986). The in vitro cytotoxicity of asbestos fibers: I. P388D1 cells. *American Journal of Industrial Medicine, 9*(4), 371–384. https://doi.org/10.1002/ajim.4700090409

Wylie, A. G., Korchevskiy, A., Segrave, A. M., & Duane, A. (2020). Modeling mesothelioma risk factors from amphibole fiber dimensionality: Mineralogical and epidemiological perspective. *Journal of Applied Toxicology, 40*(4), 515–524. https://doi.org/10.1002/jat.3923

Xu, A., Wu, L. J., Santella, R. M., & Hei, T. K. (1999). Role of oxyradicals in mutagenicity and DNA damage induced by crocidolite asbestos in mammalian cells. *Cancer Research, 59*(23), 5922–5926. PMID: 10606236.

Xu, A., Zhou, H., Yu, D. Z., & Hei, T. K. (2002). Mechanisms of the genotoxicity of crocidolite asbestos in mammalian cells: Implication from mutation patterns induced by reactive oxygen species. *Environmental Health Perspectives, 110*(10), 1003–1008. https://doi.org/10.1289/ehp.021101003

Xue, J., Patergnani, S., Giorgi, C., Suarez, J., Goto, K., Bononi, A., Tanji, M., Novelli, F., Pastorino, S., Xu, R., Caroccia, N., Dogan, A. U., Pass, H. I., Tognon, M., Pinton, P., Gaudino, G., Mak, T. W., Carbone, M., & Yang, H. (2020). Asbestos induces mesothelial cell transformation via HMGB1-driven autophagy. *Proceedings of the National Academy of Sciences, 117*(41), 25543–25552. https://doi.org/10.1073/pnas.2007622117

Yang, H., Bocchetta, M., Kroczynska, B., Elmishad, A. G., Chen, Y., Liu, Z., Bubici, C., Mossman, B. T., Pass, H. I., Testa, J. R., Franzoso, G., & Carbone, M. (2006). TNF-alpha inhibits asbestos-induced cytotoxicity via a NF-kappaB-dependent pathway, a possible mechanism for asbestos-induced oncogenesis. *Proceedings of the*

National Academy of Sciences, 103(27), 10397–10402. https://doi.org/10.1073/pnas.0604008103

Yeager, H., Jr., Russo, D. A., Yañez, M., Gerardi, D., Nolan, R. P., Kagan, E., & Langer, A. M. (1983). Cytotoxicity of a short-fiber chrysotile asbestos for human alveolar macrophages: Preliminary observations. *Environmental Research, 30*(1), 224–232. https://doi.org/10.1016/0013-9351(83)90182-2

Zolondick, A. A., Gaudino, G., Xue, J., Pass, H. I., Carbone, M., & Yang, H. (2021). Asbestos-induced chronic inflammation in malignant pleural mesothelioma and related therapeutic approaches-a narrative review. *Precision Cancer Medicine, 4*, 27. https://doi.org/10.21037/pcm-21-12

5 Cell responses to elongated mineral fibers

Multiple roles of shape and dimension

Brooke T. Mossman

BACKGROUND, OVERVIEW, AND CRITICAL QUESTIONS

An understanding of the adverse health effects of mineral fibers requires a basic understanding of the cell and tissue responses that occur after their natural route of inhalation into the body. Various mineral fibers, such as asbestos and erionite, are known to induce toxicity (a general term that encompasses cell death and decreased cell survival) and pulmonary disease. However, the chain of events in cells that give rise to these diseases, which include pulmonary and pleural fibrosis, lung cancers, and malignant mesotheliomas (MMs), is unclear. Moreover, many chemical and physical properties of mineral fibers appear to contribute to the pathogenic potential of these fibers. In past occupational settings where diseases have developed, the heterogeneity in size and other characteristics of fibers in the workplace, as well as a lack of sensitive measuring techniques (i.e., use of phase microscopy historically as opposed to electron microscopy), has hampered the determination of which fiber parameters are associated with critical events in the causation of these diseases. For these reasons, investigators have pursued *in vitro* studies on isolated cells and organ cultures to address key events in the induction of fibrosis and carcinogenesis (reviewed in Mossman, 2018). These results have been correlated, whenever possible, to events occurring after the inhalation of fibers as studied in rodents and human lungs (reviewed in Mossman et al., 2011). These latter investigations have provided information on the deposition and retention of various types of elongated fibers (defined here as a structure with a > 3:1 length-to-diameter ratio), their translocation to lung compartments and pleural sites after inhalation, and their persistence over time (reviewed in Mossman et al., 2011, 2013). In contrast, the administration of minerals by intratracheal instillation or injection into the pharynx, pleura, and peritoneum bypasses the normal clearance mechanisms in the upper and lower respiratory tracts. These models will not be described in detail here because of their artificial nature and lack of agreement with observations from inhalation studies (reviewed in Mossman et al., 2011; Drummond et al., 2016).

The pathogenicity, that is, disease potential, of elongated fibers such as amphibole asbestos has been historically linked to dose, dimension, and durability in human

DOI: 10.1201/9781003424277-6

lungs and pleura. However, chemistry and a plethora of other fiber characteristics, including surface charge and area, are also relevant and may contribute to toxicity, dose, and durability (Korchevskiy et al., 2019; Gualtieri et al., 2017). Each of these interactive parameters is difficult to assess in animals and humans. However, cell and organ culture models preserving the architecture of the lung allow examination of known concentrations of well-characterized fibers and particles over a range of doses, albeit extrapolation to airborne concentrations of minerals causing diseases in the past workplace is difficult. It should also be noted that *in vitro* experiments are generally conducted over hours or days and therefore measure acute as opposed to chronic events.

Historically, the use of various cell types in experiments on fiber and particle toxicology has evolved from early studies in the 1960s, which focused on red blood cells (RBCs) and monolayers of immortalized or malignant cell lines, to investigations using normal cell isolates from rodents and eventually human cells. Organ cultures from the trachea and bronchi were used to preserve the structure and interaction of multiple cell types in the lung over months of culture (reviewed in Mossman, 2008, 2018). It is important to emphasize that most current studies have focused on progenitor cells of diseases such as the pulmonary epithelial cell, which develops into lung or tracheobronchial cancers; the mesothelial cell, which develops into malignant mesotheliomas (MMs); and the interstitial or pleural fibroblast, which gives rise to pulmonary or pleural fibrosis. Fibroblasts are one of a number of cell types in the interstitium or supporting matrix of the airways, whereas epithelial cells line the airways and alveoli of the lung. Under normal circumstances, they are separated from underlying fibroblasts by a basement membrane (Figures 5.1, 5.3), but this is dissolved during cancer development, allowing epithelial cells to become invasive and multiply. Epithelial cells give rise to > 90% of lung cancers, that is, carcinomas.

Mesothelial cells comprise the lining surfaces of the pleural cavity (visceral and parietal mesothelium) and the peritoneal cavity (Figure 5.1). Note that these cell types differ markedly in their sensitivity, as compared to human fibroblasts and epithelial cells, to the toxic effects of asbestos fibers *in vitro,* and individual susceptibilities to the carcinogenic effects of fibers may also exist (reviewed in Kane, 1996). Moreover, responses to asbestos fibers, including cytokine (growth factor) and chemokine (secreted proteins that attract other cell types) profiles, differ between pleural and peritoneal mesothelial cells (Dragon et al., 2015).

Although longer fibers perturb cells in culture via multiple mechanisms (see below), the transport and translocation of needle-like asbestos fibers after inhalation may reflect why longer, thinner durable fibers are carcinogenic in humans (reviewed in Kane, 1996; ATSDR, 2003; Barlow et al., 2018; Nel, 2023). They are aligned with airway flow and penetrate the deep lung to gain access to the pleural space (Mossman et al., 2011; Lippmann, 2014). At high concentrations, they may be trapped and persist, avoiding clearance via stomata or pores between parietal mesothelial cells that afford drainage via lymph nodes (Figure 5.2). Thus, the dimensional characteristics of long, thin amphibole fibers are most important in modeling risk factors for MMs (Korchevskiy & Wylie, 2021; Wylie et al., 2020; Wylie & Korchevskiy, 2023).

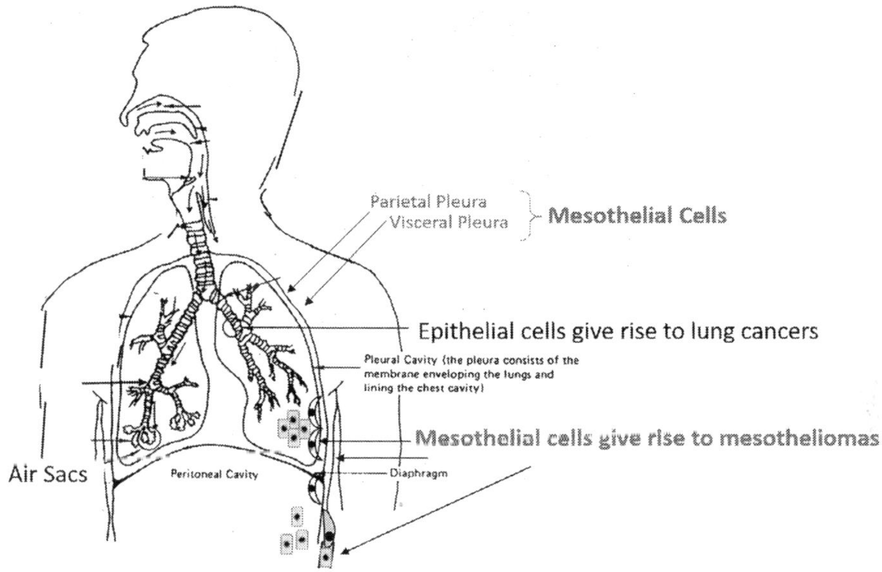

FIGURE 5.1 Location of epithelial and mesothelial cells in the human lung. Arrows indicate the inhalation pathways from the proximal nose and mouth, breathing through the tracheobronchial tree consisting of progressively smaller diameter airways to the air sacs (alveoli) of the lung where gas exchange occurs. Epithelial cells line the tracheobronchial airways and give rise to lung cancers. Pleural mesothelial cells comprise the visceral and parietal pleura that line the lungs. Normally a single-cell layer, they can multiply in the pleural space to form malignant mesotheliomas (MMs). In contrast, peritoneal mesothelial cells line the body cavity (peritoneum) encompassing the lower body organs.

Studies on 'effector cells' of the immune system, most notably isolated alveolar macrophages (AMs) and cells from pleural/peritoneal lavage, have allowed for the elucidation of key events occurring during initial fiber deposition, uptake, and clearance in the upper respiratory tract and at pleural sites. More importantly, they have indicated that chemokine and cytokine production is integral to the advent of inflammation and altered cell proliferation – early events in carcinogenicity and the development of fibrosis. Because a number of fibers and particles of diverse geometry, chemistry, and size ranges have been linked at high airborne concentrations to the development of pulmonary fibroses, including asbestosis, silicosis, coal workers' pneumoconiosis, and talc pneumoconiosis, there appears to be a nonspecific inflammatory response elicited by these particles at "overload" concentrations in human and animal lungs that fuels the development of fibrosis (reviewed in Mossman et al., 2011). Therefore, the importance of shape and size in fibrogenic minerals is not as obvious as has been documented in MMs and lung cancers. Because of the overwhelming contributions of smoking in most asbestos-induced lung cancers, it is

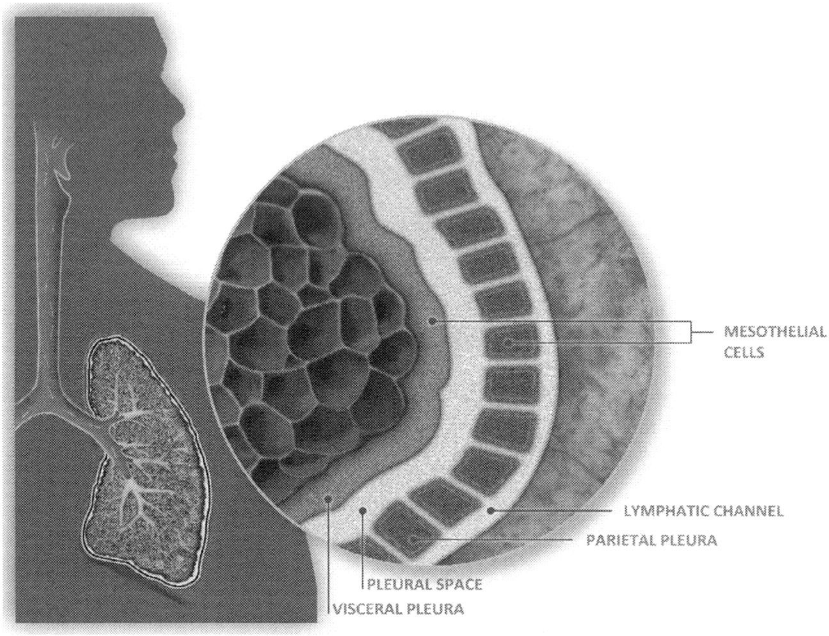

FIGURE 5.2 Translocation of elongate mineral particles after inhalation. Long, thin fibers occur in the distal lung and can penetrate or be transported by alveolar and pleural macrophages across the alveoli through the visceral pleura to the pleural space. At high fiber concentrations, they may be juxtaposed next to the parietal pleura, blocking clearance of fibers by preventing access to lymphatic channels via pores (stomata) in the parietal pleura.

difficult to dissect the roles and properties of asbestos linked to the initiation and promotion of these tumors. However, it has been acknowledged that long (> 5 microns) asbestos fibers are more potent in the induction of MMs, lung cancers, and pulmonary fibrosis (ATSDR, 2003; Barlow et al., 2018; Carbone et al., 2019; Garabrant & Pastula, 2018; Roggli, 2015; HEI, 1991; Mossman et al., 1990). For these reasons, the shape and size properties of fibers, which are important in carcinogenesis, are emphasized below with an emphasis on the development of lung cancers and MMs. In human MMs, it has been calculated that crocidolite asbestos is the most potent (500-fold), followed by amosite (100-fold), and chrysotile (1-fold risk) (Hodgson & Darnton, 2000; Darnton, 2023; Garabrant & Pastula, 2018).

The critical questions that have evolved from decades of research on carcinogenic fibers such as commercial amphibole asbestos types include the following: 1) Are their common cellular effects initiated by various pathogenic fibers that can be related primarily to their physical and chemical characteristics? 2) Can these cellular events be linked to the process of carcinogenesis? and 3) Are these effects genetic (affecting DNA), epigenetic (affecting mRNA or proteins), or both in origin?

CONCEPTS OF CANCER DEVELOPMENT

There is general consensus that most solid cancers occur through a multi-stage process over several years or decades, particularly in the case of malignant mesotheliomas (MMs) (reviewed in Mossman, 2017, 2018; Mossman & Gualtieri, 2020). In the original studies by Berenblum (1974) and others in the 1970s, mutations in DNA were commonly observed by soluble chemical carcinogens, giving rise to the mutational theory of carcinogenesis, which postulates that initiating agents give rise to critical mutations in cancer causation by acting directly on DNA to induce an irreversible effect. Initiated cells are then propagated during a long process of tumor promotion that favors cell proliferation and the acquisition of characteristics allowing their conversion to malignant cells over time. These properties include uncontrolled cell proliferation, genomic instability, invasion, and metastasis. The transformation of malignant cells was demonstrated after the injection of cells into animals and demonstration of sarcomas. Tumor-promoting agents, as opposed to initiating agents, do not interact directly with DNA and are proposed to work in a reversible epigenetic fashion using processes such as DNA methylation, histone modification, and noncoding long and short microRNAs (reviewed by Reid, 2015).

Study of various types of asbestos in hamster and human tracheobronchial epithelial cells, that is, the target cells of lung cancers, showed that amphibole types of commercial asbestos (crocidolite, amosite) had features common with classical tumor promoters in the skin, such as phorbol esters. After injection of treated tissues into syngeneic hamsters, lung carcinomas were not observed with asbestos or other particles alone, but fibers and particles, including crocidolite asbestos, Fe_2O_3, carbon particles, kaolin, etc., were effective carriers of adsorbed polycyclic aromatic hydrocarbons (PAHs) to cells without obvious effects due to particle or fiber type (Mossman & Craighead, 1979, 1982). Thus, both particles and fibers carrying PAHs were effective co-carcinogens, whereas tissues exposed to particles alone failed to cause tumors. These data are supported by studies in humans showing that lung cancers are rarely induced in nonsmokers exposed to asbestos (Craighead & Mossman, 1982; Mossman & Gee, 1989). We now know that tobacco smoke contains hundreds of chemical carcinogens, particulates, and tumor-promoting agents that contribute to the causation of lung cancer. Moreover, there are mutations and binding partners to proteins (ALK, EGFR, etc.) associated with the development of lung cancers in patients with no smoking and/or asbestos exposure history (reviewed in Mossman & Gualtieri, 2020). It is generally accepted that the combination of smoking and asbestos exposure has a more than additive effect in the development of lung cancers. Moreover, a plethora of genetic and epigenetic changes occur during the evolution of different types of lung cancers. Because tobacco smoke is an overwhelming factor and complex agent, it has been difficult to decipher the importance of asbestos type and its physicochemical properties in this disease.

In contrast to lung cancers, amphibole types of asbestos are complete carcinogens not requiring exposures to other agents in the development of MMs (reviewed in Mossman et al., 2013). Crocidolite and amosite asbestos have both initiating and tumor-promoting properties in the development of MMs in animals and humans.

Whereas a number of proto-oncogenes and tumor suppressor genes have been identified in lung tumors (albeit not unique to asbestos exposures) (reviewed in Mossman & Gualtieri, 2020), MMs have been characterized by that loss of function of one or more tumor suppressor genes, including BAP1, FBXW7, and NF2 (Badhai et al., 2020; Carbone et al., 2019). The loss of gene function governing accurate DNA repair, apoptosis (programmed cell death), and other normal processes has been linked to early and late clonal events over the long period of MM development, with an average latency of 40+ years (Zhang et al., 2021). The regulation of these genes appears to be primarily through epigenetic processes (Yuan et al., 2021). Thus, MM is considered to be a "disease of gene loss," attributed to loss of tumor suppressor genes, as no driver mutations or oncogenes have been implicated in its causation (Yoshida, 2019).

In summary, genetic and epigenetic changes may contribute to the many properties required for cell transformation to malignancy in lung cancers and MMs (Joseph et al., 2016; Lorenzini et al., 2021). As described below, it is unlikely that asbestos and other elongated fibers cause precancerous changes by interacting directly with the DNA of cells. In contrast, it is clear that the peripheral lung and tumor microenvironment contribute to the carcinogenic process to produce many of the hallmarks of cancer (Hanahan, 2022).

PARAMETERS OF TOXICITY AND CARCINOGENICITY AND EVOLUTION OF HYPOTHESES

Historically, the toxic and carcinogenic effects of mineral fibers (defined here as elongated structures with a > 3:1 length-to-diameter ratio) have been examined in hundreds of different cell types. Species and cell types have evolved from red blood cells (RBCs) to human and normal differentiated cell types, giving rise to lung cancers and MMs. Difficulties in interpretating many of these studies are 1) a single type of fiber was often introduced at a single toxic concentration; 2) studies were often performed over a single time frame; 3) when multiple fibers were compared, they were added at similar weight (milligram) concentrations, often reflecting different numbers of fibers. This is especially misleading when comparing chrysotile asbestos to amphibole types of asbestos, as many more chrysotile fibrils are observed on an equal weight basis; 4) fibers were frequently evaluated without the inclusion of a non-disease-causing particle (negative) control; 5) preparations of fibers and particles were rarely characterized by mineralogists to determine size dimensions and other properties of these materials; and 6) sources of asbestos and other materials were often not specified and may differ from location to location. Despite these shortcomings, however, data emerged from some studies on the cell organelles adversely affected by toxic and carcinogenic fibers. These cellular endpoints are listed in Table 5.1 and have been used to address the hypotheses numbered 1 through 4 below. Note that the properties of pathogenic fibers hypothetically linked to the induction of these processes are listed in Table 5.2.

For a more detailed description of assays, see Woodworth et al. (1982) and Hillegass et al. (2010a, 2010b).

For further discussion, see Gualtieri et al., 2017; Mossman & Gualtieri, 2020.

TABLE 5.1
Cellular endpoints reflecting toxicity and carcinogenicity

Toxicity	Carcinogenicity
• Hemolysis • Membrane lysis (Trypan Blue Exclusion, LDH release, release of B-glucuronidase) • Apoptosis, necrosis • DNA damage (genotoxicity) • Alterations in chromosomal structure and number • Unscheduled DNA synthesis • Alterations in chromosomal structure and number • Unscheduled DNA synthesis • Oxidant and 8-oxo-2'-deoxyguanosine release • Increased mRNA, protein, and activity of antioxidant enzymes	• Hyperplasia, metaplasia • Colony-forming efficiency (CFE) • Anchorage-independent cell growth • Morphologic transformation • Alterations in gene expression (transcriptome profiling for mRNA) • Release of inflammatory mediators and cytokines causing proliferation and aberrant cell function of "target" cells

TABLE 5.2
Features that collectively determine the toxic and carcinogenic effects of elongated fibers

- Morphology (particle vs. fiber)
- Shape (needle-like vs. tangled or curly fibers)
- Length
- Diameter
- Bulk and surface chemistry
- Iron content and availability
- Surface charge
- Adsorptive properties
- Crystal structure
- Biodurability

Hypothesis 1. Toxicity predicts carcinogenicity

The toxicity of various asbestos types was first tested in experiments documenting hemolysis or release of heme after lysis of RBCs. This simple assay did not require long-term culture of cells and revealed that chrysotile asbestos was more active than crocidolite asbestos due to its positive surface charge from Mg^{++}. Although it was initially postulated that positively charged chrysotile fibers selectively interacted with negative sialic acid residues on the cell surface by electrostatic attraction, sialic acid and other membrane components appeared to be involved (Pelé & Calvert, 1983). Studies in mammalian cells overwhelmingly suggested that on an equal weight basis, chrysotile proved to be the most toxic, regardless of toxic endpoint, more so than crocidolite or other fibers and particles (Woodworth et al., 1982; Mossman et al., 1983). Cell death reflected lysis of the extracellular membrane, as measured by the release of lactic acid dehydrogenase (LDH) and B-glucuronidase due to lysosomal rupture. These endpoints have been validated in inhalation experiments using chrysotile and crocidolite – measurement of these enzymes in bronchoalveolar lavage samples shows that they are elevated in acute and chronic mineral exposures (Mossman, 1990; Haegens et al., 2005). We now know from epidemiological studies that chrysotile asbestos is much less pathogenic in the causation of MMs than amphibole types of asbestos (reviewed in Mossman et al., 1990; Hodgson & Darnton, 2000; Darnton, 2023; Garabrant & Pastula, 2018). Simply put, a dead cell cannot give rise to a tumor, an explanation for the disconnect between the toxicity and carcinogenicity of mineral fibers. In fact, its ability to cause cell death, large-scale deletions in DNA, and aneuploidy (see below) might explain why chrysotile is not as potent a carcinogen when compared to amosite and crocidolite asbestos.

Hypothesis 2. Carcinogenic fibers interact with DNA to cause mutations and other anomalies

Despite differences in fiber potency, all types of asbestos have been classified by IARC as carcinogenic to man (WHO, 1987, 2012). Since the mechanisms of action of carcinogenic chemicals were initially linked to interactions with DNA in the form of mutations, aneuploidy, and/or DNA adduct formation, asbestos and other types of elongated particles, such as synthetic fiber glasses, were tested in models of mutagenesis in a number of cell types. As reviewed by Kane (1996), the evidence for mutagenesis and DNA damage is conflicting. In general, asbestos fibers were inactive or weakly positive in inducing point mutations, sister chromatid exchange, or DNA strand breakage. Experiments by our laboratory showed that neither crocidolite nor chrysotile asbestos bound to the DNA of hamster tracheal epithelial cells, as did the PAH benz(o)apyrene (Mossman et al., 1983; Eastman et al., 1983). In contrast, rat pleural mesothelial cells showed some effects on sister chromatid exchanges and DNA repair by chrysotile and crocidolite but not by talc (Endo-Capron et al., 1993). A hamster-human hybrid cell model was developed to examine chrysotile effects at low and high fiber concentrations (Hei et al., 1992). These experiments showed that large deletions in DNA were caused by chrysotile at lethal concentrations of fibers.

As stated by the Health Effects Institute/EPA Panel on Asbestos Research (HEI, 1991),

> One theory assumes that asbestos fibers initiate carcinogenesis by direct damage to DNA or chromosomes, so that theoretically at least one fiber would be capable of initiating the formation of a tumor. This method of carcinogenesis by fibers is not established.

Cell defense mechanisms, including the induction of antioxidant enzymes and DNA repair processes, may explain why dose-related changes occur in cell transformation assays, suggesting thresholds below which adverse effects do not occur (reviewed in Mossman, 2018; Cox et al., 2023).

Another explanation for why asbestos fibers may not interact with DNA after internalization is that intracellular fibers occur in perinuclear cytoplasmic structures encompassed by a membrane, that is, a phagolysosome (Mossman et al., 1977; MacCorkle et al., 2006). The fact that chrysotile fibers have been found free in the cytoplasm may reflect their dissolution and leaching of Mg^{++} occurring after membranolytic activity (Jaurand et al., 1984). In summary, the mutational/aneuploidy model to explain the carcinogenicity of asbestos and other pathogenic types of minerals is questionable based on the fact that large-scale gene deletions are incompatible with cell survival. Asbestos fibers do not occur in the intact cell nucleus. Moreover, it has been shown that aneuploidy is regulated by cytoplasmic proteins bound to asbestos fibers (MacCorkle et al., 2006) (see below).

Hypothesis 3. Long asbestos fibers interfere physically with chromosomes to induce carcinogenesis

Morphologic approaches show that asbestos fibers cause aneuploidy, bi-nuclei or multi-nuclei, and chromosomal damage (clastogenicity) after addition to a variety of cell types at cytotoxic concentrations *in vitro* (reviewed in Kane, 1996). These findings suggested that missegregation of chromosomes during mitosis, a process where the outer cell membrane is discontinuous, resulted in cell transformation and cancer (Hesterberg & Barrett, 1985). Studies on rodent cell lines (Syrian hamster embryo cells, Chinese hamster ovary cells, etc.) showed that long, thin fibers (> 5 microns in length and <.25 microns in diameter), including synthetic fiber glasses, as opposed to short fibers of a variety of types, were most potent in induction of chromosomal aberrations. Moreover, rodent assays demonstrated their carcinogenicity after application to the pleura (Stanton et al., 1981). Possible mechanisms were explored in normal rat pleural mesothelial cells: when comparable numbers of long, thin fibers of Canadian chrysotile and crocidolite were tested, more chromosomal abnormalities were observed with crocidolite (Yegles et al., 1993). However, on a per-weight or per-fiber basis, *in vitro* changes were similar. Genetic alterations were not observed using anatase (titanium dioxide) particles, suggesting shape, chemistry, and length were factors in cell response. For example, video-enhanced time-lapse microscopy using amphibian lung epithelial cells showed that long crocidolite asbestos fibers were entrapped in keratin microfilaments protruding into the spindle region during mitosis, whereas short fibers were more effectively encapsulated in the cytoplasm (Ault et al., 1995).

Subsequent species and cell imaging studies suggested that the hypothesis that asbestos fibers physically interacted with nuclear DNA and chromosomes during mitosis to induce cancers was incorrect. For example, cytogenetic studies on human bronchial epithelial cells showed that these cells were resistant to DNA alterations by asbestos (Kodama et al., 1993). Moreover, in human lung fibroblasts, both crocidolite and chrysotile asbestos bound a subset of cytoplasmic proteins known to govern regulation of the cell cycle and mitosis during the process of aneuploidy (MacCorkle et al., 2006). Precoating of fibers with proteins, including tubulin and bovine serum albumin, long known to reduce the cytotoxicity of asbestos (reviewed in HEI, 1991), blocked asbestos-induced aneuploidy, whereas fiber glass (Pyrex from Corning, NY) induced aneuploidy and chromosomal interference in the absence of protein binding. These authors concluded that ". . . natural mineral fibers, like asbestos, that are introduced into the cytoplasm, can effect epigenetic pathways leading to aneuploidy . . . ." (MacCorkle et al., 2006). These data, the fact that mutations observed with asbestos are lethal to cells (Hei et al., 1992), the lack of direct binding of chrysotile or crocidolite asbestos to DNA in lung epithelial cells (Mossman et al., 1983; Eastman et al., 1983), and the lack of demonstration of asbestos fibers in cell nuclei from intact cells or in cells *in vivo* using electron microscopy argue against the mutation/aneuploidy model of cancer causation by physical interference of long fibers. Others have concluded that studies extrapolating results above to human mesothelial cells and purporting that fibers mechanically interfere with the cell spindle during mitosis to cause chromosomal alterations responsible for carcinogenesis are short-term observations because cells die from extensive genetic damage (Carbone et al., 2019). Thus, these studies fail to demonstrate viable clonal cells required for the emergence and propagation of cancers.

In recent years, research emphasis on the mutagenic effects of asbestos has shifted to the elucidation of epigenetic events in mesothelioma. "Epigenetics" is regarded as the study of changes in gene function that cannot be explained solely by changes in the DNA sequence. Recent studies have identified many micro-RNAs and long non-coding RNAs as regulators of gene expression important in the pathogenesis of cancers. In addition, processes of gene and protein methylation and acetylation appear to play key roles in gene expression and chromatin remodeling (reviewed in Mossman, 2017; De Rienzo et al., 2017). In addition, genomic profiling of human MMs has demonstrated the loss of function of several tumor suppressor genes that are important in normal epigenetic regulation, that is, BAP1, SETD2, and DDX3X (Joseph et al., 2016; Zhang et al., 2021). It is likely that multiple epigenetic events control immortalization and cancer progression in mesothelial cells. Other studies suggest that responses to chronic inflammation by long fibers, the tumor microenvironment, and the immune system are "drivers" of MM development. Due to these processes, multiple growth factors and high mobility group box 1 protein (HMGB1, one of several putative carcinogenic factors stimulating the inflammasome in mesothelial cells and other cell types) (Dostert et al., 2008; reviewed in Mossman et al., 2013) are secreted (Suarez et al., 2023; reviewed in Nel et al., 2023).

Hypothesis 4. Amphibole asbestos fibers (crocidolite and amosite) cause production of oxidants that interact with DNA and other organelles to cause cancers.

Decades of research have shown that various types of asbestos cause the generation of reactive oxygen species (ROS) *in vitro* and *in vivo* (reviewed in Shukla et al., 2003). The elaboration of ROS and reactive nitrogen species (RNS) occurs through many chemical reactions, both fiber-driven and cellular. Accordingly, several properties of asbestos fibers have been linked to the generation of oxidants that cause DNA damage and cytotoxicity at high concentrations, and abnormal cell proliferation, an early event in carcinogenesis, at low concentrations. Several mechanisms support the hypothesis that pathogenic fibers generate oxidants through fiber-specific reactions and interactions with cell organelles. First, high iron-containing fibers, such as crocidolite and amosite asbestos, cause iron-catalyzed formation of ROS (reviewed in Shukla et al., 2003). Secondly, crocidolite fibers cause oxidation of membrane lipids and proteins both *in vitro* and after inhalation (Petruska et al., 1991). These changes lead to activation of cell signaling cascades and increases in gene expression (reviewed in Mossman et al., 2006, 2013). At toxic concentrations, formation of the potentially mutagenic DNA lesion, 8-oxo-2' deoxyguanosine, is released from human mesothelial cells (Chen et al., 1996). In phagocytic cells, frustrated uptake of long fibers larger than cell diameters (>20 microns in human phagocytes) is a potent stimulus for the release of ROS that may affect surrounding target cells of disease (reviewed in Mossman et al., 2011).

The induction of DNA repair enzymes, antioxidant enzymes, and elevated levels of glutathione and other naturally occurring antioxidants in cells at lower concentrations of asbestos fibers suggests that cells have a cadre of antioxidant defense responses to pathogenic fibers (reviewed in Cox et al., 2023). These phenomena may explain dose-response effects to asbestos fibers, including toxicity at high concentrations and proliferation or immortalization at low, nonlethal concentrations. It is known that oxidant release due to frustrated phagocytosis of long fibers that exceed the diameter of a cell triggers epigenetic changes and genomic changes in mesothelial cells and MMs. These, in concert with chemokines and cytokines, likely cause a multiplicity of signaling pathways linked to various stages of cell transformation (reviewed in Mossman, 2017).

The lung epithelial cell, a target cell of lung cancers, undergoes sequential changes that are characterized morphologically during its development into carcinomas. These include stages of hyperplasia (increased cell proliferation) progressing to metaplasia (altered cell function), dysplasia (more adverse cell function), carcinoma *in situ* (non-invasive cancers), and eventually invasive tumors (Figure 5.3). Surface macrophages and underlying fibroblasts and matrices of support are preserved in 3-D tracheal organ cultures over months and can be used to determine

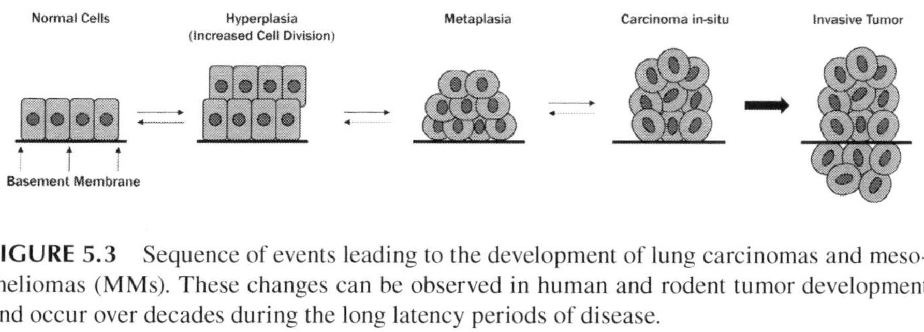

FIGURE 5.3 Sequence of events leading to the development of lung carcinomas and mesotheliomas (MMs). These changes can be observed in human and rodent tumor development and occur over decades during the long latency periods of disease.

cellular responses to fibers and particles. Changes over time and the processing of fibers and particles within and between cells can be examined by using scanning and electron microscopy. In addition, toxicity, hyperplasia, and squamous metaplasia are responses to a number of fiber types (synthetic glass, UICC crocidolite, UICC chrysotile) (Mossman et al., 1977, 1980; Woodworth et al., 1983). Particles including various synthetic glasses, fragments of riebeckite and antigorite, and short (< 5 microns) fibers of chrysotile and attapulgite were used to examine the specificity and extent of responses. Moreover, sized preparations of long fibers of chrysotile (> 10 microns) were also used to determine whether cell effects were exacerbated by long fibers. Studies revealed that the proliferation of epithelial cells significantly increased after 2 weeks of exposure to crocidolite and fiber glasses, whereas metaplasia at one month was also seen with these fiber types and long and short chrysotile. However, both chrysotile preparations caused cytotoxic alterations and loss of epithelial cells. Increases in cytotoxicity, cell proliferation, and metaplasia were not seen with the use of fragments and particles.

The striking effects of crocidolite in these experiments, in terms of increased cell proliferation, metaplasia, and accumulation of macrophages (interpreted as the advent of inflammatory lesions), led to future work comparing molecular responses to this potent asbestos type with fragment preparations of riebeckite containing both fibers and particles. These experiments elucidated the importance of fiber type, shape, and size in a number of protein signaling pathways linked to crocidolite hyperplasia and metaplasia in both lung cancers and MMs (Shukla et al., 2009; reviewed in Heintz et al., 2010). In addition, they demonstrate that many downstream cellular events are linked to oxidant stress and redox-active transcription factor proteins that influence gene expression linked to cell defense, proliferation, and carcinogenesis by crocidolite asbestos (reviewed in Mossman et al., 2013). These events are summarized in Figure 5.4. Note that chronic inflammation caused by elongated mineral fibers, to the right of this diagram, is a function of chemistry (not seen with the dissolution of chrysotile fibers due to leaching of magnesium), length, and durability that involves the persistence of crocidolite and amosite fibers over decades, that is, an average of 40–45 years, the average latency period of human MMs. The fact that amosite and crocidolite persist in human lungs over this time period, whereas chrysotile fibers dissolve into amorphous silica structures (Giacobbe et al., 2020), may explain, in part, why chrysotile is less mesotheliomagenic than amphibole types of asbestos.

CHAIN OF EVENTS IN CELL PROCESSING OF ELONGATED FIBERS

The ability to maintain rodent and human tracheobronchial organ cultures in a differentiated state over time has allowed visualization of the uptake and clearance of elongated fibers of different sizes. Figure 5.5 illustrates the differences in epithelial cell responses to long fibers that exceed the cell diameter of 5–8 microns in lung epithelial cells and shorter fibers that can be successfully phagocytized into membrane-bound phagolysosomes. The left panel shows the normal epithelium, which is characterized by ciliated cells and mucin-secreting cells with surface microvilli. Chrysotile bundles and nonpathogenic particles with wide diameters are transported upward

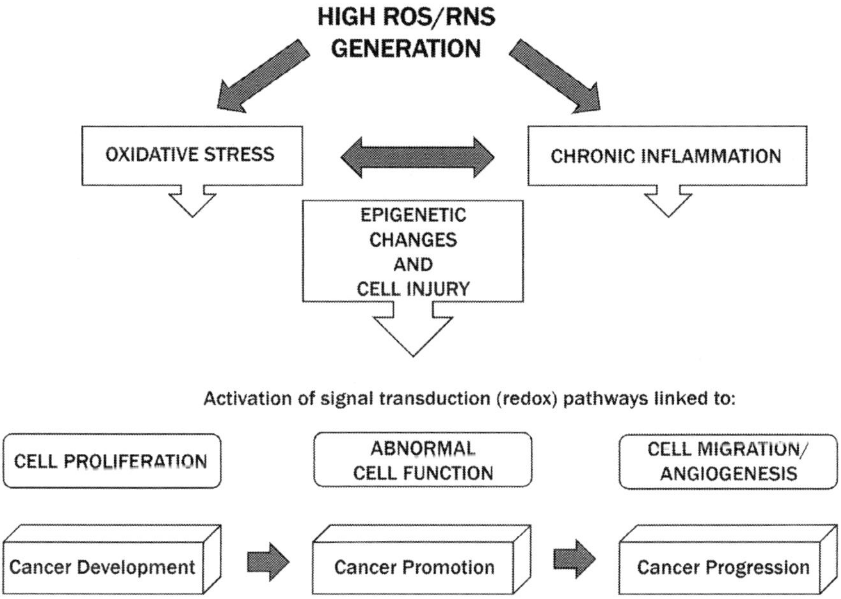

FIGURE 5.4 Mechanisms of oxidant generation and cancer development by the amphibole asbestos types, crocidolite and amosite. Reactive oxygen species (ROS) and reactive nitrogen species (RNS) at high concentrations of asbestos drive cell injury, epigenetic protein pathways, and chronic inflammation, hallmarks of tumor development.

and cleared from the lung by the mucociliary escalator, whereas thinner fibers can penetrate through this barrier and intersect with cell surfaces. Phagocytosis of longer fibers is "frustrated" and unsuccessful (upper middle panel of Figure 5.5), causing oxidant release from cells, while attempts to phagocytize shorter fibers and particles are successful and result in their encapsulation in phagolysosomes without obvious cytotoxicity (bottom middle panels of Figure 5.5). Over a period of weeks to months, the surface epithelial cells in these cultures become squamous and lose their normal differentiation, a process called metaplasia, or loss of normal function. In addition, one can see the excrescences of squamous epithelial cells, a signature of incipient tracheobronchial lung cancers (right panel of Figure 5.5). The accumulation of alveolar macrophages around long fibers signals the release of oxidants, chemokines, and cytokines from cells and the beginnings of an inflammatory response. Studies by others have shown that inflammation occurs preferentially after exposure of rodents to long (> 4–5 microns) vs short fibers of crocidolite asbestos (Goodglick & Kane, 1990), amosite asbestos, and carbon nanotubes (Murphy et al., 2011; Schinwald et al., 2012; reviewed in Nel, 2023). However, chrysotile asbestos is degraded in the acidic environment of the phagolysosome (Jaurand et al., 1984), a possible explanation for its less potent long-term carcinogenicity.

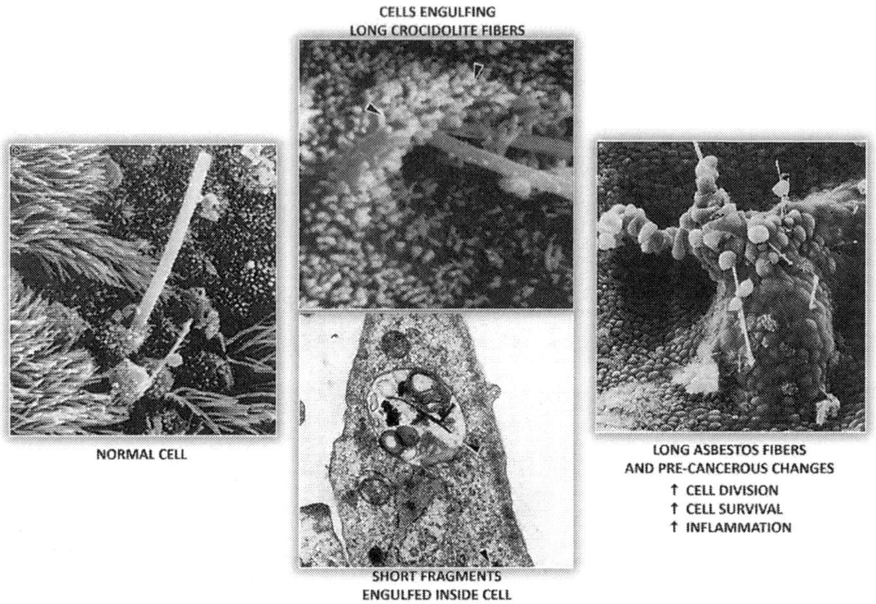

FIGURE 5.5 Epithelial cell responses to long and short crocidolite fibers. Normal mucociliary cells (left panel) proliferate and become squamous in response to long fibers over time (right panel). Increased proliferation and altered cell function are early signatures of carcinomas.

Phagocytosis is also a process by which inflammatory macrophages (Dostert et al., 2008) and mesothelial cells (Hillegass et al., 2013) activate NLRP3 inflammasomes, which are multiprotein cytoplasmic structures that, when activated, result in the secretion of cytokines, pro-inflammatory proteins, and caspases. Assembly, priming, and activation of the inflammasome are linked to oxidative stress caused by crocidolite asbestos due to frustrated phagocytosis. Moreover, actin polymerization during this process is causally linked to the spatial localization and assembly of inflammasome components within human mesothelial cells (MacPherson et al., 2016). These experiments suggest that the frustrated phagocytosis of long fibers initiates chains of events in cells that are linked to inflammation and carcinogenesis.

SUMMARY AND CONCLUSIONS

Long amphibole fibers first interact with the outer membrane of cells to induce cell signaling cascades triggered by oxidant release and possibly other chemical and physical reactions. Epigenetic pathways targeting lipids and proteins that may promote tumor development are complex and have not been exploited to determine the properties of pathogenic fibers important in their causation. Figure 5.6 provides a summary diagram indicating the chain of events in cell processing leading to the successful uptake of short fibers (Figure 5.6A) or the frustrated phagocytosis of long

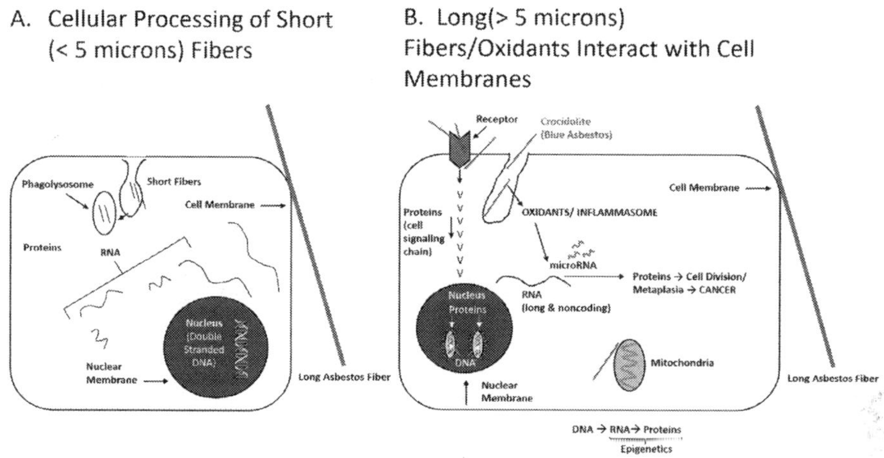

FIGURE 5.6 Cellular processing of short (< 5 microns) (A.) and long (B.) amphibole asbestos fibers and release of oxidants. These events result in oxidation of membrane proteins and lipids, increased expression of early response genes (Janssen et al., 1994a, 1994b), and modifications in cellular organelles such as the inflammasome. Micro (mi)- and long noncoding RNAs, and methylation of histone proteins may be critical to altered cell gene expression and function (reviewed in Mossman, 2017). The diagram is modified from Mossman, 2018.

fibers (Figure 5.6B). As opposed to genetic events that affect the structure of DNA directly, pathogenic fibers elaborate a myriad of oxidants through a variety of surface reactions due to their chemistry and other surface features. Fiber type, shape, and size appear to predominantly govern initial cell responses generating ROS. Oxidants may affect cell surface receptors, membrane proteins, and lipids to initiate phagocytic events after interaction with the plasma membrane and may also affect organelles or proteins and lipids within the cell. Of the features that collectively determine the carcinogenic potential of inhaled elongated fibers (Table 5.2), the shape and dimensions (both length and diameter) of fibers appear to be most important in evoking oxidant production, although iron chemistry and surface features are also critical.

One factor that deserves further exploration is the role of surface area or specific surface area in fiber toxicology. In our dose-response studies using crocidolite asbestos and fibrous talcs, this factor was associated with dose responses measuring cytotoxicity and colony-forming efficiency, a measure of increased cell survival (Wylie et al., 1997). Defining surface area per fiber by its outer surface, as we determined by a nitrogen adsorption assay, may reflect merely the amount of fiber surface interacting with the external cell membrane, but the specific surface area, which is surface area divided by weight or volume, may have a different predictive correlation with carcinogenicity or cytotoxicity.

A number of receptor-dependent and independent protein cascades have been elucidated in lung epithelial cells after exposures to crocidolite or amosite asbestos (reviewed in Mossman et al., 2011, 2013). These may also trigger oxidant formation, antioxidant defenses, and gene expression (Heintz et al., 1993; Hillegass et al., 2010b), sometimes from other organelles such as mitochondria (Kim et al., 2014).

It is generally accepted that membrane-bound asbestos fibers are perinuclear and unable to physically penetrate the nuclear membrane (Ault et al., 1995). Conversely, soluble oxidants elaborated by fibers may be "second messengers" of elongated mineral fibers in causing differences in methylation patterns of DNA and cell signaling proteins through epigenetic pathways (reviewed in Mossman, 2017). Although DNA methylation and other epigenetic signatures (profiles of noncoding RNAs) have been studied in lung cancers and MMs from patient materials (Christensen et al., 2009), only one study has reported patterns of DNA methylation by different types of asbestos fibers (chrysotile, amosite, and crocidolite) in immortalized human bronchial epithelial cells (Öner et al., 2018). DNA methylation was documented on CpG sites, as these are the most common sites of altered DNA methylation in cancers in general. Although chrysotile was the most cytotoxic fiber in these studies, global DNA methylation was only observed after exposures to crocidolite or amosite asbestos. No changes were observed at the lowest concentrations of fibers, suggesting thresholds in response. In future experiments, it will be interesting to connect these patterns to functional changes representative of precancerous alterations as well as the chemical and physical properties of elongated mineral fibers.

The elucidation of size (length and width), shape, and surface area of fibers as important parameters in asbestos carcinogenesis and risk analysis has contributed to QSAR models previously published (Korchevskiy et al., 2019; Korchevskiy & Wylie, 2021; Wylie et al., 2020; Wylie & Korchevskiy, 2023) and described in detail in other chapters of this volume. For example, a parameter called the dimensional coefficient of carcinogenicity (DCC), an excellent predictor of potency for amphiboles, erionite, chrysotile, and fibrous talc, could be coupled with additional parameters of biosolubility and rigidity to evaluate cleavage fragments and nanotube libraries.

It is clear that the development of MM is a disease characterized by epigenetic changes and deletion of tumor suppressor gene function. Epigenetic studies, including mRNA profiling to determine transcriptional changes in gene expression, methylation of DNA and histone proteins surrounding DNA, and profiling of miRNAs in response to well-characterized preparations of mineral fibers, are encouraged in human normal mesothelial and tracheobronchial epithelial cells. Fiber-type-specific alterations and those related to the chemical and physical properties of carcinogenic fibers may reveal common signatures of response that can be linked to preventive approaches to both MMs and lung cancers.

REFERENCE LIST

Agency for Toxic Substances and Disease Registry (ATSDR). (2003). *Report of the expert panel on human effects of asbestos and synthetic vitreous fibers: The influence of fiber length*. ATSDR Division of Health Assessment and Consultation. https://www.atsdr.cdc.gov/HAC/asbestospanel/finalpart1.pdf

Ault, J. G., Cole, R. W., Jensen, C. J., Bachert, L. A., & Rieder, C. L. (1995). Behavior of crocidolite asbestos during mitosis in living vertebrate lung epithelial cells. *Cancer Research*, *55*(4), 792–798. PMID: 7850791.

Badhai, J., Pandey, G. K., Song, J. Y., Krigsman, O., Bhaskaran, R., Chandrasekaran, G., Kwon, M.-C., Bombardelli, L., Monkhorst, K., Grasso, C., Zevenhoven, J., van der Vliet, J., Cozijnsen, M., Krimpenfort, P., Peeper, D., van Lohuizen, M., & Berns, A. (2020). Combined deletion of *Bap1, Nf2* and *Cdkn2ab* causes rapid onset of malignant mesothelioma in mice. *Journal of Experimental Medicine*, *217*(6), e20191257. https://doi.org/10.1084%2Fjem.20191257

Barlow, C. A., Grespin, M., & Best, E. A. (2018). Asbestos fiber length and its relation to disease risk. *Inhalation Toxicology*, *29*(12–14), 541–554. https://doi.org/10.1080/08958378.2018.1435756

Berenblum, I. (1974). *Carcinogenesis as a biological problem*. American Elsevier Publishing Company.

Carbone, M., Adusumilli, P. S., Alexander, H. R., Jr., Baas, P., Bardelli, F., Bononi, A., Bueno, R., Felley-Bosco, E., Galateau-Salle, F., Jablons, D., Mansfield, A. S., Minaai, M., de Perrot, M., Pesavento, P., Rusch, R., Severson, D. T., Taioli, E., Tsao, A., Woodard, G., . . . Pass, H. I. (2019). Mesothelioma: Scientific clues for prevention, diagnosis, and therapy. *CA Cancer Journal for Clinicians*, *69*(5), 402–429. https://doi.org/10.3322/caac.21572

Chen, Q., Marsh, J., Ames, B., & Mossman, B. (1996). Detection of 8-oxo-2'-deoxyguanosine, a marker of oxidative DNA damage, in culture medium from human mesothelial cells exposed to crocidolite asbestos. *Carcinogenesis*, *17*(11), 2525–2527. https://doi.org/10.1093/carcin/17.11.2525

Christensen, B. C., Houseman, E. A., Godleski, J. J., Marsit, C. J., Longacker, J. L., Roelofs, C. R., Karagas, M. R., Wrensch, M. R., Yeh, R-F., Nelson, H. H., Wiemels, J. L., Zheng, S., Wiencke, J. K., Bueno, R., Sugarbaker, D. J., & Kelsey, K. T. (2009). Epigenetic profiles distinguish pleural mesothelioma from normal pleura and predict lung asbestos burden and clinical outcome. *Cancer Research*, *69*(1), 227–234. https://doi.org/10.1158%2F0008-5472.CAN-08-2586

Cox, L. A., Bogen, K. T., Conolly, R., Graham, U., Moolgavkar, S., Oberdorster, G., Roggli, V. L., Turci, F., & Mossman, B. (2023). Mechanisms and shapes of causal exposure-response functions for asbestos in mesotheliomas and lung cancers. *Environmental Research*. https://doi.org/10.1016/j.envres.2023.115607

Craighead, J. E., & Mossman, B. T. (1982). The pathogenesis of asbestos-associated diseases. *New England Journal of Medicine*, *306*(24), 1446–1455. https://doi.org/10.1056/nejm198206173062403

Darnton, L. (2023). Quantitative assessment of mesothelioma and lung cancer risk based on phase contrast microcopy (PCM) estimates of fibre exposure: An update of 2000 asbestos cohort data. *Environmental Research*, *230*, 114753. https://doi.org/10.1016/j.envres.2022.114753

De Rienzo, A., Richards, W. G., & Bueno, R. (2017). Gene signature of malignant pleural mesothelioma. In J. R. Testa (Ed.), *Asbestos and mesothelioma* (Chapter 9. pp. 197–209). Springer International Publishing. https://doi.org/10.1007/978-3-319-53560-9_9

Dostert, C., Pétrilli, V., Van Bruggen, R., Steele, C., Mossman, B. T., & Tschopp, J. (2008). Innate immune activation through Nalp3 inflammasome sensing of asbestos and silica. *Science*, *320*(3876), 674–677. https://doi.org/10.1126/science.1156995

Dragon, J., Thompson, J., MacPherson, M., & Shukla, A. (2015). Differential susceptibility of human pleural and peritoneal mesothelial cells to asbestos exposure. *Journal of Cellular Biochemistry*, *116*(8), 1540–1552. https://doi.org/10.1002%2Fjcb.25095

Drummond, G., Bevan, R., & Harrison, P. (2016). A comparison of the results from intra-pleural and intra-peritoneal studies with those from inhalation and intratracheal tests for the assessment of pulmonary responses to inhalable dusts and fibres. *Regulatory Toxicology and Pharmacology*, *81*, 89–105. https://doi.org/10.1016/j.yrtph.2016.07.019

Eastman, A., Mossman, B. T., & Bresnick, E. (1983). Influence of asbestos on the uptake of benzo(a)pyrene and DNA alkylation in hamster tracheal epithelial cells. *Cancer Research*, *43*(3), 1251–1255. PMID: 6297722.

Endo-Capron, S., Renier, A., Janson, X., Kheuang, L., & Jaurand, M. C. (1993). In vitro response of rat pleural mesothelial cells to talc particles in genotoxicity assays (sister chromatid exchanges and DNA repair). *Toxicology In Vitro*, *7*(1), 7–14. https://doi.org/10.1016/0887-2333(93)90107-g

Garabrant, D. H., & Pastula, S. T. (2018). A comparison of asbestos fiber potency and elongate mineral particle (EMP) potency for mesothelioma in humans. *Toxicology and Applied Pharmacology*, *15*(361), 127–136. https://doi.org/10.1016/j.taap.2018.07.003

Giacobbe, C., Giuseppe, D. D., Zoboli, A., Gualtieri, M. L., Bonasoni, P., Moliterni, A., Corriero, N., Altomare, A., Wright, J., & Gualtieri, A. F. (2020). Crystal structure determination of a lifelong biopersistent asbestos fibre using single-crystal synchrotron X-ray micro-diffraction. *IUCrJ*, *8*, 76–86. https://doi.org/10.1107%2FS2052252520015079

Goodglick, L. A., & Kane, A. B. (1990). Cytot0oxicty of long and short crocidolite asbestos fibers in vitro and in vivo. *Cancer Research*, *50*(16), 5153–5163. PMID: 2165857.

Gualtieri, A. F., Mossman, B. T., & Roggli, V. L. (2017). Towards a general model for predicting the toxicity and pathogenicity of mineral fibres. In A. F. Gualtieri (Ed.), *Mineral fibres: Crystal chemistry, chemical-physical properties, biological interaction and toxicity* (Vol. 18, pp. 501–532). European Mineralogical Union and the Mineralogical Society of the UK and Ireland. https://www.minersoc.org/emu-notes-18-15.html

Haegens, A., van der Vliet, A., Butnor, K. J., Heintz, N., Taatjes, D., Hemenway, D., Vacek, P., Freeman, B. A., Hazen, S. L., Brennan, M. L., & Mossman, B. T. (2005). Asbestos-induced lung inflammation and epithelial cell proliferation are altered in myeloperoxidase-null mice. *Cancer Research*, *65*(21), 9670–9677. https://doi.org/10.1158/0008-5472.can-05-1751

Hanahan, D. (2022). Hallmarks of cancer: New dimensions. *Cancer Discovery*, *12*(1), 31–45. https://doi.org/10.1158/2159-8290.CD-21-1059

Health Effects Institute (HEI). (1991). *Asbestos in public and commercial buildings: A literature review and synthesis of current knowledge* (Special Report). Health Effects Institute.

Hei, T. K., Piao, C. Q., He, Z. Y., Vannais, D., & Waldren, C. A. (1992). Chrysotile fiber is a strong mutagen in mammalian cells. *Cancer Research*, *52*(22), 6305–6309.

Heintz, N. H., Janssen-Heininger, Y. M. W., & Mossman, B. T. (1993). Persistent induction of c-fos and c-jun expression by asbestos. *Proceedings of the National Academy of Sciences of the United States of America*, *90*(8), 3299–3303. https://doi.org/10.1073/pnas.90.8.3299

Heintz, N. H., Janssen-Heininger, Y. M. W., & Mossman, B. T. (2010). Asbestos, lung cancers, and mesotheliomas: From molecular approaches to targeting tumor survival pathways. *American Journal of Respiratory Cell and Molecular Biology*, *42*(2), 133–139. https://doi.org/10.1165/rcmb.2009-0206tr

Hesterberg, T. W., & Barrett, J. C. (1985). Induction by asbestos fibers of anaphase abnormalities: Mechanism for aneuploidy inducti8on and possibly carcinogenesis. *Carcinogenisis*, *6*(3), 473–475. https://doi.org/10.1093/carcin/6.3.473

Hillegass, J. M., Miller, J. M., MacPherson, M. B., Westbom, C. M., Sayan, M., Thompson, J. K., Macura, S. L., Perkins, T. N., Beuschel, S. L., Alexeeva, V., Pass, H. I., Steele, C., Mossman, B. T., & Shukla, A. (2013). Asbestos and erionite prime and activate the NLRP3 inflammasome that stimulates autocrine cytokine release in human mesothelial cells. *Particle and Fibre Toxicology*, *10*, 39. https://doi.org/10.1186/1743-8977-10-39.

Hillegass, J. M., Shukla, A., Lathrop, S. A., MacPherson, M. B., Fukagawa, N. K., & Mossman, B. T. (2010a). Assessing nanotoxicity in cells in vitro. *WIRES Nanomedicine and Nanobiotechnology*, *2*(3), 219–231. https://doi.org/10.1002/wnan.54

Hillegass, J. M., Shukla, A., MacPherson, M. B., Bond, J. P., Steele, C., & Mossman, B. T. (2010b). Utilization of gene profiling and proteomics to determine mineral pathogenicity in a human mesothelial cell line (LP9/TERT-1). *Journal of Toxicology and Environmental Health A*, *73*(5), 423–436. https://doi.org/10.1080%2F15287390903486568

Hodgson, J. T., & Darnton, A. (2000). The quantitative risks of mesothelioma and lung cancer in relation to asbestos exposure. *Annals of Occupational Hygiene*, *44*(8), 565–601. PMID: 11108782

Janssen, Y. M., Heintz, N. H., Marsh, J. P., Borm, P. J., & Mossman, B. T. (1994a). Induction of c-fos and c-jun proto- oncogenes in target cells of the lung and pleura by carcinogenic fibers. *American Journal of Respiratory Cell and Molecular Biology*, *11*(5), 522–530. https://doi.org/10.1165/ajrcmb.11.5.7946382

Janssen, Y. M., Marsh, J. P., Absher, M. P., Gabrielson, E., Borm, P. J., Driscoll, K., & Mossman, B. T. (1994b). Oxidant stress responses in human pleural mesothelial cells exposed to asbestos. *American Journal of Respiratory Critical Care Medicine*, *149*(3 Pt 1), 795–802. https://doi.org/10.1164/ajrccm.149.3.8118652

Jaurand, M. C., Gaudichet, A., Halpern, S., & Bignon, J. (1984). In vitro biodegradation of chrysotile fibres by alveoloar macrophages and mesothelial cells in culture: Comparison with a pH effect. *British Journal of Industrial Medicine*, *41*(3), 389–395. https://doi.org/10.1136%2Foem.41.3.389

Joseph, N. M., Chen, Y. Y., Nasr, A., Yeh, I., Talevich, E., Onodera, C., Bastian, B. C., Rabban, J. T., Garg, K., Zaloudek, C., & Solomon, D. A. (2016). Genomic profiling of malignant peritoneal mesothelioma reveals recurrent alterations in epigenetic regulatory genes BAP1, SETD2, and DDX3X. *Modern Pathology*, *30*(2), 246–254. https://doi.org/10.1038/modpathol.2016.188

Kane, A. B. (1996). Mechanisms of mineral fibre carcinogenesis. In A. B. Kane, P. Boffetta, R. Saracci, & J. D. Wilboum (Eds.), *Mechanisms of fibre carcinogenesis* (IARC Scientific Publication No. 140). IARC Scientific Publication. PMID: 9101315.

Kim, S.-J., Cheresh, P., Williams, D., Cheng, Y., Ridge, K., Schumacker, P. T., Weitzman, S., Bohr, V. A., & Kamp, D. W. (2014). Mitochondria-targeted Ogg1 and aconitase-2 prevent oxidant-induced mitochondrial DNA damage in alveolar epithelial cells. *The Journal of Biological Chemistry*, *289*(9), 6165–6176. https://doi.org/10.1074/jbc.m113.515130

Kodama, Y., Boreiko, C. J., Maness, S. C., & Hesterberg, T. W. (1993). Cytotoxic and cytogenetic effects of asbestos in human bronchial epithelial cells in culture. *Carcinogenesis*, *14*(4), 691–697. https://doi.org/10.1093/carcin/14.4.691

Korchevskiy, A., Rasmuson, J. O., & Rasmuson, E. (2019). Empirical model of mesothelioma potency factors for different mineral fibers based on their chemical composition and dimensionality. *Inhalation Toxicology*, *31*(5), 180–191. https://doi.org/10.1080/08958378.2019.1640320

Korchevskiy, A. A., & Wylie, A. G. (2021). Dimensional determinants for the carcinogenic potency of elongate amphibole particles. *Inhalation Toxicology*, *33*(6–8), 244–259. https://doi.org/10.1080/08958378.2021.1971340

Lippmann, M. (2014). Toxicological and epidemiological studies on effects of airborne fibers: Coherence and public [corrected] health implications. *Critical Reviews in Toxicology*, *44*(8), 643–695. https://doi.org/10.3109/10408444.2014.928266

Lorenzini, E., Ciarrocchi, A, & Torricelli, F. (2021). Molecular fingerprints of malignant pleural mesothelioma: Not just a matter of genetic alterations. *Journal of Clinical Medicine*, *10*(11), 24270. https://doi.org/10.3390/jcm10112470

MacCorkle, R. A., Slattery, S. D., Nash, D. R., & Brinkley, B. R. (2006). Intracellular protein binding to asbestos induced aneuploidy in human lung fibroblasts. *Cell Motility and the Cytoskeleton*, *63*(10), 646–657. https://doi.org/10.1002/cm.20151

MacPherson, M., Westbom, C., Kogan, H., & Shukla, A. (2016). Actim polymerization plays a significant role in asbestos-induced inflammasome activation in mesothelial cells *in vitro*. *Histochemistry and Cell Biology*, *147*(5), 595–604. https://doi.org/10.1007%2Fs00418-016-1530-8

Mossman, B. T. (1990). In vitro studies on the biologic effects of fibers: Correlation with in vivo bioassays. *Environmental Health Perspectives*, *88*, 319–322. https://doi.org/10.1289%2Fehp.9088319

Mossman, B. T. (2008). Assessment of the pathogenic potential of asbestiform vs. nonasbestiform particulates (cleavage fragments) in in vitro (cell or organ culture) models and bioassays. *Regulatory Toxicology and Pharmacology*, *52*(Suppl 1), S200–S203. https://doi.org/10.1016/j.yrtph.2007.10.004

Mossman, B. T. (2017). Cell signaling and epigenetic mechanisms in mesothelioma. In J. Testa (Ed.), *Asbestos and mesothelioma: Current cancer research*. Springer. https://doi.org/10.1007/978-3-319-53560-9_10

Mossman, B. T. (2018). Mechanistic in vitro studies: What they have told us about carcinogenic properties of elongated mineral particles (EMPs). *Toxicology and Applied Pharmacology*, *361*, 62–67. https://doi.org/10.1016/j.taap.2018.07.018

Mossman, B. T., Bignon, J., Corn, M., Seaton, A., & Gee, J. B. (1990). Asbestos: Scientific developments and implication for public policy. *Science*, *247*(4940), 294–301. https://doi.org/10.1126/science.2153315

Mossman, B. T., & Craighead, J. E. (1979). Use of hamster tracheal organ cultures for assessing the cocarcinogenic effects of inorganic particulates on the respiratory epithelium. *Progress in Experimental Tumor Research*, *24*, 37–47. https://doi.org/10.1159/000402082

Mossman, B. T., & Craighead, J. E. (1982). Comparative cocarcinogenic effects of crocidolite asbestos, hematite, kaolin, and carbon in implanted tracheal organ cultures. *Annals of Occupational Hygiene*, *26*(1–4), 553–567.

Mossman, B. T., Craighead, J. E., & MacPherson, B. V. (1980). Asbestos-induced epithelial changes in organ cultures of hamster trachea: Inhibition by retinyl methyl ether. *Science*, *207*(4428), 311–313. https://doi.org/10.1126/science.7350661

Mossman, B. T., Eastman, A., Landesman, J. M., & Bresnick, E. (1983). Effects of crocidolite and chrysotile asbestos on cellular uptake and metabolism of benzo(a)pyrene in hamster tracheal epithelial cells. *Environmental Health Perspectives*, *51*, 331–335. https://doi.org/10.1289/ehp.8351331

Mossman, B. T., & Gee, J. B. (1989). Asbestos-related diseases. *New England Journal of Medicine*, *320*(26), 1721–1730. https://doi.org/10.1056/nejm198906293202604

Mossman, B. T., & Gualtieri, A. F. (2020). Lung cancers: Mechanisms of asbestos carcinogenesis by asbestos. In S. Antilla & P. Boffetta (Eds.), *Occupational cancers* (2nd ed., pp. 236–239). Springer Nature Global. https://link.springer.com/chapter/10.1007/978-3-030-30766-0_12

Mossman, B. T., Kessler, J. B., Ley, B. W., & Craighead, J. E. (1977). Interaction of crocidolite asbestos with hamster respiratory mucosa in organ culture. *Laboratory Investigation*, *36*(2), 131–139. PMID: 839730.

Mossman, B. T., Light, W., & Wei, E. (1983). Asbestos: Mechanisms of toxicity and carcinogenicity in the respiratory tract. *Annual Review of Pharmacology and Toxicology*, *23*, 595–615. https://doi.org/10.1146/annurev.pa.23.040183.003115

Mossman, B. T., Lippman, M., Hesterberg, T. W., Kelsey, K. T., Barchowsky, A., & Bonner, J. C. (2011). Pulmonary endpoints (lung carcinomas and asbestosis) following inhalation exposures to asbestos. *Journal of Toxicology and Environmental Health, Part B*, *14*(1–4), 76–121. https://doi.org/10.1080/10937404.2011.556047

Mossman, B. T., Lounsbury, K., & Reddy, S. P. (2006). Oxidants and signaling by mitogen-activated protein kinases in lung epithelium. *American Journal of Respiratory Cell and Molecular Biology*, *34*(6), 666–669. https://doi.org/10.1165%2Frcmb.2006-0047SF

Mossman, B. T., Shukla, A., Heintz, N. H., Verschraegen, C. F., Thomas, A., & Hassan, R. (2013). New insights into understanding the mechanisms, pathogenesis, and management of malignant mesotheliomas. *American Journal of Pathology*, *182*(4), 1065–1077. https://doi.org/10.1016/j.ajpath.2012.12.028

Murphy, F. A., Poland, C. A., Duffin, R., Al-Jamal, K. T., Ali-Boucetta, H., Nunes, A., Byrne, F., Prina-Mello, A., Volkov, Y., Li, S., Mather, S. J., Bianco, A., Prato, M., Macnee, W., Wallace, W. A., Kostarelos, K., & Donaldson, K. (2011). Length-dependent retention of carbon nanotubes in the pleural space of mice initiates sustained inflammation and progressive fibrosis on the parietal pleura. *American Journal of Pathology*, *178*(6), 2587–2600. https://doi.org/10.1016/j.ajpath.2011.02.040

Nel, A. E. (2023). Carbon nanotube pathogenicity conforms to a unified theory for mesothelioma causation by elongate minerals and fibers. *Environmental Research*, *230*, 114580. https://doi.org/10.1016/j.envres.2022.114580

Nel, A. E., Pavlisko, E. N., & Roggli, V. L. (2023). The interplay between the immune system, tumor suppressor gene, and immune senescence in mesothelioma development and response to immunotherapy. *Journal of Thoracic Oncology*, *19*(4), 551–564. https://doi.org/10.1016/j.tho.2023.11.017

Öner, D., Ghosh, M., Moisse, M., Duca, R. C., Coorens, R., Vanoirbeek, J. A., Lambrechts, D., Godderis, L., & Hoet, P. H. (2018). Global and gene-specific DNA methylation effects of different asbestos fibres on human bronchial epithelial cells. *Environment International*, *115*, 301–311. https://doi.org/10.1016/j.envint.2018.03.031

Pelé, J. P., & Calvert, R. (1983). Hemolysis by chrysotile asbestos fibers. I: Influence of the sialic acid content in human, rat, and sheep red blood cell membranes. *Journal of Toxicology and Environmental Health*, *12*(4–6), 827–840. https://doi.org/10.1080/15287398309530473

Petruska, J. M., Leslie, K. O., & Mossman, B. T. (1991). Enhanced lipid peroxidation in lung lavage of rats after inhalation of asbestos. *Free Radical Biology & Medicine*, *11*(4), 425–432. https://doi.org/10.1016/0891-5849(91)90160–5

Reid, G. (2015). MicroRNAs in mesothelioma: From tumour suppressors and biomarkers to therapeutic targets. *Journal of Thoracic Disease*, *7*(6), 1031–1040. https://doi.org/10.3978/j.issn.2072-1439.2015.04.56

Roggli, V. L. (2015). The so-called short-fiber controversy: Literature review and critical analysis. *Archives of Pathology & Laboratory Medicine*, *139*(8), 1052–1057. https://doi.org/10.5858/arpa.2014-0466-ra

Schinwald, A., Murphy, F. A., Prina-Mello, A., Poland, C. A., Byrne, F., Movia, D., Glass, J. R., Dickerson, J. C., Schultz, D. A., Jeffree, C. E., MacNee, W., & Donaldson, K. (2012). The threshold length for fiber-induced acute pleural inflammation: Shedding light on the early events in asbestos-induced mesothelioma. *Toxicological Sciences*, *128*(2), 461–470. https://doi.org/10.1093/toxsci/kfs171

Shukla, A., Gulumian, M., & Hei, T. K. (2003). Multiple roles of oxidants in the pathogenesis of asbestos-induced diseases. *Free Radical Biology and Medicine*, *34*(9), 1117–1129. https://doi.org/10.1016/s0891-5849(03)00060-1

Shukla, A., MacPherson, M. B., & Hillegass, J. (2009). Alterations in gene expression in human mesothelial cells correlate with mineral pathogenicity. *American Journal of Respiratory Cell and Molecular Biology*, *41*(1), 114–123. https://doi.org/10.1165/rcmb.2008-0146oc

Stanton, M. F., Layarad, M., Tegeris, A., Miller, E., May, M., Morgan, E., & Smith, A. (1981). Relation of particle dimensions to carcinogenicity in amphibole asbestos and other fibrous minerals. *Journal of the National Cancer Institute*, *67*(5), 965–975.

Suarez, J. S., Novelli, F., & Goto, K. (2023). HMGB1 released by mesothelial cells drives the development of asbestos-induced mesothelioma. *Proceedings of the National Academy of Sciences of the United States of America*, *120*(39), e2307999120. https://doi.org/10.1073/pnas.2307999120

Woodworth, C. D., Mossman, B. T., & Craighead, J. E. (1982). Comparative effects of fibrous and nonfibrous minerals on cells and liposomes. *Environmental Research*, *27*(1), 190–205. https://doi.org/10.1016/0013-9351(82)90070-6

Woodworth, C. D., Mossman, B. T., & Craighead, J. E. (1983). Induction of squamous metaplasia in organ cultures of hamster trachea by naturally occurring and synthetic fibers. *Cancer Research*, *43*(10), 4906–4912. PMID: 6883341.

World Health Organization (WHO). (1987). *IARC monographs on the evaluation of the carcinogenic risks to humans. Overall evaluations of carcinogenicity: An updating of IARC monographs volumes 1 to 42* (IARC Monograph). WHO.

World Health Organization (WHO). (2012). *Arsenic, metals, fibres, and dusts* (IARC Monograph No. 100C, p. 465). Working Group on the Evaluation of Carcinogenic Risks to Humans.

Wylie, A. G., & Korchevskiy, A. A. (2023). Dimensions of elongate mineral particles and cancer. A review. *Environmental Research, 2300*, 114688. https://doi.org/10.1016/j.envres.2022.114688

Wylie, A. G., Korchevskiy, A. A., Segrave, A. M., & Duane, A. (2020). Modeling mesothelioma risk factors from amphibole fiber dimensionality: Mineral and epidemiological perspective. *Journal of Applied Toxicology*, *40*(4), 515–524. https://doi.org/10.1002/jat.3923

Wylie, A. G., Skinner, H. C., Marsh, J., Snyder, H., Garzione, C., Hodkinson, D., Winters, R., & Mossman, B. T. (1997). Mineralogical features associated with cytotoxic and proliferative effects of fibrous talc and asbestos on rodent tracheal epithelial and pleural mesothelial cells. *Toxicology and Applied Pharmcology*, *147*, 143–150. https://doi.org/10.1006/taap.1997.8276

Yegles, M., Saint-Etienne, L., Renier, A., Janson, S., & Jaurand, M. C. (1993). Induction of metaphase and anaphase/telophase abnormalities by asbestos fibers in rat pleural mesothelial cells in vitro. *American Journal of Respiratory Cell and Molecular Biology*, *9*(2), 186–191. https://doi.org/10.1165/ajrcmb/9.2.186

Yoshida, G. J. (2019). Letter to the editor. Beyond Stanton and Pott hypothesis: Carbon nanotubes-induced malignant mesothelioma as a disease of gene loss. *Journal of Occupational Health*, *61*, 203–205. https://doi.org/10.1002/1348-9585.12019

Yuan, L., Sun, B. M., Liangliang, X., Chen, L., & Ou, W. (2021). The updating of biological functions of methyltransferase SETDB1 and its relevance in lung cancer and mesothelioma. *International Journal of Molecular Science*, *22*, 7416. https://doi.org/10.3390/ijms22147416

Zhang, M., Luo, J.-L., Sun, Q., Harber, J., Dawson, A. G., Nakas, A., Busacca, S., Sharkey, A. J., Waller, D., Sheaff, M. T., Richards, C., Wells-Jordan, P., Gaba, A., Poile, C., Baitei, E. Y., Bzura, A., Dzialo, J., Jama, M., Le Quesne, J., . . . Fenell, D. A. (2021). Clonal architecture in mesothelioma is prognostic and shapes the tumor environment. *Nature Communications*. https://doi.org/10.1038/s41467-021-21798-w

6 Elongate mineral particles in tissue

Physical and mineralogical characteristics of retained EMPs

Ann Wylie, Andrey Korchevskiy, and Richard Attanoos

INTRODUCTION

"Asbestos" is an unusual carcinogen. The process of hazard identification, risk assessment, and classification of any carcinogen is complex, but this is particularly so when seeking to evaluate non-uniform and heterogeneous materials like asbestos. "Asbestos" refers to a specific habit of minerals from two very common groups of minerals, amphiboles and serpentine, which are known to have widely varied physicochemical properties, inhomogeneous populations of elongate mineral particles in aerosols and in respired fractions, and widely different effects in tissue, from innocuous to cytotoxic to carcinogenic. Recorded length and width dimensions range over orders of magnitude, and they change from one occurrence to another and from one elongate mineral particle (EMP) to another, all the while maintaining an aspect ratio of at least 3:1. The carcinogen is not "asbestos" as a whole, but those elongate mineral particles (EMPs) within an asbestos exposure that possess carcinogenic properties, a proportion that is variable across occurrences.

The inhomogeneity of inhaled aerosolized EMPs means that they have differing potentials for penetrating the various regions of the respiratory tract, including the tracheobronchial site, alveolar region, lung interstitium, pleura tissue, and other organs in the body. The likelihood of elongate mineral particles being found in lung burden samples depends on prior exposures and their physical and chemical properties. If carcinogenic EMPs must be in physical contact with the target tissue to initiate a tissue reaction, whether inflammation or a complex series of processes resulting in cancer, then that contact will depend on the characteristics of the EMP. It is essential to differentiate carcinogenic EMPs from other mineral dusts based on the properties that govern an EMP's ability to reach target tissues (along with other factors and processes impacting the carcinogenicity of EMPs). Mesothelioma is the most specific and important cancer for analysis because of its reported close association

DOI: 10.1201/9781003424277-7

with amphibole asbestos, difficulty in diagnosis, aggressive clinical course, and poor prognosis. Also, although cancer is the most critical type of EMP-related health outcome, other conditions are related to asbestos exposure.

The properties of the particles that govern their ability to be deposited and then translocated elsewhere in the body include such interrelated characteristics as biopersistence, rigidity, dimension, density, and potential for disaggregation. These properties affect all parts of the journey from exposure to target tissue and include transportation in the airways, deposition in the pulmonary system, translocation, and clearance. If an EMP must translocate from the lung to the parietal and peritoneal pleura to cause mesothelioma, which most accept as highly probable (Cook et al., 2016; Donaldson et al., 2010), or be retained in the lung over a long period for lung cancer or lung fibrosis (asbestosis) to develop, then better understanding the characteristics of particles deposited in the lung or capable of reaching the pleura and other organs would clarify the nature of mineral EMP carcinogens generally. In addition, dimensions and mineral composition govern the ability of EMPs to penetrate the membrane of target cells and potentially damage cell nuclei, another element of dose delivery that may be an important characteristic of an EMP carcinogen. Cell dimensions also impact the interaction between elongate mineral particles and macrophages.

This chapter looks at the particles that make up so-called lung burden, meaning EMPs that have been inhaled and retained. The physical and chemical properties that are likely to enhance or limit EMP inhalation, deposition, and translocation are discussed. There is an examination of what is precisely known about the nature of elongate mineral particles recovered from lungs and other tissues in an attempt to understand the characteristics of deposited and translocated EMPs and to define a carcinogenic EMP. Further, this chapter addresses the characteristics of particle populations that can be used as surrogate aerosols to which lung burden can be compared. Such an analysis sheds light on the properties of particles that, when inhaled, can lead to the development of fibrosis, lung cancer, mesothelioma, and other cancers, and it could also enable more effective worker protection against asbestos-related diseases by enhanced monitoring of EMPs with high carcinogenic potential.

DEFINITIONS FOR INHALABLE AEROSOL-SIZED PARTICLES

Inhalable means particles that can enter the nose or mouth during breathing. Thoracic means particles that also enter the large airways and the ciliated portion of the airways. Respirable means particles that can reach the alveolar region of the lung beyond the ciliated airways and enter the lung interstitium. Only respirable elongate particles are likely to translocate to the pleura.

PROCESSES THAT AFFECT TISSUE BURDEN OF EMPS

To better understand the relevance of the dimensions of EMPs found in lung burden to the dimension of inhalable EMPs in the aerosol or of EMPs that ultimately cause mesothelioma, we will first review the processes that affect the dimensional characteristics of EMPs.

Respirability

First, as noted above, EMPs that enter the body through respiration must be "respirable" to gain access to the lung interstitium. If Brown et al. (2013) are correct, all will have average aerodynamic diameters < 4 μm. Although particles with 4 <AD < 10 μm can be inhaled, they will be largely deposited prior to entering the deep lung. For rigid EMPs traveling parallel to the airstream, the aerodynamic diameter is largely influenced by the width.

Deposition

Various parameters affect the ability of particles to be deposited in human lungs.

According to Fernández Tena and Casan Clarà (2012), the particles can be deposited by means of four mechanisms:

1. *Impaction*. This is the phenomenon by which the particles of an aerosol continue on a trajectory when they travel through the airway, instead of conforming to the curves of the respiratory tract. Tena and Clara suggested that particles with enough momentum are affected by centrifugal force at the points where the airflow suddenly changes direction, colliding with the airway wall. This mainly happens in the first 10 bronchial generations, where the air speed is high and the flow is turbulent. This phenomenon apparently affects particles larger than one micron, which are mostly retained in the oropharyngeal region.
2. *Interception*. This mechanism was suggested as especially relevant to elongated particles. The particles are assumed to be deposited as soon as they contact the airway wall.
3. *Sedimentation*. This is the physical phenomenon by which particles with sufficient mass are deposited due to the force of gravity when they remain in the airway for a sufficient length of time. This apparently predominates in the last five bronchial generations, where the air speed is slow and the residence time is longer.
4. *Suspension*. This is the process by which the particles of aerosol move erratically from one place to another in the airways. This happens as a consequence of the Brownian diffusion of particles with an aerodynamic diameter smaller than 0.5 μm when they reach the alveolar spaces, where the air speed is practically zero. Based on Tena and Clara, these particles are generally not expected to be deposited, and they are expelled once again upon exhalation.

It was suggested that spherical particles with an aerodynamic diameter larger than 10 μm are mostly deposited in the oropharynx, those with aerodynamic diameter between 5 and 10 μm in the central airways, and those from 0.5 to 5 μm in the small airways and alveoli. However, it can be expected that elongated particles behave differently than spherical ones when entering the respiratory system of humans or animals.

According to the multiple-path particle dosimetry (MPPD) model developed by the United States Environmental Protection Agency (U.S. EPA), the likelihood of an inhaled EMP with an aspect ratio of 10:1 being deposited in the pulmonary region is lowest when the diameter is 0.30 μm, increasing until the diameter reaches about 2 μm (Asgharian et al., 2018). If the aspect ratio is 50:1, the lowest deposition takes place at a diameter of about 0.1 μm and the maximum retention at a diameter of 1 μm. The model also predicts that any EMP narrower than 0.30 μm (or 0.1 μm) should be deposited in increasing proportions, reaching almost 20% of the 0.02 μm particles in the aerosol. However, lung burden EMP populations do not just mirror the likelihood of one EMP size over another depositing in the deep lung. The dimensional composition of lung burden also reflects the abundances of the various EMP sizes in the aerosol.

As we will demonstrate in this chapter, there is an obvious discrepancy between the size-resolved deposition model by the EPA and observed populations of elongate particles in lungs. It should be remembered that validation of the lung deposition model for elongate mineral particles is quite limited, and further studies are needed to fully see how dimensional parameters affect the modeled estimations of the deposition rate. In this chapter, we will explore what dimensional characteristics of EMPs deposited in human lungs can tell us about the deposition process and the probability that EMPs will be deposited and translocated to the pleura. Also, EMP transport to the pleura is not covered by the U.S. EPA model. The correlation between the biological effects of EMPs and the MPPD-predicted pulmonary lung deposition of EMPs appears to be low.

Disaggregation

Because asbestos forms in bundles of individual single crystals (*fibrils*) that are not bonded to each other chemically and are easily separable by hand pressure, these bundles may separate or *disaggregate* into their constituent fibrils after they have been inhaled and deposited. Animal evidence for the breakup or disaggregation following deposition in the lung of asbestiform bundles of mineral fiber of all types is abundant, although results on the degree appear somewhat conflicting, in part because of the heterogeneity of "asbestos" source samples, specimen preparation, and differences among *in vivo* methods of analysis. For example, Coffin et al. (1982) exposed rats to amosite and ferro-actinolite asbestos by intratracheal and intraperitoneal injection, and then sequentially sacrificed the animals. After all exposure ceased, the number of EMPs per gram of lung tissue with narrow widths rose for 200 days for amosite and 400 days for ferro-actinolite asbestos, before clearance outpaced disaggregation and the EMP number began slowly decreasing to approximately the initial number at two years. Coin et al. (1992) concluded that the number of chrysotile fibers greater than 16 μm in length that appeared to clear slowly were actually increasing in number due to longitudinal splitting of bundles. It should be noted that Bernstein et al. (2013) criticized the publication by Coin for certain methodological discrepancies. Bellman et al. (1986) report that following rat lung instillation, the number of chrysotile fibers longer than 5 μm doubled over a year. Single, short chrysotile fibrils ($L < 2$ μm) are very common in tissue (see Table 6.1 and Figure 6.1).

TABLE 6.1
Chrysotile

	Notes	Reference	Width			Length			Length
			GM (µm)	Mean (µm)	Median (µm)	GM (µm)	Mean (µm)	Median (µm)	Restriction (µm)
Lung		Pooley and Clark (1980)		0.07			1.8		
	Cement	Pooley and Mitha (1986)	0.06			1.1			
	Textile	Pooley and Mitha (1986)	0.06			2.4			
	Control C	Pooley and Mitha (1986)	0.06			1.2			
	Control t	Pooley and Mitha (1986)	0.06			0.9			
		Warnock (1989)			0.05			1.7	
		Warnock (1989)	0.09 (1.89)			10.88 (1.79)			L > 5
	Charleston	Sebastien et al. (1989)		0.1			7.9		L > 5
	Thetford	Sebastien et al. (1989)		0.07			8.3		L > 5
		Dodson et al. (1990)	0.05			1.51			
		Dodson et al. (1990)	0.06			0.85			
		Gibbs et al. (1990)	0.06			1.1			
	Fibrosis upper	Gibbs et al. (1991)	0.06 (0.13)			1.39 (0.89)			
	Fibrosis central	Gibbs et al. (1991)	0.07 (0.22)			1.32 (0.89)			
		Tuomi (1992)		0.05	0.05		1	0.9	
	Normal	Friedrichs et al. (1992)	0.05 (1.7)			1.4 (2.1)			L > 1
	Lung cancer	Friedrichs et al. (1992)	0.07 (1.8)			2.3 (2.6)			L > 1
	Asbestosis	Friedrichs et al. (1992)	0.07 (1.9)			1.7 (1.9)			L > 1
		Friedrichs et al. (1992)	0.06 (1.6)			2 (2.3)			L > 1
	Other industry	Dufresne et al. (1996)	0.05 (1.6)			1.5 (1.8)			L < 5

(*Continued*)

TABLE 6.1 *(Continued)*
Chrysotile

			Width			Length			Length
	Notes	Reference	GM (μm)	Mean (μm)	Median (μm)	GM (μm)	Mean (μm)	Median (μm)	Restriction (μm)
	Asbestos	Dufresne et al. (1996)	0.05 (1.4)			1.9 (1.6)			L < 5
	Thetford	Dufresne et al. (1996)	0.05 (1.5)			1.9 (1.7)			L < 5
	Other industry	Dufresne et al. (1996)	0.06 (1.9)			7.8 (1.5)			L > 5
	Asbestos	Dufresne et al. (1996)	0.05 (1.7)			7.2 (1.5)			L > 5
	Thetford	Dufresne et al. (1996)	0.05 (1.3)			7.6 (1.4)			L > 5
	Background	Dodson et al. (1999)	0.06			1.81			
		Suzuki and Yuen (2002)	0.04 (1.46)			0.42 (2.26)			
		Dodson et al. (2005)	0.064			5.53			
		Cardiff audit information (see this chapter)	0.12 (1.62)			9.48 (1.71)			L > 5
Pleura	Lung cancer	Dodson et al. (2004)	0.06			5.58			
	Visceral pleura	Gibbs et al. (1991)	0.06 (0.13)			0.96 (0.79)			
	Plaque	Suzuki and Kohyama (1991)	0.04 (1.46)			0.39 (2.37)			
	Tumor	Suzuki and Kohyama (1991)	0.04 (1.36)			0.35 (1.97)			
Lymph node		Dodson et al. (1990)	0.06			0.94			

(a)

(b)

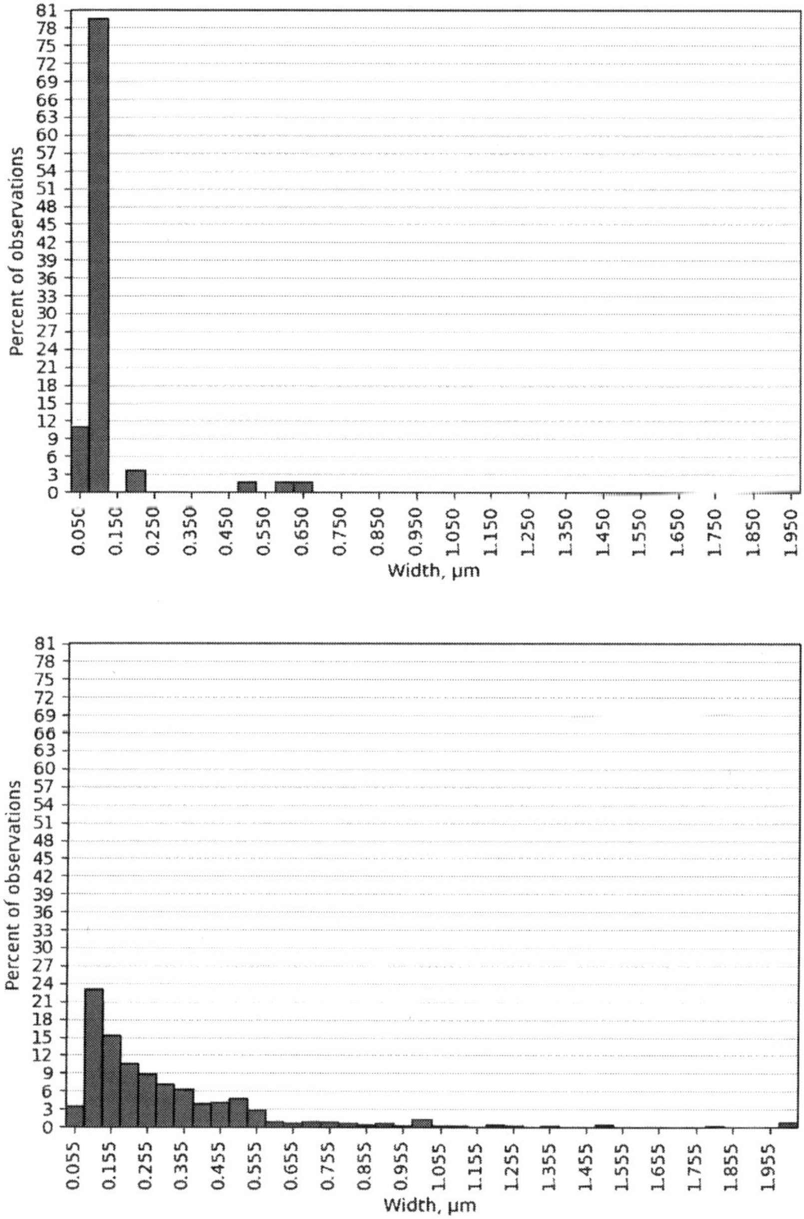

FIGURE 6.1 Chrysotile frequencies of width and length. a) Cardiff audit data. Width for L > 5 µm. N = 54, Bin width = 0.05 µm, GM width = 0.14 µm, range 0.05–0.66 µm. b) "Aerosol" (airborne TEM data from Swift Creek, CA, El Dorado, CA, Quebec, NC textiles, European textile, cement plant, and friction plant). Width for L > 5 µm. N = 2022, GM width = 0.29 µm, range 0.03–2.0 µm. c) Cardiff audit data. Length < 50 µm (longer than 50 µm not shown = 0% of all EMP). N = 276, Bin width = 1 µm, GM length = 4.0 µm, range 0.6–48 µm. d) "Aerosol." Length < 50 µm (longer than 50 µm not shown = 0.2% of all EMP). N = 27612, Bin width = 1 µm, GM length = 2.23, range 0.045–115.7 µm. Proportion of lengths greater than 5 µm = 19.6% for Cardiff audit data and 7% of aerosol comparison.

(c)

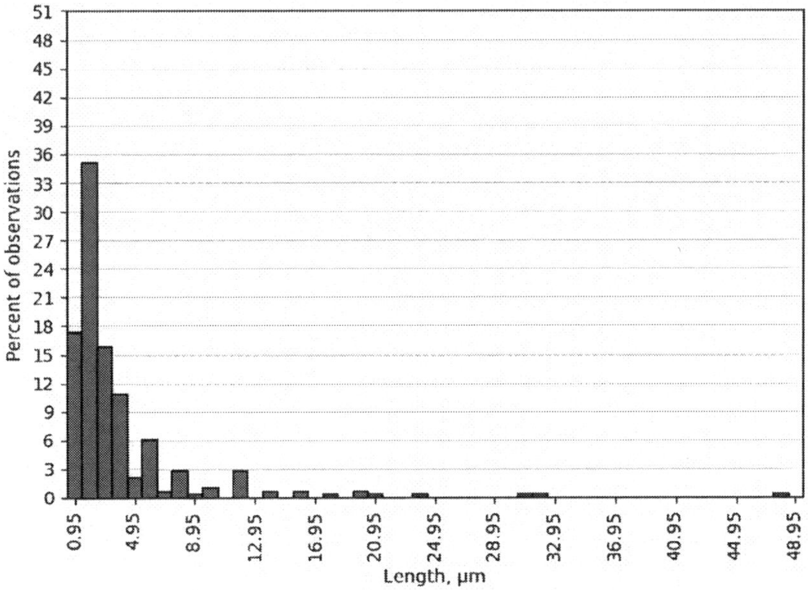

(d)

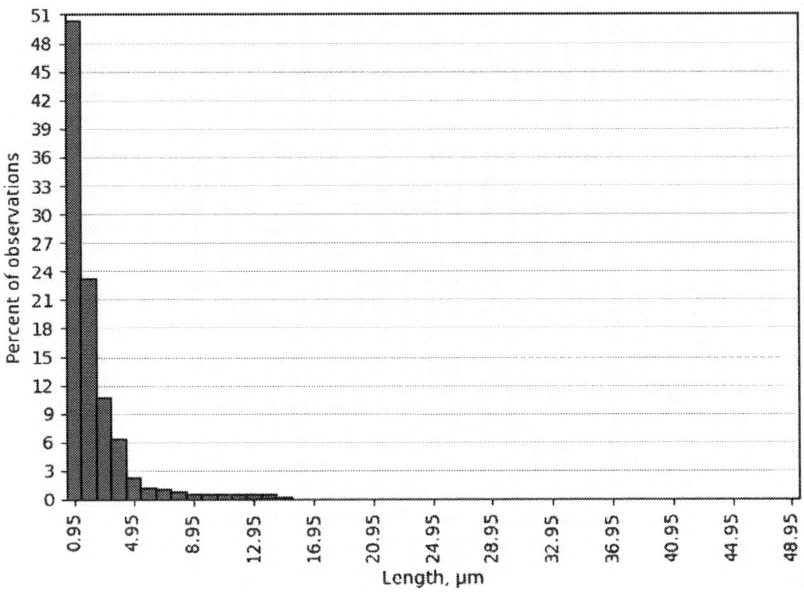

FIGURE 6.1 (Continued)

It is not uncommon to find them in lymph tissue many years after exposure ceased (Velasco-García et al., 2017).

If the disaggregation process continues throughout the residency of fiber bundles in the lung, a renewing supply of "new" very narrow fibers would be available, increasing the dose measured by fiber number abundance and altering fiber dimensions following exposure (Langer et al., 1970; Uibu et al., 2009). It is likely that the frequency of "new" fibers would decrease over decades, even among the most friable asbestos occurrences. Nonetheless, there exist opposing effects; the process of disaggregation increasing fiber number is counter to clearance, which seeks to reduce EMP number, thereby complicating our understanding of both processes and, in turn, the interpretation of observed EMP content and its relation to disease.

Inhaled chrysotile EMPs are subject to rapid disaggregation into fibrils in the host acidic microenvironment. Macrophage phagolysosomes at pH 4.5 readily deplete the magnesium layer, dissociating the crystalline integrity of serpentine. Ingested macrophages cleared by the mucociliary apparatus are subsequently cleared into the gastrointestinal system and face gastric (hydrochloric) acid (pH 1). Inhaled chrysotile bundles are thereby rapidly disaggregated into fibrils and are biosoluble in such acidic host settings (Oze & Solt, 2010). Chrysotile fibrils found in human tissue are commonly reported as < 0.04 μm in diameter (see Table 6.1). These are rolled tubes whose outer diameter is limited by the geometry of the tube; only rarely do fibrils have diameters with widths > 0.10 μm. The geology of asbestiform amphiboles is different: bundles of crocidolite fibrils from South Africa and Australia disaggregate readily, while South African amosite fibrils are somewhat more resistant. Nonetheless, one can see from the lung burden data that a large portion of the deposited EMPs have the widths of nanofibers.

Due to its unique crystalline habit, only asbestiform mineral EMPs will separate into populations of narrow, high aspect ratio fibrils following inhalation. Elongate mineral particles that are formed from the breakage of rock are not aggregates of fibrils, but instead are single crystals, covalently bonded solids that take considerable force to break into smaller particles. There is no evidence that any biological process mechanically reduces the size of inhaled particles except through enhancing the disaggregation of bundles and agglomerates.

Clearance

It is generally accepted that the retention of EMPs, or the inability for their clearance, correlates with cancer risk. Once inhaled and deposited in the pulmonary system, clearance processes begin to sort out the EMP burden. The largest particles deposited in or near the ciliated portions of the airways move along the mucociliary escalator toward the esophagus and are swallowed, providing a potential pathway to the peritoneal cavity.

EMPs deposited outside the mucociliary escalator in deeper parts of the lung can remain or be removed by other processes. Phagocytes can engulf them if they are smaller than about 10 μm in length and deposit them in the lymph nodes, where they enter the blood; although particles longer than 5 μm can cause impairment of phagocyte function (Schinwald et al., 2012). EMPs can remain in the pulmonary interstitium, where some are coated, forming the core of asbestos bodies. Some, such as wollastonite, chrysotile, and fibrous glass, may dissolve. Some of the EMPs will translocate through the lung interstitium, migrating toward the lung periphery and eventually to the pleura, probably through the blood and lymph systems.

EMPs of different minerals and different occurrences of the same mineral can be cleared at different rates because of the differences in their physical and chemical properties. While chrysotile was the most abundant fiber type used in commercial applications, in almost all reports, amphibole EMPs outnumber chrysotile in lung burden, widely interpreted as evidence for the more rapid clearance of chrysotile over amphibole. Early work on the more rapid clearance of chrysotile is summarized in WHO (1986). Berry et al. (2009) showed that over time, among mesothelioma patients from a gas mask factory, the concentration in lung burden of EMPs longer than 6 μm increased from < 10% in 1965 to almost 40% in 1988. There was no significant change in width over time, with 85 to 95% of the EMPs having W< 0.125 μm. They interpret this change in length frequency as more effective clearance of short EMPs.

Different types of mineral EMPs vary by their clearance rate. Korchevskiy and Wylie (2022) reviewed literature sources regarding the clearance rate of EMPs and developed a model for the estimation of lung burden concentrations based on exposure. See Chapter 4 of this book for more information.

Phagocytosis

The macrophage clearance mechanism, phagocytosis, is believed to have a length threshold. Phagocytosis appears to be effective for EMPs that are less than about 10 μm in length (Lippmann, 1990; Vigliaturo et al., 2024; Donaldson et al., 2010; Schinwald et al., 2012), although the largest EMP possible should be closer to 21 μm given the size of macrophages (Krombach et al., 1997). Macrophages probably evolved to manage natural atmospheric aerosols, which have very few particles larger than 20 μm (Mahowald et al., 2014).

Morgan and Holmes (1980) estimated that the longest rigid EMP that could be mechanically cleared by phagocytosis is 17 μm; Lippmann (1990) estimated this maximum as 30 μm, but clearance of such long EMPs by phagocytosis is unlikely given the high probability of cell death associated with very long EMPs. Phagocytosis increases in efficiency as particle size decreases to a few micrometers, so even EMPs 5 to 10 μm in length that can be phagocytized are not done so efficiently. In a study of asbestos found in the kidney, liver, spleen, pancreas, and gastrointestinal tract by Huang et al. (1988), all EMPs were < 20 μm in length. The longest EMPs reported from the pleura are less than 30 μm in length. If EMPs lack biological rigidity, their effective length could be less than their actual length, making it easier for macrophages to internalize them, as Lehmann et al. (2019) demonstrated for silver nanowires.

However, in addition to length limitations, phagocytes are not well adapted to dealing with particles < 0.30 μm in diameter but prefer particles 2 to 3 μm in scale

(Fröhlich, 2012; Geiser et al., 2008). Geiser et al. (2008) examined the role of macrophages in the clearance of particles with widths <0.100 μm and observed that macrophage uptake was sporadic and nonspecific. They concluded that macrophages play an insufficient role in the clearance of these very small particles from the peripheral lung.

EMPs that are internalized by phagocytes are taken to the lymph nodes where they can remain or enter the blood stream, potentially to disperse throughout the body. Wang et al. (2020) hypothesized that macrophages carry EMPs into the pleural cavity directly as part of the inflammatory process. EMPs internalized by macrophages that die are released, perhaps to be taken up by other phagocytes. EMPs that are only partially engulfed will result in so-called frustrated phagocytosis, a process that is thought to be a step in the development of fibrosis, and perhaps mesothelioma and lung cancer.

Internalization of EMPs by other means

While EMPs can enter cells by phagocytosis, an active cellular process, they can also enter passively, a process known generally as endocytosis (Bernareggi et al., 2015). There are many possible pathways for particulate to enter cells by endocytosis, and they are only beginning to be understood (Rennick et al., 2021). Endocytosis is limited by length. Vigliaturo et al. (2024) showed that non-asbestiform elongate particles of grunerite and anthophyllite shorter than about 5 μm with W < 0.9 μm are easily internalized by alveolar epithelial cells through endocytosis. The efficiency of endocytosis also drops off for EMPs with widths below 0.05 to 0.06 μm (Lehmann et al., 2019), the size at which virus capsids can enter the cells without specific molecular interactions.

Nagai et al. (2011) suggested that not all EMPs behave like asbestos. For example, they showed that multi-walled carbon nanotubes (MWCNT) are not internalized by endocytosis in the way that asbestos is, suggesting that these two materials are internalized by fundamentally different processes. They also showed that MWCNT penetrated both the plasma and nuclear membranes of macrophages by directly piercing cell membranes in a diameter-dependent manner. Strong, rigid MWCNT of 0.050 μm diameter were able to pierce mesothelial membranes, but not similarly strong MWCNT that were 0.145 μm in diameter. The same force applied to two very different materials would result in greater force/area for the smaller diameter EMPs. EMPs that penetrate the nuclear membranes may interfere with mitosis, leading to carcinogenesis.

Internalized EMPs that are enclosed by lysosomal vesicles may also cause damage and cell death (Zhu et al., 2016; Lehmann et al., 2019). In this case, damage also depends on length because length determines contact time between the EMP and the enclosing membrane; and the longer the contact time, the greater the chance of damage to the lysosomal membranes, resulting in cell death. It also depends on the width, which, if small enough, causes the rigidity of the EMP to decrease such that a force of 20–100 pN exerted by the enclosing membrane will bend it and render it nontoxic (Lehmann et al., 2019; Zhu et al., 2016).

Formation of asbestos bodies

Some respirable biopersistent EMPs will remain in the lung and be coated by ferritin, an amorphous material of Fe, Ca, Mg, P, protein, and mucopolysaccharides. The proportion of respirable EMP that is coated is generally small and subject to EMP type, size, and tissue iron content. This coating is referred to as an "asbestos body," although it can form on other EMPs, for example, erionite. Asbestos bodies rarely form on EMPs shorter than 20 μm (Morgan & Holmes, 1980; Vorwald et al., 1951; Case, 1994; Roggli, 2014), and those that are longer than 80 μm are almost always coated (Roggli, 2014). Because of the high dissolution of inhaled chrysotile, asbestos bodies are rare. Roggli demonstrated that 96% of asbestos bodies form on commercial amphibole asbestos cores, 2% on non-commercial amphibole asbestos cores, and 2% on chrysotile cores. Roggli also observed that thicker EMPs are more often coated than thinner EMPs, and that a core of amphibole was more common than a core of chrysotile, even though exposure to chrysotile was more common. In their cohort, Churg and Warnock (1977) report amosite as by far the most common mineral forming the core of asbestos bodies among those environmentally exposed to asbestos. They also report that while amosite and crocidolite made up 86% of the asbestos body cores in men, in women, anthophyllite and tremolite make up 57%, likely reflecting different sources of EMP aerosols.

Studies have shown loose correlations between asbestos ferruginous bodies identified by light microscopy and retained amphibole asbestos EMPs on electron microscopy. For example, Warnock (1989) reported that if asbestos bodies exceed 2000 per gram of dry lung, then there will be greater than 500,000 amphibole EMPs/g dry lung, and that the number of asbestos bodies is proportional to amphibole exposure. There is observed variability in asbestos body formation subject to host factors, with some persons having inherited macrophage lysosomal deficiencies and an inability to process and coat inhaled EMPs. In addition, intrinsic elemental iron content in the tissue microenvironment impacts coating, as do technical sample preparation methods. Warnock showed that if asbestos bodies are extracted from the tissue before counting, their number is greater than expected based on counts in tissue. This is related to the use of acid-alkali digestion steps in mineral digests of biological samples.

In historical settings, reflecting extensive asbestos use, asbestos bodies were commonly identified by routine light microscopy in lungs among the general population. Today, in Western societies, asbestos body detection in such subjects with no known occupational history of exposure or disease is exceptionally rare. The finding of an asbestos body in the lung would likely reflect significant above-background exposure, likely to commercial amphibole asbestos (Attanoos et al., 2016).

With the asbestos industry moving its activities to Eastern Europe, Asia, and Central and South America, it is in these settings that asbestos bodies are now more commonly seen in worker and non-worker populations, reflecting a different and often continued use of mixed commercial asbestos forms. For example, in a recent study by Incharoen et al. (2019), it was shown that about half the general population of Thailand, on autopsy, had asbestos bodies in their lungs.

The role of asbestos bodies and/or the process of their formation in asbestos-related disease is unknown (Pooley, 1972). Apparently, when asbestos bodies form on EMPs, the EMP does not translocate readily, and it would not likely be involved in tumorigenesis outside the lung. Asbestos bodies have been found in the lymph nodes and omentum, where they could have been formed locally. There is consistency showing that for persons with detected asbestos bodies in peritoneal tissue, omentum, or lymph nodes, there are clear correlations with elevated commercial amphibole asbestos EMP content in the lung (Dodson et al., 1996, 2000; Roggli & Benning, 1990).

It also would seem that an encased EMP would no longer be biologically active, so in a sense, it is "cleared" from the category of a carcinogen. However, Ghio et al. (2023) propose that the biological effects of asbestos develop in response to and are associated with the disruption of iron homeostasis, which is augmented by the formation of asbestos bodies drawing iron from both the cell, resulting in iron deficiency, and from mineral particles. They suggest that the processes that form asbestos bodies occur even in cases when large, visible asbestos bodies do not develop, as evidenced by the common presence of very thin layers of ferritin on many EMPs.

Clearance by dissolution

Dissolution is an important mechanism for the removal of mineral particles from the body, although minerals have a wide range of solubilities under biological conditions. Quartz is the most insoluble common silicate mineral (Gualtieri et al., 2018; summarized by Wylie, 2024). Once inhaled, it will remain in the lung for a lifetime unless it is physically removed. Other minerals have a short half-life because they will dissolve once deposited in the lung or engulfed by a macrophage. Carbonates generally fall into this category, but silicates may also. For example, wollastonite, a soluble calcium silicate, injected into the peritoneum of mice caused inflammation, but by 6 months, < 2% of the instilled EMP remained, and the inflammation had resolved (MacDonald & Kane, 1997). Gibbs and Pooley (1996) report that on autopsy, in a case occupational exposure to wollastonite, no wollastonite was found in the lung burden.

There is no recognized protocol for expressing dissolution rates that occur within macrophages or the lung interstitium. There are experiments in the literature that provide dissolution constants under pH conditions that EMPs might encounter in the lung or macrophage interior, but the exact chemical conditions governing the dissolution of nanoparticles within the body are not known. Utembe et al. (2015) review the many factors that impact dissolution experiments. These variables can make comparisons among solubility experiments difficult. Relative solubilities can be used by controlling as many variables as possible. Wylie (2024) summarizes studies on the half-life of many elongate mineral particles in several different types of fluids and the size of the particles whose dissolution half-lives are calculated. Despite all the variability in estimating solubility rates, overall, they show that chrysotile EMPs have an expected half-life in the human lung that is measured in days, while amphibole has a half-life measured in years.

Chrysotile has a very short half-life under conditions of low pH, such as within the macrophage phagolysosome (pH = 4–4.5) or even in the extracellular fluid (pH 7.4) (Gualtieri et al., 2018). In this setting, there is dissolution of chrysotile fibrils, which has been shown in experiments to occur in fluids with pH > 8 (Bales & Morgan, 1985), with consequent clearance. For this reason, many chrysotile fibers with long residence times *in vivo* show alterations of the outer MgOH layer that likely modulate their biological activity (Morgan et al., 1977); in some cases, only a Si-rich residue can be left (Seshan, 1983). Almost always, when exposure was to amphibole and chrysotile, it is the case that chrysotile abundance in lung burden is much less than that of amphibole. Even in those exposed to tremolite asbestos, which occurs only in trace amounts intergrown with chrysotile in Canada, amphibole dominates in lung burden, and chrysotile levels are often similar to controls (Pooley & Wagner, 1988), so it is reasonable to conclude that chrysotile could dissolve after a very short time. Amphibole, on the other hand, is essentially insoluble following deposition in the lung.

Despite the evidence for the dissolution of chrysotile, it has been reported in tissue from cases many years following occupational exposure. Either a slower than expected dissolution of chrysotile is taking place, or larger fibers continue to release the component fibrils, or, in some cases, ongoing environmental exposure is continuing to take place. In a set of experiments with monkeys, Hiroshima et al. (1993) found chrysotile fibers in lung tissue 11.5 years following exposure. Feder et al. (2016) studied lung burden at two points with a median interval of about 8 years (range 4–21 years). The pulmonary asbestos fiber burden was stable between both examinations (median 1623/4269 asbestos bodies per gram wet lung); however, no measurements were taken to determine changes in width or length. While electron microscopy demonstrated a preponderance of chrysotile (median 80%), even after 20 years following exposure, these could be smaller and narrow EMPs as larger bundles disintegrate.

Despite these limitations, biosolubility indices can be constructed by using a method that measures dissolution rates across different minerals under the same conditions that are comparable to those in the human body. We have used dissolution rates provided by Gualtieri et al. (2018) at pH 4, the pH expected in the interior of a macrophage, as an index of solubility, but others could also be used. For example, Brantley (2003) estimates the mean lifetime of many minerals at pH 5. Published solubility rates for the same mineral may vary due to different experimental conditions or from real differences between two samples of the same mineral, especially chemical composition. These uncertainties may explain reported variances in solubility estimates for the same mineral from different locations.

Translocation

Mossman et al. (2011) describe translocation as the movement of intact EMP from the non-ciliated airspaces where they were deposited, either 1) along the epithelial surface to the ciliated epithelium to be removed, **or** 2) into and through the epithelium, migrating to the interstitial sites in the lung where they may move along lymphatic drainage pathways toward the pleura. The thinnest and shortest EMPs gain access to the blood capillaries and to distribution throughout the body.

EMP distribution within the lung

To the extent that translocation of deposited EMPs takes place, sorting by size during the process would be expected, and we might expect to see systematic changes in the dimension and abundance of EMP burden as a function of the position in the lung. At the same time, removal of EMPs by macrophages can take place, EMP may migrate in response to fluid flow, and in some cases, dissolution is underway, so that more than one process shaping the dimensions of EMP lung burden can be at work.

In humans, Warnock (1989) showed that the longest EMPs of all mineral types are found in the lower lobes of the lung, in the direction of the strongest fluid flow out of the lung. In a careful study of a single lung, Pooley (2018) demonstrated that EMPs are most abundant in the center of the lung corresponding to airway clearance sites, diminishing in abundance toward the periphery and the visceral pleura. He also found that the width of the EMPs decreased from the lung center to the periphery while length increased slightly. In the Pooley study, most of the amosite fibers found near the pleura were 7 to 10 μm in length and $W < 0.175$ μm. Others have also shown that EMP populations show a decrease in average width toward the periphery of the lung (Oberdörster & Graham, 2018; Bignon et al., 1979; Churg & Wiggs, 1989). Churg and Wiggs (1989) showed EMP size differences among lung locations in cases of mesothelioma vs. cases of lung cancer, suggesting that disease likely impacts deposition and translocation.

EMPs could decrease in average width across the lung for several possible reasons as described at the beginning of this chapter: narrow EMPs are more capable of penetrating the lung interstitium and moving toward the visceral pleura in response to fluid flow; EMPs separate into component fibrils; or wider EMPs are selectively removed by phagocytes that favor micron over nanoscale objects.

Only limited information is available on the distribution of fibers in the lungs of animals. Hiroshima et al. (1993) in their primate study showed no difference in the size distributions among four sampling locations in the lungs of animals exposed to either amosite, chrysotile, or crocidolite. However, they concluded that fragmentation, separation, and translocation of inhaled EMPs are important contributory factors that control the size and size distribution of lung burden.

Migration into the pleural space

The exact path or paths that EMPs follow as they translocate into the pleura is unknown. Several hypotheses have been put forward, but whatever the path, it sorts for width and, in most cases, length. Gualtieri (2022) discusses the hypotheses in detail.

Macrophage dependent. The first hypothesis is that macrophages carry and deposit EMPs directly into the pleura. This would be size determined. If this is the path, as already discussed, the sizes and capacities of the macrophage would place limitations on the sizes of EMPs reaching the pleura. Rigid MWCNT translocated to the pleura following exposure of rats to carbon nanotubes, and most were observed in macrophages (Xu et al., 2014), so it seems likely that at least some EMPs could reach the pleura by macrophage transport. Nonetheless, given the difficulty reported for macrophages managing narrow fibrils and the abundance of narrow EMPs in all reports of EMPs found in pleural tissue, and the increasing inefficiency of EMP removal as length increases above a few micrometers, it seems highly *unlikely* that the path to the pleura would be macrophage transport.

Macrophage independent. A second hypothesis is that EMPs move in and out of the lung as a component of a moving fluid, so-called paracellular transport (Gualtieri,

2022). Excess fluid in the pleural space is common in many diseases of the lung. This fluid may arise within the lung interstitium in response to inflammation induced by inhaled EMPs. As fluid accumulates, a pressure gradient develops between the lung and the pleura, reversing the normal gradient, pushing fluid out of the lung and into the pleural space, probably through the permeable pleural membranes (Broaddus et al., 2011; Donaldson et al., 2010) and perhaps conveying it from the pulmonary lymphatic drainage system to systemic lymphatic flow (Hojo et al., 2022) and the blood stream. Oberdörster and Graham (2018) conclude that EMPs 6 to 9 μm in length are cleared directly into the lymphatic system.

To move with fluids, EMPs must be rigid but narrow. Biologically rigid EMPs with nanoscale widths will align with their long axis parallel to the fluid flow and be able to move with these fluids directly through the lung interstitium and visceral pleura into the pleural cavity, provided they are not too long. These same EMPs have the capacity to penetrate tissue directly. Rigid, narrow MWCNT (length 8 μm, width 0.150 μm) have been observed penetrating both the visceral pleura and the parietal mesothelium in rats (Xu et al., 2014). Lentz et al. (2003) concluded that EMPs must be thinner than 0.4 μm and shorter than 10 μm to be translocated to the pleura; Lippmann (2014) places the thinness of translocated EMP closer to < 0.15 μm, more consistent with the EMP reported from the pleura (see Tables 6.1 through 6.7).

Suzuki and Yuen (2002) found different types of asbestos in pleural and peritoneal tissue (plaque or tumor) compared to that found in the lungs of the same cases. In the pleural group, chrysotile was more abundant on a weight basis than amosite (no other amphibole found). It should be noted that Sporn and Roggli (2013) criticized the results of this study for apparent methodological shortcomings. Similarly, Bignon et al. (1979) found amphibole common in the lung, but chrysotile was almost the only EMP found in the pleura. On the other hand, Caraballo-Arias et al. (2022a) reviewed the literature for reports of asbestos in normal and pathological pleural tissue. They found that when occupational exposure was known, asbestos was commonly reported, but not always.

Consistently, high aspect ratio, Stanton dimension EMPs are amphiboles and not chrysotile (Roggli, 2014). EMPs were identified in pleural plaque, pleural fibrosis tissue, and tumor tissue. Both amphibole and chrysotile were reported with approximately equal frequency and with relative abundances reflecting occupational exposure. In a similar review of peritoneal tissue, Caraballo-Arias et al. (2022b) also found that the abundance of chrysotile and amphibole were not systematically different but rather reflected exposure. It is possible that the reports prior to about 2000 reflect ongoing exposure to chrysotile, which could still be detected in the air in most major cities of the world during that time.

Translocation to the pleura of MWCNT in animal experiments is rapid. It has been shown to pierce the visceral pleura and penetrate the parietal mesothelium in rats 6 hours after exposure (Xu et al., 2014). Xu et al. also showed that when two CNTs of differing sizes were compared, only the material with an average width of 0.15 μm and an average length of 8 μm translocated to the pleura. Shorter (3 μm) EMP and EMP narrow enough to lack biological rigidity (0.015 μm) did not.

Clearance from the pleural space through the parietal pleura

The fate of an EMP once it reaches the pleural space is also not well characterized in the literature. Many researchers support the hypothesis that mesothelioma develops from failed peritoneal and pleural cavity clearance of EMPs (Donaldson et al., 2010; Kane et al., 2018; Moalli et al., 1987; Boutin et al., 1996). Once an EMP enters the pleural space, it can only exit by direct penetration of the parietal pleura or via its lymphatic stomata that are about 3 to 10 μm in diameter (Donaldson et al., 2010). EMPs and other particulates have been observed to pile up around these openings, producing black spots (Boutin et al., 1996) (see Table 6.7b). The peritoneal cavity also has stomata through the diaphragm, which are less than 10 μm in diameter. CNTs installed in the peritoneal cavity have also been observed to accumulate in the diaphragm, suggesting flow across the diaphragm.

EMPs in pleural tissue are not abundant. Perhaps they are unevenly distributed, and sampling has been unrepresentative. EMPs are known to pile up around stomata and impregnate plaques, but many others leave, probably through lymphatic flow. EMPs could also pass through the parietal pleura and enter the lymphatic system that surrounds the pleura. It may be that it is the tissue damage resulting from the passage through or into this very thin layer of mesothelial cells that initiates carcinogenicity.

Translocation to other locations

Asbestos, man-made mineral fiber (MMMF), and multi-walled carbon nanotubes (MWCNT) have all been demonstrated in animals to travel to almost every organ in the body shortly after exposure. This is true whether the exposure was through inhalation or instillation, pleural or peritoneal.

Asbestos has been detected in all abdominal organs, and in many cases, both amphibole and chrysotile occur in equal proportions. In humans, the EMPs found outside of the pulmonary system are almost exclusively chrysotile or crocidolite; amosite is rare or absent (Suzuki & Kohyama, 1991). In a study of stillborn fetuses of mothers exposed to asbestos occupationally, more than a third had asbestos, with 95% chrysotile and 5% crocidolite plus tremolite (Haque et al., 1996). It is clear that small, thin EMPs entering the body through respiration can travel to every organ through the circulatory system.

LUNG BURDEN, EXPOSURE, AND DISEASE

Tissue burden is one method of establishing an individual's past exposure to dusts, and it can be a predictor of lung fibrosis, lung cancer, and mesothelioma risk (Sporn & Roggli, 2013; Rasmuson et al., 2014; Korchevskiy & Wylie, 2022). In animal experiments, an increase in lung burden correlated with increased fibrosis (Fukushima et al., 2017).

In human studies, Visonà et al. (2023) showed that both asbestos bodies and EMPs in lung burden were an order of magnitude higher in cases than in controls. Gilham et al. (2016) demonstrated that lung EMP content of commercial amphibole asbestos is linearly proportional to the risk for mesothelioma and lung cancer. Rasmuson et al. (2014) demonstrated that lung concentration of asbestos EMPs correlated with the level of exposure.

Lung burden, however, has limitations in understanding exposure. Warnock (1989), in her extensive study of lung burden in asbestos-exposed cases of asbestos-related disease, showed that the lung burden type and amount appeared unrelated to illness. The same lung burden level could be found in mesothelioma patients with no fibrosis, lung cancer patients with and without fibrosis, and fibrosis patients with no mesothelioma or lung cancer. This observation suggests that there is a large variability in how individuals respond to the same exposure. Individual variability in response to asbestos exposure was recently addressed by Barlow and Mossman (2025). Also, parameters other than the lung concentration of asbestos (such as size distribution of EMPs) may affect mesothelioma risk even when the lung burden values are identical.

In addition, workers in a single cohort may have had quite different individual exposures. For example, Pooley and Wagner (1988) describe the mineral makeup of 5 mesothelioma cases from a Pennsylvania textile plant. Two were dominated by crocidolite (64 and 69%), in 2 others, chrysotile was the most abundant EMP (54 and 40%), and in one case, the amounts of tremolite, amosite, and crocidolite were approximately the same. They also describe the lung burden from 12 mesothelioma cases from a British textile plant and 4 asbestosis cases from a South Carolina textile plant. While it is possible to generalize about the mineralogy, such as that amosite is low in all cases at all plants, the mineralogy among each group is highly variable. Among the cases from the British textile plant, the % chrysotile ranged from 9.3 to 93.7, the % crocidolite ranged from 86.9 to 2.1, and the % tremolite ranged from 1.0 to 26.4%. Among the 4 asbestosis cases from South Carolina, the % ranged from 27.5 to 91.5% chrysotile, 0.4 to 26.8% crocidolite, and 8.1 to 70.7% tremolite/actinolite.

Lung burden will also vary from mining the same mineral in different locations. Dufresne et al. (1996) demonstrated that lung burden from mesothelioma cases among Thetford miners and millers contained a much higher proportion of tremolite than did the same occupations at Asbestos Townships. This corresponded to a higher mesothelioma rate in workers at Thetford mines.

Despite these limitations, in general, lung burden has been demonstrated to relate to both exposure and disease. Concentrations of EMPs in lungs are not a full reflection of a "dose" of asbestos that was inhaled because they have the quality of a temporal "snapshot" rather than playing the role of a universal metric of the amount of EMPs entering the body and causing the disease. The predictability of lung burden for disease risk is also limited, though it has been demonstrated to be correlated with the risk. Exposure, lung burden, and disease comprise a triangle that is extremely important for understanding the mode of action for asbestos. More studies are needed to fully understand the relationship between these three elements of the process, but even now it is possible to reconstruct cumulative exposure from lung burden and predict mesothelioma risk from both exposure and lung burden, considering all possible uncertainties and limitations.

LUNG BURDEN: COMPARABILITY OF DATA

The methods used to extract EMPs from tissue include chemical methods such as treatment with KOH, low-temperature oxygen plasma ashing, or a combination of the two methods together. Recently, Somigliana (2025) proposed a method of plasma ashing of freeze-dried tissue.

Some methods used for EMP extraction can alter the size distribution of the extracted EMPs, however. For example, Stettler et al. (2008) report dimensions derived from lung burden on rats and monkeys. The samples of tissue were treated either by ashing or by chemical digestion. In two sets of experiments, the lengths of EMPs from the ashed samples were significantly shorter than those recovered by chemical digestion.

Gaudichet et al. (1980) sampled lung tissue from three cases and prepared nucleopore filters that had been carbon-coated and sent to two highly experienced laboratories. One repeatedly reported more anthophyllite, and the other was more likely to identify uncommon minerals. Large variations in mullite, crocidolite, and iron oxide between the labs on some samples suggest that the samples themselves were inhomogeneous, despite their best efforts at uniformity.

Most of the data on lung burden has been collected by a small number of laboratories. Each uses its own sample preparation methods, and it seems clear from discussions with those who run laboratories that there are advantages and disadvantages to each method. Despite these differences, the data for each mineral shown in Tables 6.1 through 6.6 are remarkably consistent, with few exceptions.

In addition to issues of how tissue samples are prepared and EMPs counted, there is also a large variability reported in how individuals respond to the same exposure conditions, affecting both characteristics of lung burden and its association with disease. Because of the high variance, general observations from lung burden studies that are sustained across reports and observations from data derived from large numbers of subjects are the most reliable indicators of the factors that control the dimensions and mineralogy of lung burden EMPs.

CHARACTERISTICS OF EMPS FOUND IN LUNG, PLEURA, AND AIR BY MINERAL TYPE

Cardiff lung burden study audit

We performed a quality audit of the lung materials analyzed at the Cardiff laboratory (U.K.) (unpublished preliminary results). The audit included the systematization of the size distribution of the fibers in the anonymized acellular samples in comparison to similar data from other published sources. The Cardiff audit data came from analytical TEM measurements made on more than 300 cases of mesothelioma throughout the U.K. along with controls between 2018 and 2023. For all minerals except tremolite, width frequencies are reported for EMPs longer than 5 µm in bins that are 0.050 µm in width (±0.025 µm), approximately twice the measurement error expected when measurements are made at 40,000 magnification. For tremolite, because of the small number of particles measured, bin widths were doubled, reflecting an error of (± 0.05 µm). Length frequencies are given in bins that are approximately 1 µm in width, reflecting an assumed measurement uncertainty of ± 0.5 µm and for a range of lengths from > 0.5 to 50 µm. The full range of lengths is given in the figure captions.

Frequency distributions of potential aerosols

For each of the minerals for which we have length and width measurements from lung burden, we have provided a frequency distribution of length and width for reference of what might represent an aerosol. To produce the "aerosol," we have combined sets of data from the NSSGA database from airborne particles and/or from particle populations elutriated to represent an "aerosol." It contains a high proportion of inhalable particles made up of a mixture of all of those sources; the frequencies do not therefore represent a single exposure, but the range and relative abundances are a reasonable first approximation in the absence of other information. Descriptions of the data sources are provided in the figure captions. Only particles sized by Transmission Electron Microscopy (TEM) were included.

Dimensional descriptions of pulmonary EMPs by mineral type

The level and composition of lung burden have been shown to be predictors of lung cancer and mesothelioma mortality, although each mineral associated with asbestos-related disease displays somewhat different dimensional characteristics in the aerosol, in lung tissue, and in tissue outside the lung, providing insight into properties that govern tissue-specific penetration and retention. EMP occurrences in many studies of asbestos-related diseases have been reported. Tables 6.1 through 6.7 provide dimensional descriptions of lung burden by mineral type from representative studies. The data are organized by tissue location and year of publication.

Chrysotile

Chrysotile is commonly reported in the literature from tissue of individuals occupationally exposed to asbestos. In human tissues from organs other than the lungs, it is often the most abundant. In the lung, however, because of the low biopersistence of chrysotile, amphibole normally dominates despite the fact that its use was much less common in North America and Europe, where most exposures of the lung burden cases occurred.

Even among chrysotile ore miners in Canada, amphibole abundance in lung tissue exceeds that of chrysotile, while making up less than 1% of the EMP from the mine (see discussion of tremolite below). For example, Dufresne et al. (1996) report ratios of the number of tremolite EMPs ($L > 5$ μm) to chrysotile EMPs ($L > 5$ μm) among cases of mesothelioma among Canadian chrysotile workers to range from about 4 to 20. In both Asbestos Township and Thetford mesothelioma cases, tremolite was the most abundant mineral EMP found.

Among the studies in Table 6.1 (see pages 159–160), the measured EMP width of chrysotile is very uniform. The average GM width reported in Table 6.1 for EMPs of all lengths is 0.060 μm, with a range of 0.04 to 0.07 μm; the average width for EMPs longer than 5 μm is 0.070 μm. This uniformity extends across laboratories and tissue types, and even mine air.

This uniformity in width should not be surprising because chrysotile forms in nature as tubes that vary little among locations around the world, and tissue burden data reflect that uniformity. Single chrysotile fibrils in *nature* are reported to range from 0.010 to 0.085 µm, with most between 0.020 and 0.040 µm (Chisholm, 1983). The mean width reported for fibrils in lung tissue shown in Table 6.1 is slightly wider than the reported width for single fibrils. Either wider fibrils are more likely to survive and are preserved preferentially, or many EMPs in lung tissue are composed of two or more fibrils. It might also be that only wider (more rigid) chrysotile fibrils will penetrate lung tissue.

An exception to the common average widths in Table 6.1 is several chrysotile analyses by Suzuki and Yuen, where the mean width was given as 40 nm. Given the inherent constraints on chrysotile fibril sizes, a mean of 0.040 µm would suggest that large proportions of the population must be single fibrils. The differences in the results of Suzuki and Yuen and others may reflect counting rules, sample preparation, or exposure source, and we note that the paper by Suzuki and Yuen was criticized in the literature because of possible methodological shortcomings.

Another exception is lung burden chrysotile from exposures to textile-grade EMP, which is slightly wider than other grades. For example, Sebastien et al. (1989) report an average width of 0.1 µm from the textile factories in Charleston, but only 0.07 µm from the chrysotile mines at Thetford.

Chrysotile exists in all tissue almost exclusively as very short EMPs. For most analyses, mean lengths are less than or equal to 2 µm, and when provided, the standard deviation is also about 2 µm (see Table 6.1). The average length of chrysotile lung burden from exposure to textiles described by Pooley and Mitha (1986) is 2.4 µm, longer than all other comparable studies. Given the fragility of chrysotile EMPs, experimental technique may account for some of the differences in mean lengths among laboratories, but it is also possible that mine source and EMP treatment may result in dimensional differences reflected in lung burden.

For populations of EMPs with lengths greater than 5 µm, average lengths may be as high as 8 µm (reported for Charleston and Thetford by Sebastien et al., 1989). These data demonstrate the presence of long EMPs despite the overwhelming number of short ones reported in most studies.

In the Cardiff audit data, approximately 90% of chrysotile EMPs with lengths greater than 5 µm have measured widths < 0.13 µm, with about 80% measuring between 0.075 and 0.125 µm (0.100 ± 0.025), and about 11% with widths < 0.075 µm (Figure 6.1a on page 161); the geometric mean width is 0.027 µm, slightly larger than reported elsewhere (Table 6.1). As shown in Figure 6.1a and 6.1b (see page 161), both lung burden and airborne width frequencies for EMPs longer than 5 µm have a modal frequency at 0.100(0.025). One significant difference is that the aerosol shown in Figure 6.1b has a much greater range in width than found in lung burden.

The modal width from the Cardiff audit dataset (0.14 µm) is somewhat larger than might be expected from the averages given from other analyses of lung burden in the literature in Table 6.1 for L > 5 µm. Most of those sources are for Canadian chrysotile. In Charleston, South Carolina, where exposure was to textile-grade Thetford chrysotile, the mean width found in lung burden (L>5 μm) was 0.10 μm, close to that found in Cardiff audit data, while among miners, the average width was 0.07 μm. The wider widths from Cardiff audit data could be explained by a source somewhat different from most Canadian exposures and more similar to textile-grade chrysotile. It may also be, however, that, unlike many of the studies which were conducted during a time of high background levels of chrysotile, there was no continuing background exposure in the Cardiff audit data, and it is possible that the narrowest EMPs have been removed.

Shown in Figure 6.1c and 6.1d (see page 162) are the distributions of the frequency of length from the Cardiff audit data set and from the "aerosol." The most obvious difference is in EMPs less than 2.0 (±0.5) μm in length. For the lung burden, these short EMPs make up about 52% of all EMPs, but in the possible aerosol, they make up more than 72%. EMPs with L > 5 μm make up 20% of the total EMP in the Cardiff audit data but only 7% of the EMPs in the "aerosol." As is the case for all types of asbestos, there are higher proportions of longer EMPs in lung burden than in the "aerosol."

Although data are limited, chrysotile has been found to be the most abundant EMP in pleural tissue but not in lung tissue. This may simply reflect size, with mostly short chrysotile particles being present in the size range that is not expected to cause pathology. Indeed, small carbon dust particles are also commonplace in pleural tissue. Gibbs et al. (1991) found that chrysotile made up less than 20% of the EMP found in the lungs of cases with asbestos-related asbestosis but more than 95% of the EMP found in the pleura. Others have had similar findings.

The reports of chrysotile from tissue outside the lung are for EMPs of about the same width as found in lung burden, but with an average length of about < 1 μm, slightly shorter than lung burden chrysotile. This includes EMPs from pleural tumors, fibrosis, plaques, and lymph nodes.

Given the efficiency of removal of short particles and the chemical solubility of serpentine, the abundance of short chrysotile EMPs in tissue long after occupational exposure has ceased is problematic. It could arise from breaking up long EMPs during tissue digestion. Because most long chrysotile EMPs are composed of many shorter fibrils, over time they will disaggregate, supplying short EMPs to the lymph system and explaining the ubiquity of chrysotile in most tissue reports. Given that many of the cases lived during a time when chrysotile was widespread in urban environments, in some cases, chrysotile could be from recent exposure. However, for the Cardiff audit cases (for 2018 to 2023), recent exposure is less likely given declining background abundances.

Amosite (grunerite asbestos)

Virtually all amosite in commerce comes from a single mining district in South Africa referred to as the Transvaal. Within the district, some variation in characteristics might be expected, especially in minor element chemistry. For example, ferro-actinolite asbestos (Ca-bearing) is known to occur in the same district, indicating a chemical environment slightly different from that forming riebeckite asbestos (Na-bearing) or grunerite asbestos (Mg-bearing amosite), both also found together in the Transvaal district. (Nearby is the Cape Asbestos province, where riebeckite also forms blue asbestos [crocidolite], but this is a different mining district, and the fiber displays different dimensional characteristics.) Asbestos from the same mining district formed by the same process might be expected to display some uniformity in fibril length and width.

Mineralogical investigations have shown that amosite fibers are formed from fibrils with a wider range in diameter than chrysotile, although the smallest reported from lung burden have a similarly sized diameter of about 0.020 μm. Cressey et al. (1982) examined bundles of amosite fibrils by ion milling to create a cross-sectional view. The images show fibrils with widths ranging from about 50 to more than 200 nm. It also appears that the narrower fibrils occur in clusters, a feature that may influence their toxicity.

Amosite fibrils have been reported to display weak intra-fibral bonding, which would discourage disaggregation and maintain bundle structures. Amosite is known as a "harsh" asbestos because of its resistance to disaggregation. However, among different commercial uses, amosite is sometimes "fiberized." This process is designed to break up fiber bundles and free fibrils. If this happens, the aerosol may be quite different from a mine aerosol. Given the uniformity of the material, and if laboratory techniques are comparable, differences among the average widths could reflect the degree of fiberization in the exposure.

Among lung burden studies shown in Table 6.2, geometric mean widths for EMPs of all lengths range from 0.140 to 0.250 μm, with an average of 0.180 μm; for EMPs longer than 5 μm, the average width is 0.230 μm.

In Figure 6.2a, the frequency distribution of width for EMPs longer than 5 μm from Cardiff Audit Data shows a well-developed mode at 0.250 (0.025) μm and abundant (>20%) EMPs ≤ 0.150(0.025) μm. The modal width for amosite from the "aerosol" L > 5 μm shows a broad mode centered at about 0.20(0.075) μm; although given the large number of measurements (N = 1853), the smaller modes at 0.155(0.025) and 0.255(0.025) μm may reflect two fibril subpopulations, one corresponding to the Cardiff Audit Data mode. The proportion of EMPs L > 5 μm that have widths ≤ 0.155(0.025) μm is 15% in the database, which is less than Cardiff Audit Data lung burden with more than 20%; and in general, there are more, wider EMPs available for respiration than are deposited in the lung.

Amosite is the longest asbestos EMP found in human tissue. The average lengths range from 2 to 7 μm in the studies from Table 6.2, with an average of 4.2 μm in the lung and 3.5 μm in the pleura. Amosite EMPs of more than 300 μm in length are reported in the Cardiff Audit Data sets, but the average length is only 7.3 μm.

A comparison of the length distribution of Cardiff Audit Data lung burden (Figure 6.2c) and aerosol comparison (Figure 6.2d) shows the same clear differences found for chrysotile: a very low abundance of EMPs < 2 μm in length and a higher proportion of long EMPs. For Cardiff Audit Data, the proportion of EMPs with L <

TABLE 6.2
Amosite

			Width			Length			Length
	Notes	Reference	GM (μm)	Mean (μm)	Median (μm)	GM (μm)	Mean (μm)	Median (μm)	Restriction (μm)
Lung		Pooley and Clark (1980)		0.28			5.5		
		Churg et al. (1984)	0.19	0.23 (0.18)		3.9	5.8 (6.0)		
		Warnock (1989)	0.23 (1.92)			14.12 (1.91)			L > 5
		Warnock (1989)			0.17			3.9	
		Gibbs et al. (1990)	0.2			5.1			
		Gibbs et al. (1991)	0.17			3.6			
		Suzuki and Kohyama (1991)	0.19 (2.47)			5.08 (3.12)			
	Other industry	Dufresne et al. (1996)	0.14 (2.0)			2.0 (1.7)			L < 5
	Asbestos	Dufresne et al. (1996)	0.19 (2.0)			2.9 (1.6)			L < 5
	Other industry	Dufresne et al. (1996)	0.21 (1.9)			8.6 (1.7)			L > 5
	Asbestosis	Dufresne et al. (1996)	0.25 (1.8)			8.7 (2.1)			L > 5
		Dodson et al. (2004)	0.2			6.97			
		Dodson et al. (2005)	0.185			6.3			
		Cardiff audit data (2025) (See this chapter)	0.27 (1.76)			9.83 (1.79)			L > 5
Pleura	Plaque	Suzuki and Kohyama (1991)	0.14 (2.61)			2.83 (3.62)			
	Tumor	Suzuki and Kohyama (1991)	0.21 (2.19)			4.55 (3.50)			

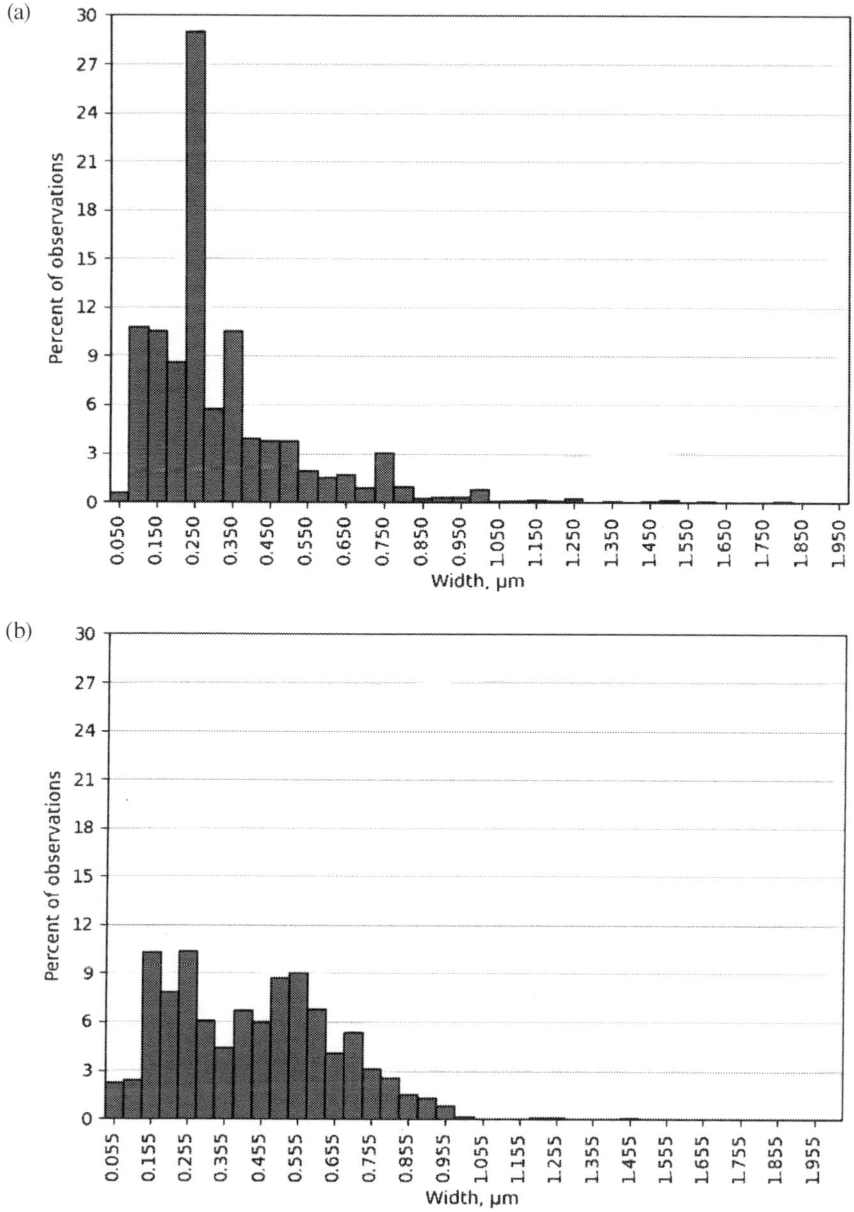

FIGURE 6.2 Amosite frequencies of width and length. a) Cardiff Audit Data. Width for L > 5 µm. N = 2081, Bin width = 0.05 µm, GM width = 0.32 µm, range 0.01–1.81. b) "Aerosol" (airborne TEM data from South African mines and during pipe insulation fabrication). Width for L > 5 µm. N = 1853, GM width = 0.43 µm, range 0.03–1.43 µm. c) Cardiff Audit Data. Length < 50 µm (longer than 50 µm not shown = <1% of all EMP). N = 4407, Bin width = 1 µm, GM length = 6.76 µm, range 0.51–355 µm. d) "Aerosol." Length > 5 µm. N = 5930. (Longer than 50 µm not shown = <1% of all EMP). GM length = 4.20, range 0.45–377.8. Proportion of lengths greater than 5 µm = 42.7% for Cardiff Audit Data lung burden and 31.2% of the aerosol comparison.

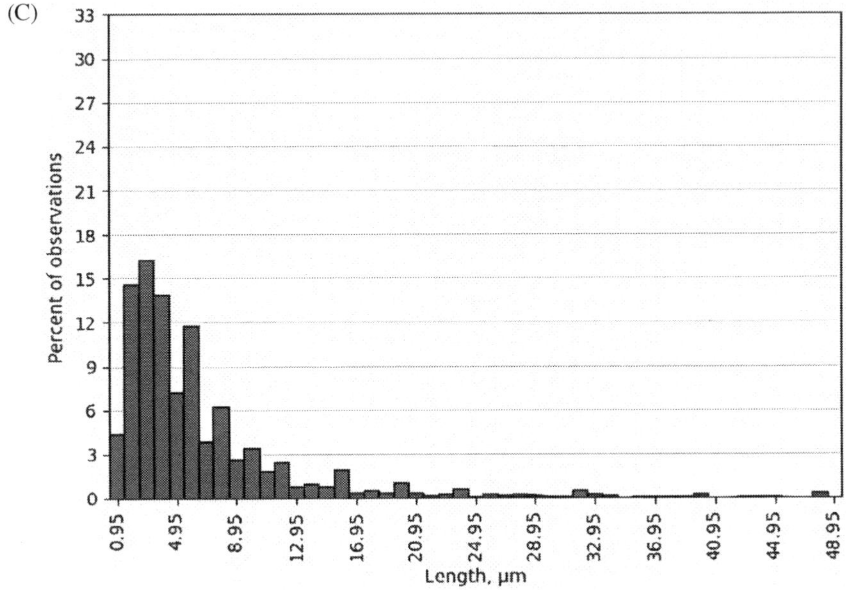

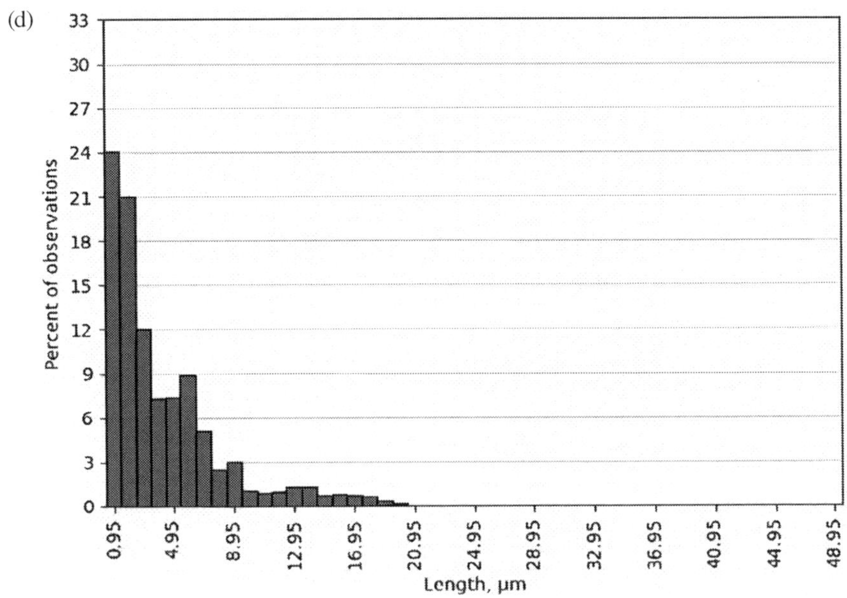

FIGURE 6.2 (Continued)

2 μm is about 19%, while in our "aerosol," almost 45% are of this length. The differences are consistent with the idea that long EMPs are preferentially retained in the lung, and short EMPs are preferentially cleared or not deposited in the first place, conforming to the fiber retention factors from the Timbrell model developed from anthophyllite asbestos burden (Burdett et al., 1988), which show a very low retention of fibers thinner than 0.2 and shorter than 5 μm.

As was the case for chrysotile, the limited data on amosite dimensions found outside the pleura is consistent with the conclusion that, on average, EMPs that translocated out of the lung are narrower and shorter than lung burden.

Crocidolite (riebeckite asbestos)

Crocidolite is common in the lungs of mesothelioma cases, and it is the most commonly reported amphibole outside the lung. Most of the world's crocidolite was mined in the Cape Province of South Africa; the production from the Hamersley Range in Australia was about 1/10th of that from the Cape (Gibbons, 2000). Geologically, the occurrences share a common formation history. It is likely that most of the crocidolite EMPs from lung tissue shown in Table 6.3 come from the Cape, given the scope and scale of exports from South Africa. According to the study of samples of crocidolite from four locations in the world, the modal widths for all lengths of crocidolite from the Cape and from the Hamersley Range are the same: 0.060 to 0.100 μm (Shedd, 1985), so it would not likely be possible to distinguish these two locations from lung burden alone. However, if the Shedd data are representative, crocidolite from other sources might be different enough to detect. For example, the modal width for Transvaal and crocidolite mined in Bolivia is 100 to 160 nm, significantly wider and slightly longer than the Cape and Hamersley crocidolite.

Alario Franco et al. (1977) ion-milled a Cape crocidolite EMP bundle to produce a cross-section that clearly demonstrated its fibrillar structure. The individual crocidolite fibril widths range from about 0.010 to 0.100 μm, are unattached to each other, and their crystallographic directions perpendicular to the EMP axis are randomly or semi-randomly arranged around the EMP axis. It is likely that the abundances of the fibrils in this width range will vary within mining districts and over time, perhaps accounting for the range in average widths for all lengths shown in Table 6.3, from 0.090 to 0.140 μm. The GM average width for all lengths is 0.110 μm; it is 0.120 μm for lengths greater than 5 μm.

The frequency distribution of width from Cardiff Audit Data has a well-developed mode at about 0.100 (0.025) μm and perhaps a second mode at about 0.250 (0.025) μm, which has the highest percentage of EMPs in the crocidolite aerosols from the NSSGA database. Despite this similarity, there is a higher proportion of EMPs narrower than about 0.250 (0.025) μm in lung burden than might be expected from the aerosol.

With respect to length, Cardiff Audit Data lung burden differs from the "aerosol" in ways similar to other forms of asbestos: while 54% of the aerosol is ≤ 1.95 (0.025) μm, only about 21% of the lung burden falls into this category; 45% of the lung burden EMPS are longer than 5 μm, while only 21% make up the "aerosol."

TABLE 6.3
Riebeckite asbestos (crocidolite)

	Notes	Reference	Width GM (μm)	Width Mean (μm)	Width Median (μm)	Length GM (μm)	Length Mean (μm)	Length Median (μm)	Length Restriction (μm)
Lung	Cape	Pooley and Clark (1980)		0.14			3.3		
		Warnock (1989)			0.09			3.8	
		Warnock (1989)	0.17 (2.15)			11.78 (1.81)			L > 5
		Dodson et al. (2005)	0.11			5.6			
		Gibbs et al. (1990)	0.08			5.2			
		Dodson et al. (2004)	0.1			3.65			
	Fibrosis upper	Gibbs et al. (1991)	0.10 (0.63)			3.17 (0.88)			
	Fibrosis central	Gibbs et al. (1991)	0.09 (0.61)			3.07 (0.83)			
	Cement	Pooley and Mitha (1986)	0.1			2.1			
	Textile	Pooley and Mitha (1986)	0.13			8.4			
	Control c	Pooley and Mitha (1986)	0.09			1.5			
	Control t	Pooley and Mitha (1986)	0.09			0.5			
		Churg et al. (1984)	0.1			2.8	4.0 (4.3)		
	Other industry	Dufresne et al. (1996)	0.1 (2.0)			1.8 (1.7)			L < 5
	Asbestos	Dufresne et al. (1996)	0.1 (2.0)			2.1 (1.6)			L < 5
	Other industry	Dufresne et al. (1996)	0.11 (2.0)			7.7 (1.6)			L > 5
	Asbestos	Dufresne et al. (1996)	0.13 (2.0)			6.8 (1.4)			L > 5
		Suzuki and Yuen (2002)	0.14 (1.96)			4.63 (2.34)			
	Korea	Jung et al. (2020)	0.132			7.7			L > 5
	Background	Dodson et al. (1999)	0.17			2.11			
		Cardiff audit data (2025) (see this chapter)	0.16 (1.56)			8.78 (1.59)			L > 5
Pleura		Gibbs et al. (1991)	0.08 (0.45)			2.30 (0.94)			
	Tumor	Suzuki and Kohyama (1991)	0.4 (1.37)*			3.53 (1.09)			

* Two fibers

(a)

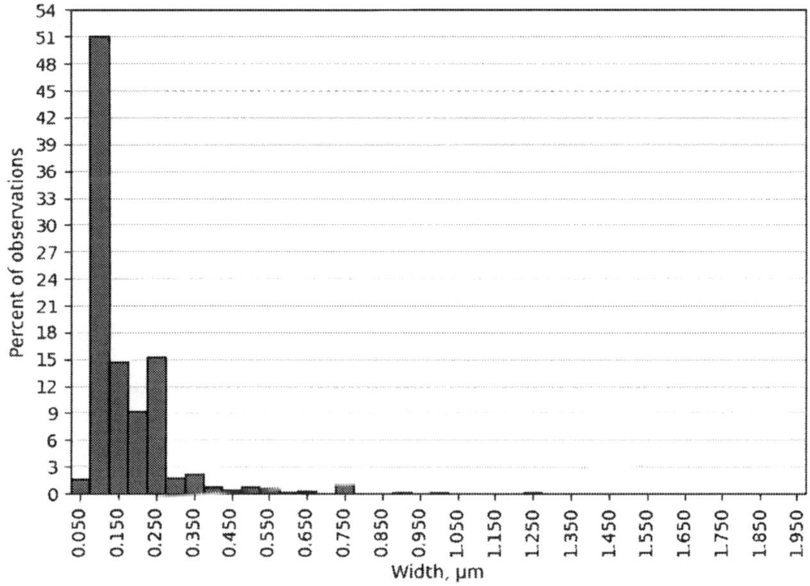

(b)

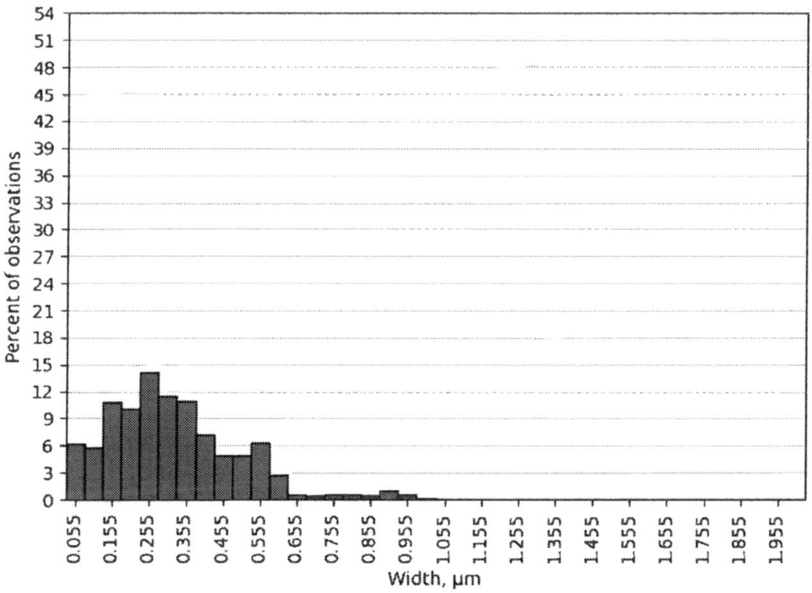

FIGURE 6.3 Crocidolite frequencies of width and length. a) Cardiff Audit Data. Width for L > 5 µm. N = 794, Bin width = 0.05 µm, GM Width = 0.18 µm, range 0.03–1.25. b) "Aerosol" (airborne TEM data from South African mines and analysis of bulk elutriated UICC sample). Width for L > 5 µm. N = 1538, GM width = 0.32 µm, range = 0.03–1.61. c) Cardiff Audit Data. Length < 50 µm (longer than 50 µm not shown = <1% of all EMP). N = 1781, Bin width = 1 µm, GM length = 5.95 µm, range 0.62 to 87.9 µm. d) "Aerosol." Length. N = 7484 (longer than 50 µm not shown = 1.2% of all EMP), GM length = 3.49 µm, range 0.45–1485 µm. Proportion of all lengths greater than 5 µm = 44.6% for Cardiff Audit Data and 20.6% of the aerosol comparison

(c)

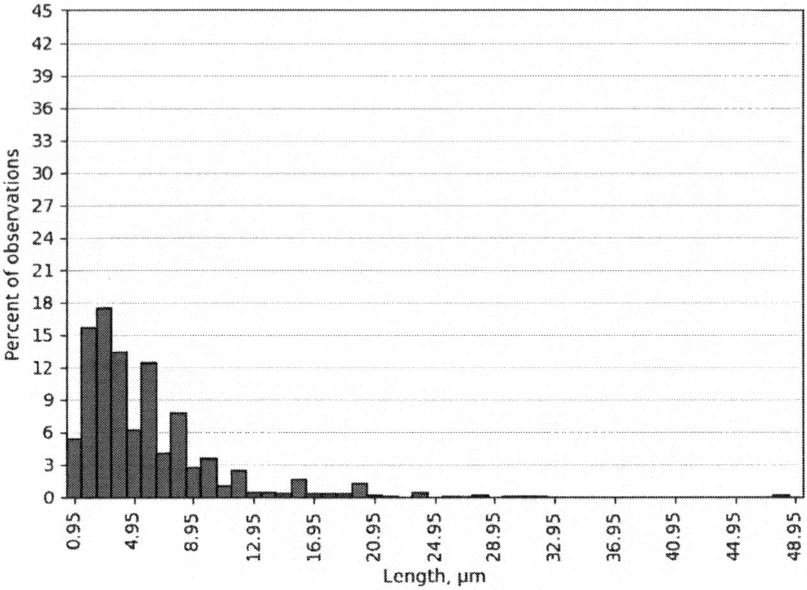

(d)

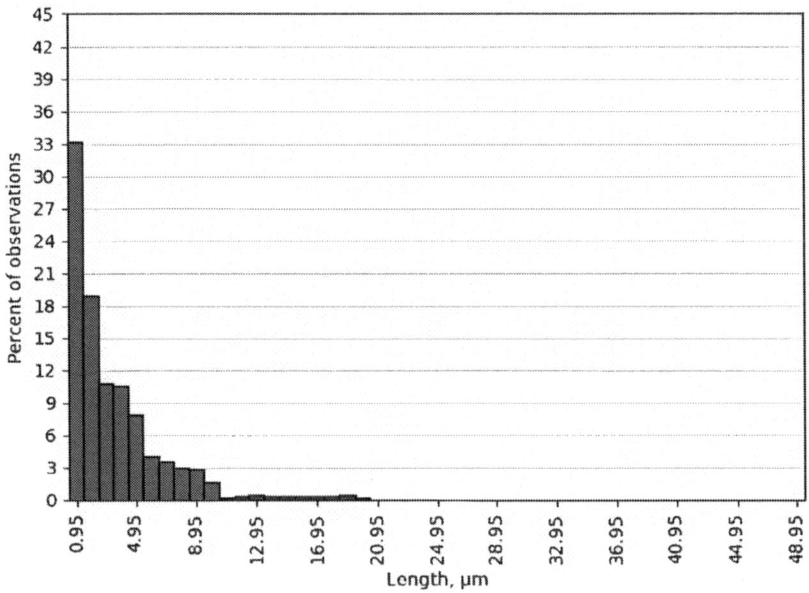

FIGURE 6.3 (Continued)

As was the case for amosite and chrysotile, EMPs found in the pleura are narrower than average for lung burden (0.080 vs. 0.110 μm) and also shorter (2.9 vs. 3.1 μm).

Tremolite

Tremolite is surprisingly common in lung burden, and most tremolite particles are rather uniform (Table 6.4). For all lengths, average geometric mean width ranges from 0.37 to 0.20 μm, with an average of 0.25 μm. For the category of EMP L > 5 μm, the average geometric mean width is 0.43 μm. Geometric mean lengths range from over 5 μm to less than 2, with an average of 2.6 μm. Tremolite in the lungs appears to have characteristics of asbestiform habit (see below).

These studies have led many to assume that tremolite asbestos does not have fibrils comparable to crocidolite in width. What is true is that there are many more occurrences of *tremolite,* both asbestiform and non-asbestiform, in surface rock than there are of amosite or crocidolite, which only occur in rocks of very restricted geographic distribution that formed more than a billion years ago with uncommon chemical composition. Tremolite and actinolite occur in a much greater variety of environments and, as such, display a much wider variety of habits. In some occurrences in the asbestiform habit, tremolite forms in fibrils as narrow as crocidolite; in others, it is brittle and looks like fiber glass. Recently, Pacella et al. (2024) demonstrated tremolite fibrils of widths less than 0.100 μm from a sample described as displaying a silky luster, a particular characteristic of asbestos with EMPA-sized fibrils.

One source of asbestiform tremolite is chrysotile ore, in which it is found as an accessory mineral. The ubiquitous association of this form of *tremolite* and chrysotile in the lungs of miners and millers from Quebec, especially from the mines near Asbestos, suggests an intimate intergrowth between fibers of these two minerals within the ore, although the physical relationship has never been described in the literature. Given the ubiquity of the association, most of the *tremolite* recorded in lung burden from asbestos workers is probably from this source and likely asbestiform, given the fact that asbestiform particles have a high likelihood of retention (Roggli, 2018). Other sources include industrial carbonates, industrial talc, crushed stone, and general mining.

The width distribution of tremolite L > 5 μm from Cardiff Audit Data has a mode at 0.35 μm with a possible second mode at about 0.65 μm. These modes are not repeated in the "aerosol," although the mode at 0.6 to 0.7 was found frequently by Wylie (2016) in amphibole cleavage populations. Like all forms of asbestos, the EMPs found in lung burden have fewer of the narrowest EMPs; in this case, the narrowest bin (<0.1 μm) is empty. This absence makes its identification as asbestiform or non-asbestiform more difficult. Another characteristic that is consistent across all minerals and very evident in the case of tremolite is that there is a higher proportion of longer EMPs retained in lung tissue than found in either asbestiform or non-asbestiform elutriated tremolite.

Figure 6.4b and 6.4c show the width frequency of elongated particles of tremolite found in our database in either an asbestiform or non-asbestiform habit. The samples used were either elutriated to reproduce an aerosol or were collected directly on air

TABLE 6.4
Tremolite

			Width			Length			Length
	Notes	Reference	GM (μm)	Mean (μm)	Median (μm)	GM (μm)	Mean (μm)	Median (μm)	Restriction (μm)
Lung	Cement SW	Pooley and Mitha (1986)	0.2			2.2			
	Textile U.S.	Pooley and Mitha (1986)	0.24			2.8			
	Control c	Pooley and Mitha (1986)	0.2			1.8			
	Control t	Pooley and Mitha (1986)	0.2			1.8			
		Warnock (1989)			0.3			2.5	
		Warnock (1989)	0.61 (1.98)			9.87 (1.58)			L > 5
	Charleston	Sebastien et al. (1989)		0.35			7.4		L > 5
	Thetford	Sebastien et al. (1989)		0.32			6.9		L > 5
		Suzuki and Kohyama (1991)	0.33 (2.6)			5.80 (2.75)			
		Tuomi (1992)		0.28	0.27		1.5	1.6	
	Other industry	Dufresne et al. (1996)	0.22 (2.2)			1.9 (1.7)			L < 5
	Asbestos	Dufresne et al. (1996)	0.24 (2.0)			2.1 (1.6)			
	Thetford	Dufresne et al. (1996)	0.22 (2.1)			1.9 (1.6)			
	Other industry	Dufresne et al. (1996)	0.35 (2.2)			6.9 (1.5)			L > 5
	Asbestos	Dufresne et al. (1996)	0.45 (2.0)			6.1 (1.4)			L > 5
	Thetford	Dufresne et al. (1996)	0.40 (2.1)			7.0 (1.5)			L > 5
	Background	Dodson et al. (1999)	0.26			2.4			
	Lung cancer	Dodson et al. (2004)	0.37			5.15			
		Dodson et al. (2005)	0.28			3.8			
		Cardiff audit data (2025) (see this chapter)	0.53 (2.01)			9.01 (1.83)			
Pleura	Tumor	Suzuki and Kohyama (1991)	0.19 (2.37)			1.61 (2.18)			

(a)

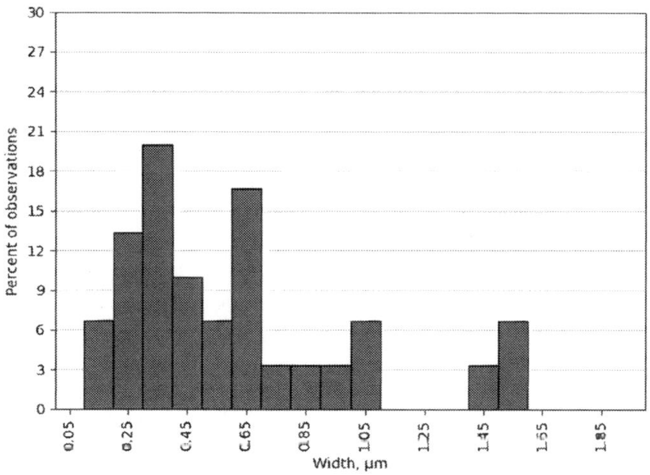

(b)

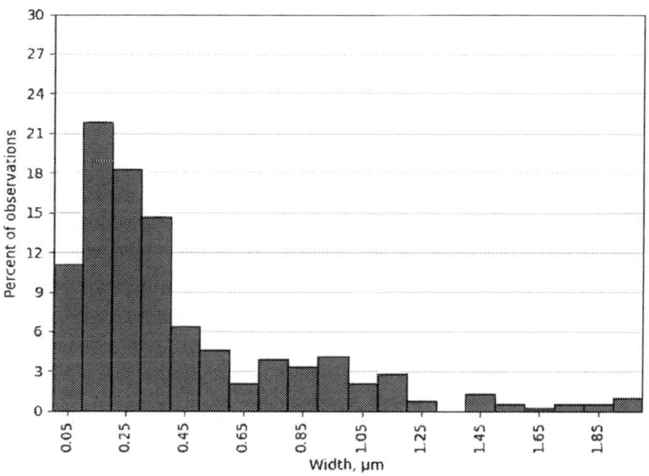

FIGURE 6.4 Tremolite frequencies of width and length. a) Cardiff Audit Data. Width for L > 5 µm. N = 30, bin width = 0.1 µm, GM width = 0.60 µm, range 0.125–1.55. b) "Aerosol" asbestiform tremolite (elutriated samples from Jamestown, CA, and Korea). Width for L > 5 µm. N = 389, bin width = 0.1 µm, GM width = 0.46 µm, range 0.09–1.9 µm. c) "Aerosol" non-asbestiform tremolite (elutriated samples from Shinness, Dornie, Ali da Stura, and airborne tremolite from El Dorado, CA). Width for L > 5 µm, N = 506, GM = 0.96 µm, range 0.16–2.0 µm. d) Cardiff Audit Data. Length < 50 µm (longer than 50 µm not shown = 1.3% of all EMP L > 5 µm). N = 76, bin width = 1 µm, GM length = 5.57 µm, range 0.99–53.4 µm. e) "Aerosol" asbestiform tremolite length. N = 13179, GM = 1.49, range 0.45–135.9 (longer than 50 µm not shown = < 1% of all EMP). f) "Aerosol" non-asbestiform tremolite length. N = 43020, GM length = 1.4 µm, range 0.51–57.2 µm (longer than 50 µm not shown = <0.1% of all EMP). Proportion of all lengths greater than 5 µm = 39.5% for Cardiff Audit Data, 3% for the asbestiform "aerosol," and 1.1% for the non-asbestiform aerosol comparison.

(c)

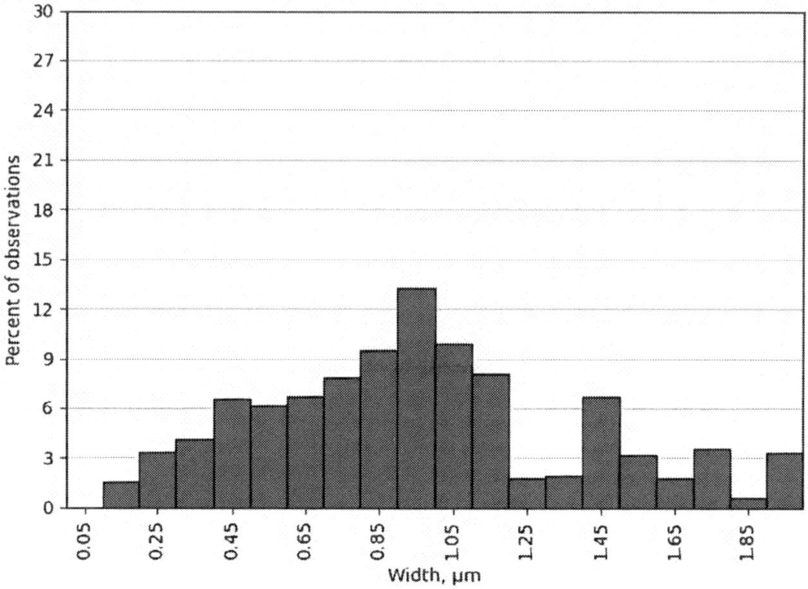

(d)

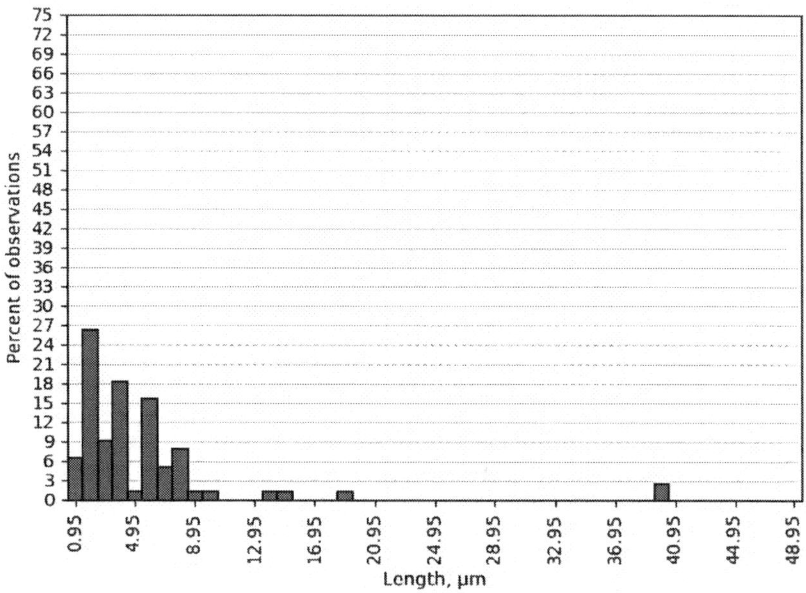

FIGURE 6.4 (Continued)

(e)

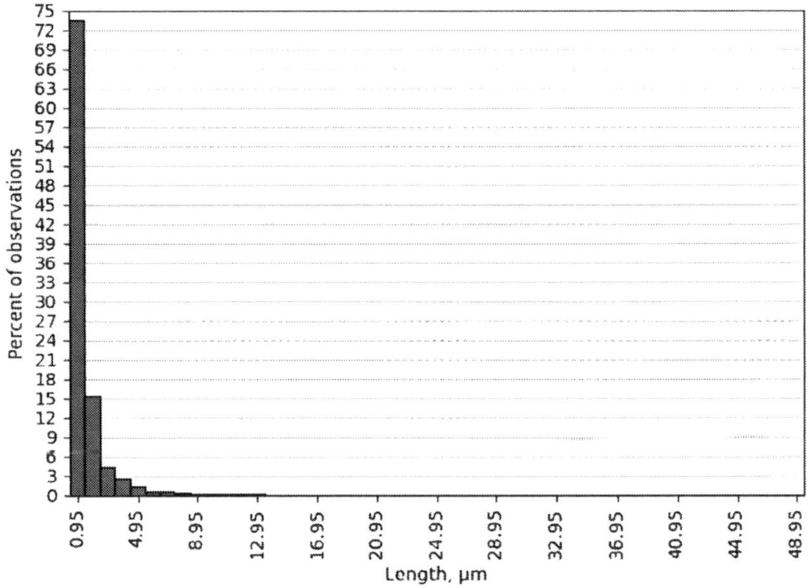

(f)

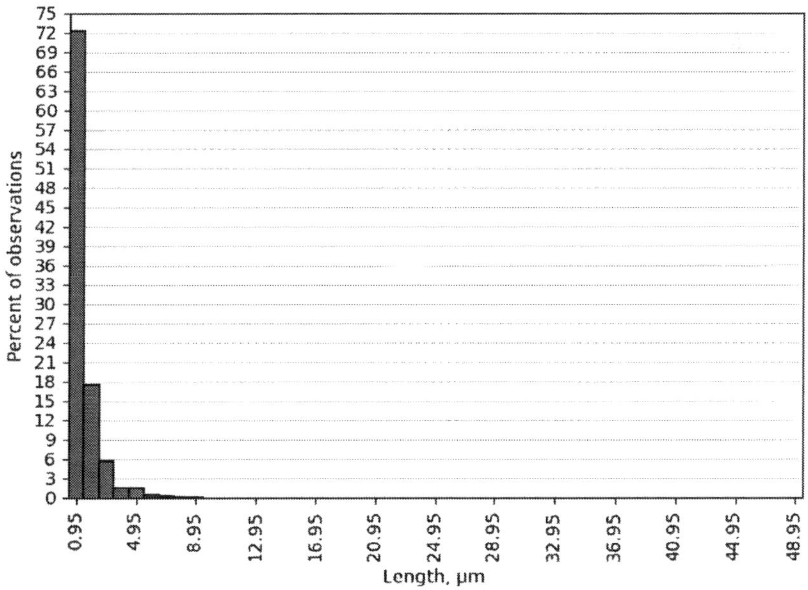

FIGURE 6.4 (Continued)

filters. The asbestiform tremolite is characterized by very abundant particles with width less than 0.50 μm, including abundant particles with width less than 0.150 μm; these EMP sizes are uncommon, and those with widths < 0.150 μm are almost absent among cleavage fragments.

In 2023, Wylie and Korchevskiy determined that the lung burden from Warnock (1989) is similar to other asbestiform minerals based on the low Pearson Index and high proportion of criteria particles. For the Cardiff Audit Data, the fraction of criteria tremolite is 0.645, and the Pearson index is 0.357. These values are typical for asbestiform tremolite. Non-asbestiform tremolite samples in our database all have a Pearson index above 0.4 and a criteria fraction smaller than 0.3 (Korchevskiy & Wylie, 2025).

Data on tremolite in the pleura are limited to a single study, and the EMP was from the tumor itself, so they may not be representative. Based on that study (see Table 6.5), the average length is about 1.6 μm and the average width is 0.190 μm.

Anthophyllite/talc

EMPs whose chemical composition and morphology are the only information on the mineral identity may not be identifiable without electron diffraction. For example, the Mg/Si ratio of chrysotile is quite different from that of anthophyllite, cummingtonite, and talc, so even though all four minerals are magnesium silicates, it can normally be used to distinguish chrysotile from amphibole or another sheet silicate. However, the Mg/Si ratio of pure Mg anthophyllite is identical to that of cummingtonite and so close to that of pure Mg talc that, without extraordinary measures not normally taken, these minerals cannot be reliably distinguished on the basis of Mg/Si alone. In some environments, however, variations in the amount of iron normally distinguish amphibole from talc. To complicate the identification further, there are the biopyriboles, Mg-rich silicate minerals jimthompsonite, clinojimthompsonite, and chesterite, which could be indistinguishable from anthophyllite by qualitative EDXA alone unless differences in the Fe/Mg among them from the mine source are known. All these chemically similar minerals can normally be distinguished if two or more zone axis electron diffraction patterns can be obtained and indexed. If reliance is only on a generic amphibole pattern with 5.3 A spacing between layer lines, the identification could be incorrect.

Studies of asbestiform anthophyllite samples from many locations in the world show that talc is always found with asbestiform anthophyllite (Watson, 1999; Cressey et al., 1982). In every case, talc EMP accompanied EMPs of anthophyllite asbestos. Therefore, it would be reasonable to find both anthophyllite and talc following exposure to anthophyllite asbestos. On the other hand, if an EMP is identified as talc, that does not mean that anthophyllite is also present because talc occurs as EMPs in rocks that lack anthophyllite.

The EMP distributions used to establish the "aerosol" came from asbestiform anthophyllite samples from the NSSGA databases. There are three characterizations of anthophyllite asbestos, each from Finland and India, and one each from Russia and Canada. The aerosol-sized particles were used for comparison, but there were no air samples in the simulated aerosol.

TABLE 6.5
Anthophyllite

		Width			Length			Length
	Notes	Reference	GM (µm)	Mean (µm)	Median (µm)	GM (µm)	Mean (µm)	Median (µm)	Restriction (µm)
Lung		Timbrell (1982)			0.57–0.76			3.4–19.4	Max = 100
		Warnock (1989)			0.23			2	
		Warnock (1989)	0.49 (2.18)			11.69 (1.72)			L > 5
		Suzuki and Kohyama (1991)	0.54 (2.37)			5.57 (3.11)			
		Tuomi (1992)		0.4	0.35		7.1	5	
	Other industry	Dufresne et al. (1996)	0.43 (1.8)			2.0 (1.7)			L < 5
	Asbestos	Dufresne et al. (1996)	0.30 (2.0)			2.0 (1.6)			L < 5
	Thetford	Dufresne et al. (1996)	0.34 (2.2)			2.1 (1.6)			L < 5
	Other industry	Dufresne et al. (1996)	0.97 (2.0)			7.0 (1.7)			L > 5
	Asbestos	Dufresne et al. (1996)	0.57 (2.5)			7.0 (1.5)			L > 5
	Thetford	Dufresne et al. (1996)	0.93 (2.0)			7.3 (1.5)			L > 5
	Background	Dodson et al. (1999)	0.25			2.97			
		Dodson et al. (2004)	0.29			4.1			
		Dodson et al. (2005)	0.35			5.7			
		Uibu et al. (2009)	0.26			9			L > 5
		Suzuki and Kohyama (1991)	0.23 (2.08)			2.3 (2.26)			
		Suzuki and Kohyama (1991)	0.39 (1.78)			4.4 (3.01)			

EMPs identified as anthophyllite are, in general, wider than amosite, chrysotile, crocidolite, and tremolite (Table 6.5). For the lung burden studies reported in Table 6.5, the geometric mean widths for all lengths average 0.36 μm, making it the widest EMP listed. With an average geometric mean length of 4.16 μm, it is within error of the geometric mean length of the other very long EMP, amosite (GML = 4.22μm).

Data on anthophyllite in the pleura are limited to two observations from a single study, so they may not be representative. Based on that study (see Table 6.5), the average length drops to about 3.3 μm; in the lymph nodes, the average EMP length is reported by Uibu et al. (2009) to be 9.

There are insufficient anthophyllite particles identified in the Cardiff Audit Data to produce a frequency distribution, but we can compare the data in Table 6.5 with data from the database for asbestiform anthophyllite. The database does not contain any data sets collected from aerosols, so we must compare the aerosol-sized portions of the TEM characterizations of bulk materials that include anthophyllite asbestos from India, Finland, and Russia in Figure 6.5. Although there is a wide range in width in the aerosol, there are EMPs that meet EMPA criteria. The averages of width reported in Table 6.5 range from 0.9 to 0.3, covering the rather uniform distribution of widths between these two limits among natural anthophyllite asbestos.

It should be noted that if the EMPs identified as anthophyllite in lungs are, in reality, talc (as we can hypothesize in many cases based on our experience and the literature), they should lack the biological potential to produce cancer because of their low rigidity (see Chapter 7).

Actinolite

There are very limited data on lung burden that specify actinolite (Table 6.6). There are no actinolite EMPs reported from tissue outside the lung. The four studies that report actinolite from lung burden show that it is very uniform in width, with geometric means ranging from 0.23 to 0.29 μm. Notably, the width is slightly less than that of tremolite, which differs from actinolite only in the amount of iron (vs. magnesium) (Verkouteren & Wylie, 2000). Prieskite is an asbestiform actinolite from South Africa.

Amphibole unspecified

The chemical signature of amosite and crocidolite appears very much the same to the energy-disperse X-ray detector, with the exception of the often hard-to-detect element sodium, a necessary component of crocidolite. In some studies, they are lumped together. Several researchers report their results by combining these two minerals under the label amphibole. As Table 6.7 shows, the EMPs are similar in dimension to crocidolite and amosite.

Mineral unspecified

Boutin et al. (1996) discussed the importance of Black Spots found around parietal pleura stomata, where EMPs pile up if they are too long to easily leave the pleural

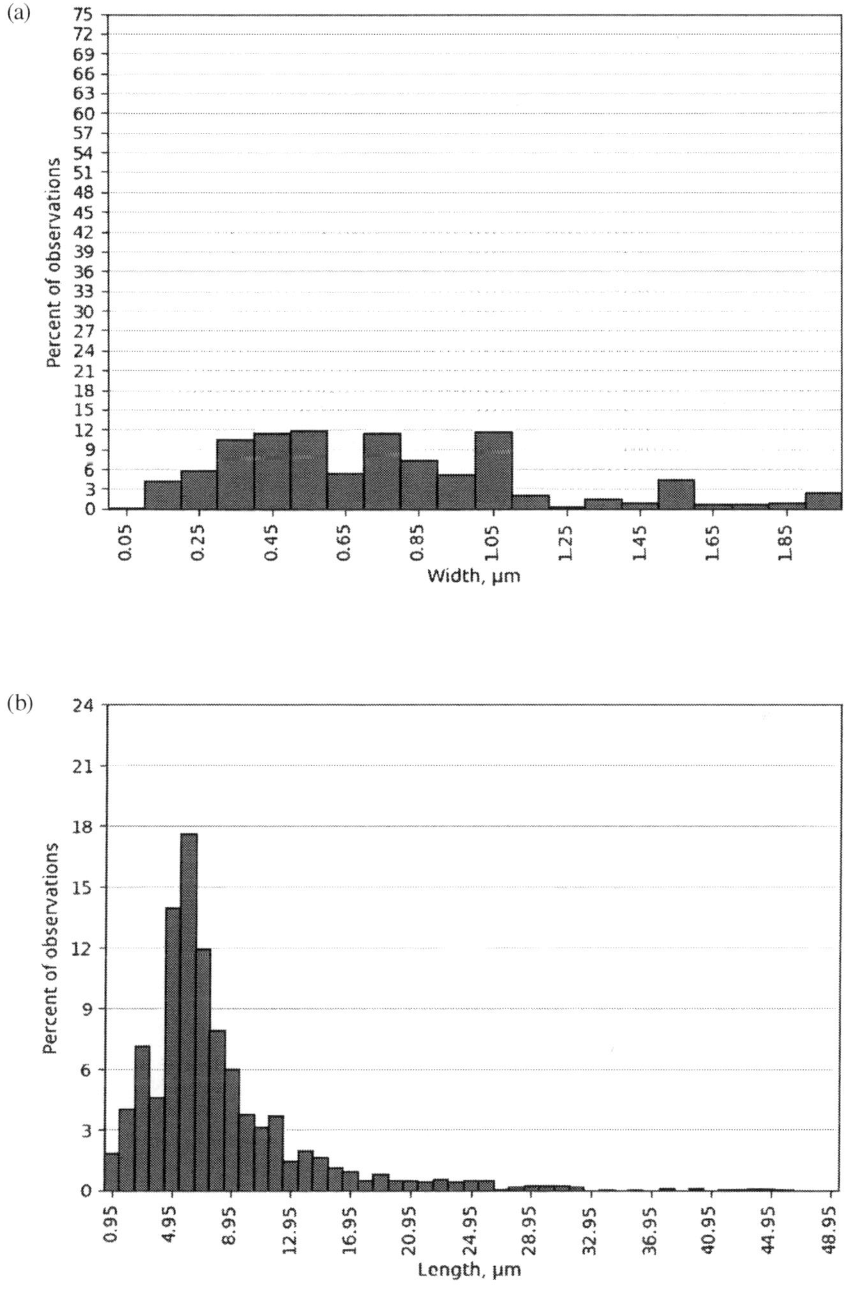

FIGURE 6.5 "Aerosol" Asbestiform Anthophyllite. a) Width distribution for L > 5 μm, TEM Database (India, Finland, Russia bulk, TEM). Bin width = 0.1 μm, N = 1056, GM width = 0.75 μm, range 0.05–2.0 μm. b) Length distribution Database, bulk TEM (Number of obs. 1501, Average 8.25 μm, range 0.7–45.8 μm)

TABLE 6.6
Actinolite

		Width			Length			Length
	Reference	GM (μm)	Mean (μm)	Median (μm)	GM (μm)	Mean (μm)	Median (μm)	Restriction (μm)
Lung	Warnock (1989)			0.25			2.1	
	Dodson et al. (2005)	0.23			5			
	Dodson et al. (2004)	0.29			4			

space through the 10 μm stomata. They compared "EMP" in the lung with that of the Black Spots and found that they are slightly wider in the Black Spots (0.13 μm) than in the lung (0.10 μm) and slightly longer (3.0 vs. 2.9 μm) (Table 6.7). These findings differ from other lung-pleura size comparisons, which generally show narrower EMP in the pleura than in the lung.

For four decades, Victor Roggli and associates recorded compositional information obtained from scanning electron microscopy and energy dispersive X-ray analysis (EDXA) examination of lung burden from mesothelioma and control cases. Roggli's data (2018) demonstrate that many different silicate minerals can form particles longer than 5 μm in length with a minimum elongation of 3:1 that are inhaled and deposited in the lung. Among this group are oxides such as rutile and other metal oxides, alumino-silicates, sulfates, talc, quartz, and a variety of silicates with variable amounts of Ca, Mg, Fe, Na, and K, as well as manufactured fibers such as rock wool and carbon nanotubes. The variety of minerals reflects exposures that are highly variable among individuals, reflecting exposure to specific dusts in each case, and varying with age, occupation, gender, and location.

Other tissue sites

Heller et al. (1999) studied the minerals found in ovarian tissue of 13 women who had experienced household contact with family members who were asbestos workers. They identified almost 400 EMPs, of which all but 2% were chrysotile or crocidolite; chrysotile made up 70% and crocidolite, 28%. In total, 77% of the crocidolite and 82% of the chrysotile had widths less than 0.100 μm, and the rest had widths less than 0.200 μm. Of the 8 tremolite particles found, 6 had widths < 0.2 μm. Of particular note is that almost all the EMPs were longer than 3 μm, and about 15% were longer than 10 μm. Normally abundant short EMP was largely absent. In a follow-up study of asbestos in fallopian tubes associated with the ovarian tissue examined earlier, they found the same two dominant minerals: chrysotile and crocidolite, as well as identifying amosite in one fallopian tube sample only (Heller et al., 1999). Langseth et al. (2007) report the dimensions of 7 EMPs from two cases of ovarian cancer among household exposure to asbestos in Norway. The

TABLE 6.7
Amphibole and unspecified mineralogy

	Notes	Reference	Width GM (μm)	Width Mean (μm)	Width Median (μm)	Length GM (μm)	Length Mean (μm)	Length Median (μm)	Length Restriction (μm)
a) Amphibole									
Lung		Dodson et al. (1990)	0.14			3.39			
	Normal	Friedrichs et al. (1992)	0.17			2.6			
	Lung cancer	Friedrichs et al. (1992)	0.19			4.4			
	Asbestosis	Friedrichs et al. (1992)	0.17			6.3			
		Friedrichs et al. (1992)	0.16			6			
Pleura		Dodson et al. (1990)	0.14			1.05			
	Node	Dodson et al. (1990)	0.18			1.55			
b) No mineral specified									
	Lung	Boutin et al. (1996)*	0.1			2.9			
	Black spot	Boutin et al. (1996)*	0.13			3.03			

* Maximum lengths were 90 and 26 μm lung and black spot, respectively.

lengths ranged from 2.5–10 μm, and the widths from 0.2–0.4 μm. Such long fibers of chrysotile and crocidolite are inconsistent with dimensions reported elsewhere for tissue burden, and additional work is needed to substantiate and understand these findings.

GENERAL CHARACTERISTICS OF LUNG BURDEN VS. AEROSOLS

Tissue burden is not a replica of an individual's exposure over a lifetime. Particle sizes in the aerosol are deposited in different proportions and cleared from the lung in different proportions, and while lung burden does not duplicate the exposure exactly, it has many characteristics in common because lung burden is a subset of the inhalable aerosol.

The dimensional characteristics of lung burden reflect both the lungs as a filter that retains certain portions of an inhalable aerosol and the mineralogical characteristics of that aerosol, which govern the availability of particular particle sizes.

The "aerosols" we have shown in Figures 6.1 to 6.5 are a composite of many samples of the same mineral in the same habit. In the case of tremolite, both an asbestiform and non-asbestiform "aerosol" were used for comparison. These "aerosols" are not the actual aerosol for the exposed individuals, but they do represent a reservoir from which inhaled particles were derived.

Comparing the "aerosol" to the lung burden frequency distributions in Figures 6.1 to 6.5 shows that

1. Lung burden has a higher proportion of EMPs ≤0.15(±0.05) μm in width, although the narrowest width category contains very few EMPs.
2. EMPs with $L > 5$ μm are more abundant in lung burden.
3. EMPs with $L < 2$ μm are less abundant in lung burden.

While there is a wide range among particle size frequencies of EMPs deposited in lungs because of individual variability, the consistency of the observations suggests that width and length frequency differences between aerosol and lung burden are reproducible and real for amosite, chrysotile, and crocidolite. For tremolite, the narrowest width category is absent, but the widest EMPs are more abundant than in tremolite asbestos but less abundant than for non-asbestiform tremolite.

The higher proportion of long EMPs in lung burden is consistent with several hypotheses:

1. Short EMPs are deposited at a lower frequency than long EMPs because they have a smaller aerodynamic diameter and are exhaled preferentially.
2. Short EMPs are deposited as agglomerates in the mucociliary portion of the airways.
3. Short EMPs are cleared more easily, and longer EMPs are more biopersistent.
4. Short EMPs are not counted for some other reason (though this option was not demonstrated practically).

That lung burden EMPs are narrower than aerosol EMPs is consistent with several hypotheses:

1. Narrow width favors the ability of long rigid EMPs to enter the lung interstitium.
2. Wider EMPs break apart (disaggregate) into component fibrils during inhalation and following deposition.
3. Wider EMPs are more readily removed than narrow ones.
4. Long narrow EMPs lack rigidity, cannot translocate out of the lung, and are preferentially retained.
5. Macrophages are less efficient at clearing the narrowest EMPs.

EMPs in lung vs. pleura

Although the data are very limited, the data in Tables 6.1 through 6.7 show that EMPs found in the pleural region are narrower than is typical of lung burden, and where the data are available, they are shorter. However, not evident in the averages is the fact that EMPs longer than about 30 µm are unknown from the pleura, but not lung burden, which may contain EMPs of 300 µm or more. It is important to highlight that areas rich in stomata do contain preferentially longer EMPs, and amphibole asbestos is common.

Several hypotheses can be proposed to explain these observations:

1. The processes that favor translocation to the pleura favor the narrowest, rigid EMPs.
2. Long EMPs may lack rigidity and cannot translocate within the lung readily.
3. EMPs are transported to the pleura by macrophages, which have an upper limit on the length they can phagocytize (10 µm).
4. EMPs translocate to the pleura as a component of lymphatic fluids, which favor narrow, rigid EMPs < 20 µm in length.

The limited number of measurements of EMP in the pleura gives some caution in interpreting differences with lung burden. Most of these measurements are from tumors and pleural plaques; however, so even though limited, they could have significance for understanding the initiation of mesothelial carcinogenicity.

In the parietal pleura, chrysotile is more commonly reported than amphibole. Amphibole is more common in the thoracic lymph nodes, explained by the observation that amphibole is better able to penetrate the alveolar wall (Bignon et al., 1979). It certainly seems clear that long amphibole EMPs, 5 to 20 µm in length, are abundant in lung burden (see Figures 6.1 to 6.5). If they are rigid and narrow enough, they can translocate to the pleura.

Lung burden studies show that, on average, tremolite, anthophyllite, and actinolite are wider than reported for chrysotile, crocidolite, and amosite. These three minerals are rarely reported in the pleura or anywhere outside the lung, with the exception of cases exposed occupationally to anthophyllite asbestos, where very narrow EMPs (< 0.150 μm) are a component of the aerosol. Others have also pointed out that mineral EMPs of all types are shorter and narrower in the pleura (Dodson et al., 1990; Bignon et al., 1979) than in the lung. Overall, studies are consistent with the hypothesis that translocation favors narrow EMPs (< 0. 2 μm) and EMPs that are < 20 μm in length.

Chrysotile EMPs are usually reported as abundant in the pleura. Thought to readily break into shorter component fibrils following inhalation and deposition, increasing numbers of chrysotile fibrils are available for translocation. The abundance of short EMPs does not rule out the potential for longer chrysotile EMPs with properties similar to amphibole. Long chrysotile EMPs could be biologically rigid if their widths are greater > 60 nm (Brobell et al., 2020; Wylie & Korchevskiy, 2025).

DISCUSSION

The mineral EMP found in human lungs and other tissues following exposures to asbestos and the development of asbestos-related diseases contains large proportions of long, very narrow fibrils. Removed from lung burden are the EMPs that migrate to the pleura, creating conditions for the development of mesothelioma. Although all particles that are longer than 5 μm and meet the minimum aspect ratio criterion of 3 are counted in assessing asbestos exposure following protocols of the National Institutes of Occupational Safety and Health (NIOSH), only a small portion of these make up lung EMP burden, and only a portion of these are responsible for mesothelioma. The strongest evidence for a "mesotheliomagenic EMP" as a subset of the NIOSH EMP is that the same exposure intensities and durations result in very different incidences of mesothelioma, differences that can be explained by the characteristics of the EMPs in the exposure.

Some investigators have suggested that it is EMPs longer than 20 μm that are most likely involved in asbestos-related cancers. It is true that very long EMPs, once inhaled and deposited, can participate in the development of lung cancer, but very long EMPs are uncommon outside the lung interstitium. For thin EMPs of most concern in mesothelioma, $W \leq 0.15$ μm, on rigidity considerations alone, very long thin EMPs (e.g., $L > 40$ μm, $W < 0.10$ μm) would lack biological rigidity and would not likely translocate. Longer EMPs are also trapped in the lungs when they become encased by asbestos bodies, which favor long, wide EMPs that do not translocate.

If we analyze the dimensional coefficient of carcinogenicity (DCC), as described in Chapter 4, it is noteworthy that DCC generally increases with length for elongate mineral particles, but the strength of the relationship drops significantly when the length range increases. In particular, for length > 40 μm, the correlation R between DCC and length is just 0.18, R^2=0.03, while for length < 40 μm, R = 0.42, R2 =0.18.

EMPs less than about 20 μm in length reach the pleura and other organs outside the lung. The length-limiting factors of narrow EMPs include rigidity and the maximum length of EMP that can be engulfed by a macrophage without killing it (10 μm) or at least delaying its death until it is transported to the pleura. The alternate route to the pleura, direct penetration through the visceral pleura or passage through the visceral pleura as part of the drainage system of the lung, must depend on length and width (as a proxy for cross-sectional area) and probably rigidity. In the case of asbestos, the mass of the EMP is determined primarily by length.

Since experiments exposing animals were first conducted, it has been recognized that there is a maximum width for mesotheliomagenic mineral EMP that is probably around 0.150 μm (±0.050), as suggested by Lippmann (2014). It is consistent with the work of Korchevskiy and Wylie (2022), who have shown that the highest predictor of mesotheliomagenicity is the proportion of EMPs with widths < 0.2 (±0.050) μm. These are the dimensions of EMPs most commonly found toward the periphery and outside the lung. If EMPs must be able to translocate to the pleura to induce mesothelioma, narrow rigid EMPs of 5 to 20 μm are probably those most able to make that journey and damage mesothelial cells.

In closing, it should be noted that there is a significant discrepancy between the size distribution of EMPs in the lungs and pleura and the results of the MPPD model developed by the EPA. In particular, there is no evidence that the expected minimum deposition rate of elongate particles can be detected at the diameter of about 0.1 μm as predicted. As demonstrated in Korchevskiy et al. (2025), there is a negative correlation between the observed pulmonary deposition rate of EMPs and the estimations by MPPD. Further studies are needed to develop an updated computer model for EMP deposition and translocation in the lungs that would better reflect observations.

REFERENCE LIST

Alario Franco, M., Hutchison, J. L., Jefferson, D. A., & Thomas, J. M. (1977). Structural imperfection and morphology of crocidolite (blue asbestos). *Nature*, *266*, 520–521. https://doi.org/10.1038/266520a0

Asgharian, B., Owen, T. P., Kuempel, E. D., & Jarabek, A. M. (2018). Dosimetry of inhaled elongate mineral particles in the respiratory tract: The impact of shape factor. *Toxicology and Applied Pharmacology*, *361*, 27–35. https://doi.org/10.1016/j.taap.2018.05.001

Attanoos, R. L., Alchami, F., & Gibbs, A. R. (2016). A correlative analysis of asbestos fibers, bodies, fibrosis and controls: Predictions on mineral analysis from tissue sections. *Archives of Pathology & Laboratory Medicine*, *140*(3), 262–263. Abstracts From the Pulmonary Pathology Society 2015 Biennial Meeting. https://doi.org/10.5858/arpa.2015-0409-AB

Bales, R. C., & Morgan, J. J. (1985). Dissolution kinetics of chrysotile at pH 7–10. *Geochimica et Cosmochimica Acta*, *49*(11), 2281–2288. https://doi.org/10.1016/0016-7037(85)90228-5

Barlow, C. A., & Mossman, B. T. (2025). Cellular defense mechanisms against asbestos fibers. *Frontiers in Public Health*, *13*. https://doi.org/10.3389/fpubh.2025.1566473

Bellman, B., Konig, H., Muhle, H., & Pott, F. (1986). Chemical durability of asbestos and of man-made mineral fibers in vivo. *Journal of Aerosol Science*, *17*, 341–345.

Bernareggi, A., Ren, E., Borelli, V., Vita, F., Constanti, A., & Zabucchi, G. (2015). Xenopus laevis oocytes as a model system for studying the interaction between asbestos fibres and cell membranes. *Toxicological Sciences*, *145*(2), 263–272. https://doi.org/10.1093/toxsci/kfv050

Bernstein, D., Dunnigan, J., Hesterberg, T., Brown, R., Velasco, J. A., Barrera, R., Hoskins, J., & Gibbs, A. (2013). Health risk of chrysotile revisited. *Critical Reviews in Toxicology*, *43*(2), 154–183. https://doi.org/10.3109/10408444.2012.756454

Berry, G., Pooley, F., Gibbs, A., Harris, J. M., & McDonald, J. C. (2009). Lung fiber burden in the Nottingham gas mask cohort. *Inhalation Toxicology*, *21*(2), 168–172. https://doi.org/10.1080/08958370802291304

Bignon, J., Monchaux, G., Sebastien, P., Hirsh, A., & Lafuma, J. (1979). Human and experimental data on translocation of asbestos fibers through the respiratory system. *Annals of the New York Academies of Science*, *330*, 745–750. https://doi.org/10.1111/j.1749-6632.1979.tb18778.x

Boutin, C., Dumortier, P., Rey, F., Viallat, J. R., & De Vuyst, P. (1996). Black spots concentrate oncogenic asbestos fibers in the parietal pleura: Thorascopic and mineralogic study. *American Journal of Respiratory and Critical Care Medicine*, *153*, 444–449. https://doi.org/10.1164/ajrccm.153.1.8542156

Brantley, S. L. (2003). 5.03 – reaction kinetics of primary rock-forming minerals under ambient conditions. In H. D. Holland & K. K. Turekian (Eds.), *Treatise on geochemistry* (pp. 73–117). Pergamon. https://doi.org/10.1016/B0-08-043751-6/05075-1

Broaddus, V. C., Everitt, J. I., Black, B., & Kane, A. B. (2011). Non-neoplastic and neoplastic pleural endpoints following fiber exposure. *Journal of Toxicology and Environmental Health, Part B*, *14*(1–4), 153–178. https://doi.org/10.1080/10937404.2011.556049

Brobell, D., Meyer-Plath, A. A., Kampf, K., Plitzko, S., Wohlleben, W., Stahlmecke, B., Wiemann, M., & Haase, A. (2020). A human risk banding scheme for high aspect-ratio materials. In R. M. Wagtervelci, J. C. M. Marynissen, L. Gradon, & A. Moskai (Eds.), *Synthetic nano-and microfibers* (Chapter 7). Westim European Center of Excellence for Sustainable Water Technology. www.wetsus.nl

Brown, J. S., Gordon, T., Price, O., & Asgharian, B. (2013). Thoracic and respirable particle definitions for human health risk assessment. *Particle and Fibre Toxicology*, *10*, 12. https://doi.org/10.1186/1743-8977-10-12

Burdett, G. J., Firth, J. G., Rood, A. P., & Streeter, R. R. (1988). Application of fibre retention and carcinogenicity curves to fibre size distributions of asbestos. *The Annals of Occupational Hygiene*, *32*(Inhaled Particles, VI), 341–351. https://doi.org/10.1093/annhyg/32.inhaled_particles_VI.341

Caraballo-Arias, Y., Caffaro, P., Boffetta, P., & Violante, F. S. (2022a). Quantitative assessment of asbestos fibers in normal and pathological pleural tissue: A scoping review. *Life*, *12*(2), 296. https://doi.org/10.3390/life12020296

Caraballo-Arias, Y., Zunarelli, C., Caffaro, P., Roccuzzo, F., Nocilla, M. R., Imperiale, M. C., Romano, C., Boffetta, P., & Violante, F. S. (2022b). Quantitative assessment of asbestos fibers in normal and pathological peritoneal tissue: A scoping review. *Life*, *12*, 1969. https://doi.org/10.3390/life12121969

Case, B. W. (1994). Biological indicators of chrysotile exposure. *The Annals of Occupational Hygiene*, *38*(4), 503–518. https://doi.org/10.1093/annhyg/38.4.503

Chisholm, J. E. (1983). Transmission electron microscopy of asbestos. In S. S. Chissick & R. Derricott (Eds.), *Asbestos: Properties, applications and hazards* (Vol. 2, pp. 86–167). John Wiley and Sons.

Churg, A., & Warnock, M. L. (1977). Analysis of the cores of ferruginous (asbestos) bodies from the general population. I: Patients with and without lung cancer. *Laboratory Investigation*, *37*(3), 280–286. PMID: 895070.

Churg, A., & Wiggs, B. (1989). The distribution of amosite asbestos fibers in the lungs of workers with mesothelioma or carcinoma. *Experimental Lung Research*, *15*(5), 771–783. https://doi.org/10.3109/01902148909062860

Churg, A., Wiggs, B., Depaoli, L., Kampe, B., & Stevens, B. (1984). Lung asbestos content in chrysotile workers with mesothelioma. *The American Review of Respiratory Disease*, *130*(6), 1042–1045. https://doi.org/10.1164/arrd.1984.130.6.1042

Coffin, D. L., Palekar, L. D., & Cook, P. M. (1982). Tumorigenesis by a ferroactinolite mineral. *Toxicology Letters*, *13*(3–4), 143–149. https://doi.org/10.1016/0378-4274(82)90202-8

Coin, P. G., Roggli, V. L., & Brody, A. R. (1992). Deposition, clearance, and translocation of chrysotile asbestos from peripheral and central regions of the rat lung. *Environmental Research*, *58*(1–2), 97–116. https://doi.org/10.1016/S0013-9351(05)80207-5

Cook, P. M., Swintek, J., Dawson, T. D., Chapman, D., Etterson, M. A., & Hoff, D. (2016). Quantitative structure-mesothelioma potency model optimization for complex mixtures of elongated particles in rat pleura: A retrospective study. *Journal of Toxicology and Environmental Health, Part B*, *19*(5–6), 266–288. https://doi.org/10.1080/10937404.2016.1195326

Cressey, B. A., Whittaker, E. J. W., & Hutchison, J. L. (1982). Morphology and alteration of asbestiform grunerite and anthophyllite. *Mineralogical Magazine*, *46*(338), 77–87. https://doi.org/10.1180/minmag.1982.046.338.13

Dodson, R. F., Brooks, D. R., O'Sullivan, M., & Hammar, S. P. (2004). Quantitative analysis of asbestos burden in a series of individuals with Lung cancer and a history of exposure to asbestos. *Inhalation Toxicology*, *16*, 637–647. https://doi.org/10.1080/08958370490464652

Dodson, R. F., Graef, R., Shepherd, S., O'Sullivan, M., & Levin, J. (2005). Asbestos burden in cases of mesothelioma from individuals from various regions of the United States. *Ultrastructural Pathology*, *29*(5), 415–433. https://doi.org/10.1080/019131290945682

Dodson, R. F., Huang, J., & Bruce, J. R. (2000). Asbestos content in the lymph nodes of nonoccupationally exposed individuals. *American Journal of Industrial Medicine*, *37*(2), 169–174. https://doi.org/10.1002/(SICI)1097-0274(200002)37:2%3C169::AID-AJIM2%3E3.0.CO;2-V

Dodson, R. F., O'Sullivan, M., & Corn, C. J. (1996). Relationships between ferruginous bodies and uncoated asbestos fibers in lung tissue. *Archives of Environmental Health*, *51*(6), 462–466. https://doi.org/10.1080/00039896.1996.9936047

Dodson, R. F., Williams, M. G., Corn, C. J., Brollo, A., & Bianchi, C. (1990). Asbestos content of lung tissue, lymph nodes, and pleural plaques from former shipyard workers. *American Review of Respiratory Disease*, *142*, 843–847. https://doi.org/10.1164/ajrccm/142.4.843

Dodson, R. F., Williams, M. G., Huang, J., & Bruce, J. R. (1999). Tissue burden of asbestos in nonoccupationally exposed individuals from east Texas. *American Journal of Industrial Medicine*, *35*(3), 281–286. https://doi.org/10.1002/(sici)1097-0274(199903)35:3%3C281::aid-ajim8%3E3.0.co;2-o

Donaldson, K., Murphy, F. A., Duffin, R., & Poland, C. A. (2010). Asbestos, carbon nanotubes and the pleural mesothelium: A review of the hypothesis regarding the role of long fibre retention in the parietal pleura, inflammation and mesothelioma. *Particle and Fibre Toxicology*, *7*, 5. https://doi.org/10.1186/1743-8977-7-5

Dufresne, A., Bégin, R., Churg, A., & Massé, S. (1996). Mineral fiber content of lungs in patients with mesothelioma seeking compensation in Québec. *American Journal of Respiratory and Critical Care Medicine*, *153*(2), 711–718. https://doi.org/10.1164/ajrccm.153.2.8564122

Feder, I. S., Tischoff, I., Theile, A., Schmitz, I., Merget, R., & Tannapfel, A. (2016). The asbestos fibre burden in human lungs: New insights into the chrysotile debate. *The European Respiratory Journal*, *48*(6), 1602534. https://doi.org/10.1183/13993003.02534-2016

Fernández Tena, A., & Casan Clarà, P. (2012). Deposition of inhaled particles in the lungs. *Archivos de Bronconeumologia*, *48*(7), 240–246. English, Spanish. https://doi.org/10.1016/j.arbres.2012.02.003

Friedrichs, K. H., Brockmann, M., Fischer, M., & Wick, G. (1992). Electron microscopy analysis of mineral fibers in human lung tissue. *American Journal of Industrial Medicine*, *22*, 49–58. https://doi.org/10.1002/ajim.4700220105

Fröhlich, E. (2012). The role of surface charge in cellular uptake and cytotoxicity of medical nanoparticles. *International Journal of Nanomedicine*, *7*, 5577–5591. https://doi.org/10.2147/IJN.S36111

Fukushima, S., Kasai, T., Umeda, Y., Ohnishi, M., Sasaki, T., & Matsumoto, M. (2017). Carcinogenicity of multi-walled carbon nanotubes: Challenging issue on hazard assessment. *Journal of Occupational Health*, *60*, 10–30. https://doi.org/10.1539/joh.17-0102-RA

Gaudichet, A., Sebastien, P., Clark, N. J., & Pooley, F. D. (1980). Identification and quantification of asbestos fibres in human tissues. *IARC Scientific Publication*, *30*, 61–62. PMID: 7239671.

Geiser, M., Casaulta, M., Kupferschmid, B., Schulz, H., Semmler-Behnke, M., & Kreyling, W. (2008). The role of macrophages in the clearance of inhaled ultrafine titanium dioxide particles. *American Journal of Respiratory Cell and Molecular Biology*, *38*(3), 371–376. https://doi.org/10.1165/rcmb.2007-0138OC

Ghio, A. J., Stewart, M., Sangani, R. G., Pavlisko, E. N., & Roggli, V. L. (2023). Asbestos and iron. *International Journal of Molecular Sciences*, *24*(15), 12390. https://doi.org/10.3390/ijms241512390

Gibbons, W. (2000). Amphibole asbestos in Africa and Australia: Geology, health hazard and mining legacy. *Journal of the Geological Society*, *157*, 851–858. https://doi.org/10.1144/jgs.157.4.851

Gibbs, A. R., Griffiths, D. M., Pooley, F. D., & Jones, J. S. (1990). Comparison of fibre types and size distributions in lung tissues of paraoccupational and occupational cases of malignant mesothelioma. *British Journal of Industrial Medicine*, *47*(9), 621–626. https://doi.org/10.1136/oem.47.9.621

Gibbs, A. R., & Pooley, F. D. (1996). Analysis and interpretation of inorganic mineral particles in "lung" tissues. *Thorax*, *31*, 327–334. https://doi.org/10.1136/thx.51.3.327

Gibbs, A. R., Stephens, M., Griffiths, D. M., Blight, B. J. N., & Pooley, F. D. (1991). Fibre distribution in the lungs and pleura of subject with asbestos related diffuse pleural fibrosis. *British Journal of Industrial Medicine*, *48*, 762–770. https://doi.org/10.1136/oem.48.11.762

Gilham, C., Rake, C., Burdett, G., Nicholson, A. G., Davison, L., Franchini, A., Carpenter, J., Hodgson, J., Darnton, A., & Peto, J. (2016). Pleural mesothelioma and lung cancer risks in relation to occupational history and asbestos lung burden. *Occupational & Environmental Medicine*, *73*(5), 290–299. https://doi.org/10.1136/oemed-2015-103074

Gualtieri, A. F. (2022). Journey to the centre of the lung: The perspective of a mineralogist on carcinogenic effects of mineral fibres in the lungs. *Journal of Hazardous Materials* https://doi.org/10.1016/j.jhazmat.2022.130077

Gualtieri, A. F., Pollastri, S., Gandolfi, N. B., & Gualtieri, M. L. (2018). In vitro acellular dissolution of mineral fibres: A comparative study. *Scientific Reports*, *8*, 7071. https://doi.org/10.1038/s41598-018-25531-4

Haque, A. K., Vrazel, D. M., Burau, K. D., Cooper, S. P., & Downs, T. (1996). Is there transplacental transfer of asbestos? A study of 40 stillborn infants. *Pediatric Pathology & Laboratory Medicine*, *16*(6), 877–892. https://doi.org/10.1080/15513819609168711

Heller, D. S., Gordon, R. E., & Katz, N. (1999). Correlation of asbestos fiber burdens in fallopian tubes and ovarian tissue. *American Journal of Obstetrics and Gynecology*, *181*(2), 346–347. https://doi.org/10.1016/s0002-9378(99)70559-4

Hiroshima, K., Mural, Y., Suzuki, Y., Goldstein, B., & Webster, I. (1993). Characterization of asbestos fibers in lungs and mesotheliomatous tissues of baboons following long-term inhalation. *American Journal of Industrial Medicine*, *23*, 883–901. https://doi.org/10.1002/ajim.4700230606

Hojo, M., Maeno, A., Sakamoto, Y., Ohnuki, A., Tada, Y., Yamamoto, Y., Ikushima, K., Inaba, R., Suzuki, J., Taquahashi, Y., Yokota, S., Kobayashi, N., Ohnishi, M., Goto, Y., Numano, T., Tsuda, H., Alexander, D. B., Kanno, J., Hirose, A., Inomata, A., & Nakae, D. (2022). Two-year intermittent exposure of a multiwalled carbon nanotube by intratracheal instillation induces lung tumors and pleural mesotheliomas in F344 rats. *Particle and Fibre Toxicology*, *19*(1), 38. https://doi.org/10.1186/s12989-022-00478-7

Huang, J., Hisanaga, N., Sakai, K., Iwata, M., Ono, Y., Shibata, E., & Takeuchi, Y. (1988). Asbestos fibers in human pulmonary and extrapulmonary tissues. *American Journal of Industrial Medicine*, *14*(3), 331–339. https://doi.org/10.1002/ajim.4700140310

Incharoen, P., Hama, T., Arsa, L., Kamprerasart, K., Wongwichai, S., & Bovornkitti, S. (2019). Asbestos bodies burden in the autopsy lung tissue from general Thai population. *The Open Respiratory Medicine Journal*, *13*, 5–10. https://doi.org/10.2174/1874306401913010005

Jung, H. S., Park, E. K., Cha, J. S., Lee, J. W., Lee, J. C., Jang, J., Kim, S., Oak, C., Yates, D. H., & Kim, H. (2020). Characteristics of asbestos fibers in lung tissue from occupational and environmental asbestos exposure of lung cancer patients in Busan, Korea. *Scientific Reports*, *10*, 20359. https://doi.org/10.1038/s41598-020-77291-9

Kane, A. K., Hurt, R. H., & Gao, H. (2018). The asbestos-carbon nanotube analogy: An update. *Toxicology and Applied Pharmacology*, *361*, 68–80. https://doi.org/10.1016/j.taap.2018.06.027

Korchevskiy, A., Attanoos, R., & Wylie, A. G. (2025). Size-dependent retention of elongate mineral particles in human lungs: Modeling and implications for risk assessment. *Frontiers in Public Health*, *13*. https://doi.org/10.3389/fpubh.2025.1646016

Korchevskiy, A. A., & Wylie, A. G. (2022). Dimensional characteristics of the major types of amphibole mineral particles and the implications for carcinogenic risk assessment. *Inhalation Toxicology*, *34*(1–2), 24–38. https://doi.org/10.1080/08958378.2021.2024304

Korchevskiy, A. A., & Wylie, A. G. (2025). Habit of elongate amphibole particles as a predictor of mesothelial carcinogenicity. *Toxicology Reports*, *14*, 101908. https://doi.org/10.1016/j.toxrep.2025.101908

Krombach, F., Münzing, S., Allmeling, A. M., Gerlach, J. T., Behr, J., & Dörger, M. (1997). Cell size of alveolar macrophages: An interspecies comparison. *Environmental Health Perspectives*, *105*(Suppl 5), 1261–1263. https://doi.org/10.1289/ehp.97105s51261

Langer, A. M., Badin, V., Hammond, E. C., & Selikoff, I. J. (1970). Inorganic fibers including chrysotile in lungs at autopsy: Preliminary report. *Inhaled Particles*, *2*, 683–694. PMID: 4129666.

Langseth, H., Johansen, B. V., Nesland, J. M., & Kjaerheim, K. (2007). Asbestos fibers in ovarian tissue from Norwegian pulp and paper workers. *International Journal of Gynecological Cancer*, *17*(1), 44–49. https://doi.org/10.1111/j.1525-1438.2006.00768.x

Lehmann, S. G., Toybou, D., Prades del Real, A-E., Arndt, D., Tagmount, A., Viau, M., Safi, M., Pacureanu, A., Cleotens, P., Bohic, S., Salomé, M., Castillo-Michel, H., Omaña-Sanz, B., Hofmann, A., Vulpe, C., Simonato, J. P., Celle, C., Charlet, L., & Gilbert,

B. (2019). Crumpling of silver nanowires by endolysosomes strongly reduces toxicity. *Proceedings of the National Academy of Sciences, United States of America*, *116*(30), 14893–14898. https://doi.org/10.1073/pnas.1820041116

Lentz, T., Rice, C. H., Succop, P. A., Lockey, J. E., Dement, J. M., & LeMasters, G. K. (2003). Pulmonary deposition modeling with airborne fiber exposure data: A study of workers manufacturing refractory ceramic fibers. *Applied Occupational and Environmental Hygiene*, *18*(4), 278–288. https://doi.org/10.1080/10473220301404

Lippmann, M. (1990). Effects of fiber characteristics on lung deposition, retention, and disease. *Environmental Health Perspectives*, *88*, 311–317. https://doi.org/10.1289/ehp.9088311

Lippmann, M. (2014). Toxicological and epidemiological studies on effects of airborne fibers: Coherence and public health implications. *Critical Reviews in Toxicology*, *44*, 643–695. https://doi.org/10.3109/10408444.2014.928266

MacDonald, J. L., & Kane, A. B. (1997). Mesothelial cell proliferation and biopersistence of wollastonite and crocidolite asbestos fibers. *Fundamental and Applied Toxicology*, *38*(2), 173–183. https://doi.org/10.1093/toxsci/38.2.173

Mahowald, N., Albani, S., Kok, J. F., Engelstaeder, S., Scanza, R., Ward, D. S., & Flanner, M. G. (2014). The size distribution of desert dust aerosols and its impact on the Earth system. *Aeolian Research*, *15*, 53–71. https://doi.org/10.1016/j.aeolia.2013.09.002

Moalli, P. A., MacDonald, J. L., Goodlick, L. A., & Kane, A. B. (1987). Acute injury and regeneration of the mesothelium in response to asbestos fibers. *American Journal of Pathology*, *128*(3), 426–445.

Morgan, A., Davies, P., Wagner, J. C., & Holmes, A. (1977). The biological effects of magnesium-leached chrysotile asbestos. *British Journal of Experimental Pathology*, *58*(5), 465–473.

Morgan, A., & Holmes, A. (1980). Concentrations and dimensions of coated and uncoated asbestos fibres in the human lung. *British Journal of Industrial Medicine*, *37*(1), 25–32. https://doi.org/10.1136/oem.37.1.25

Mossman, B. T., Lippmann, M., Hesterberg, T. W., Kelsey, K. T., Barchowsky, A., & Bonner, J. C. (2011). Pulmonary endpoints (lung carcinomas and asbestosis) following inhalation exposures to asbestos. *Journal of Toxicology and Environmental Health, Part B, Critical Reviews*, *14*(1–4), 76–121. https://doi.org/10.1080/10937404.2011.556047

Nagai, H., Okazaki, Y., Chew, S. H., Misawa, N., Yamashita, Y., Akatsuka, S., Ishihara, Y., Yamashita, K., Yoshikawa, Y., Yasui, H., Jiang, L., Ohara, H., Takahashi, T., Ichihara, G., Kostarelos, K., Miyata, Y., Shinohara, H., & Toyokuni, S. (2011). Diameter and rigidity of multiwalled carbon nanotubes are critical factors in mesothelial injury and carcinogenesis. *Proceedings of the National Academy of Sciences*, *108*(49), E1330–E1338. https://doi.org/10.1073/pnas.1110013108

Oberdörster, G., & Graham, U. (2018). Predicting EMP hazard: Lessons from studies with inhaled fibrous and non-fibrous nano- and micro-particles. *Toxicology and Applied Pharmacology*, *361*, 50–61. https://doi.org/10.1016/j.taap.2018.05.004

Oze, C., & Solt, K. (2010). Biodurability of chrysotile and tremolite asbestos in simulated lung and gastric fluids. *American Mineralogist*, *95*(5–6), 825–831. https://doi.org/10.2138/am.2010.3265

Pacella, A., Ballirano, P., Di Carlo, M. C., Altieri, A., Paccapelo, M., Skogby, H., Campopiano, A., Bruno, M. R., Croce, A., Piersante, C., Apollaro, C., Malvasi, G., Bruni, B. M., & Bloise, A. (2024). Geological and mineralogical characterization of fibrous tremolite from Iacolinei quarry (Basilicata, Italy). *Environmental Geochemistry and Health*, *46*(11), 429. https://doi.org/10.1007/s10653-024-02196-9

Pooley, F. D. (1972). Asbestos bodies, their formation, composition and character. *Environmental Research*, *5*(4), 363–379. https://doi.org/10.1016/0013-9351(72)90039-4

Pooley, F. D. (2018). Characterization of lung burden E.M.P.S. *Toxicology and Applied Pharmacology*, *361*, 18–20. https://doi.org/10.1016/j.taap.2018.10.019

Pooley, F. D., & Clark, N. J. (1980). A comparison of fibre dimensions in chrysotile, crocidolite and amosite particles from samples of airborne dust and from post-mortem lung tissue specimens. *IARC Scientific Publications*, *30*, 79–86.

Pooley, F. D., & Mitha, R. (1986). Fiber types, concentrations and characteristics found in lung tissues of chrysotile-exposed cases and controls. *Accomplishments in Oncology*, *1*(2). NIOSH/00176880.

Pooley, F. D., & Wagner, J. C. (1988). The significance of the selective retention of mineral dusts. *The Annals of Occupational Hygiene*, *32*(Inhaled Particles VI), 187–194. https://doi.org/10.1093/annhyg/32.inhaled_particles_VI.187

Rasmuson, J. O., Roggli, V. L., Boelter, F. W., Rasmuson, E. J., & Redinger, C. F. (2014). Cumulative retrospective exposure assessment (REA) as a predictor of amphibole asbestos lung burden: Validation procedures and results for industrial hygiene and pathology estimates. *Inhalation Toxicology*, *26*(1), 1–13. https://doi.org/10.3109/08958378.2013.845273

Rennick, J. J., Johnston, A. P. R., & Parton, R. G. (2021). Key principles and methods for studying the endocytosis of biological and nanoparticle therapeutics. *Nature Nanotechnology*, *16*, 266–276. https://doi.org/10.1038/s41565-021-00858-8

Roggli, V. L. (2014). Asbestos bodies and non-asbestos ferruginous bodies. In T. Oury, T. Sporn, & V. Roggli (Eds.), *Pathology of asbestos associated diseases* (pp. 25–51). Springer. https://doi.org/10.1007/978-3-642-41193-9_3

Roggli, V. L. (2018). Measuring EMPs in the lung what can be measured in the lung: Asbestiform minerals and cleavage fragments. *Toxicology and Applied Pharmacology*, *361*, 14–17. https://doi.org/10.1016/j.taap.2018.06.026

Roggli, V. L., & Benning, T. L. (1990). Asbestos bodies in pulmonary hilar lymph nodes. *Modern Pathology*, *3*(4), 513–517. PMID: 2217155.

Schinwald, A., Murphy, F. A., Prina-Mello, A., Poland, C. A., Byrne, F., Movia, D., Glass, J. R., Dickerson, J. C., Schultz, D. A., Jeffree, C. E., MacNee, W., & Donaldson, K. (2012). The threshold length for fiber-induced acute pleural inflammation: Shedding light on the early events in asbestos-induced mesothelioma. *Toxicological Sciences*, *128*(2), 461–470. https://doi.org/10.1038/s41565-021-00858-8

Sebastien, P., McDonald, J. C., McDonald, A. D., Case, B., & Harley, R. (1989). Respiratory cancer in chrysotile textile and mining industries: Exposure inferences from lung analysis. *British Journal of Industrial Medicine*, *46*(3), 180–187. https://doi.org/10.1136/oem.46.3.180

Seshan, K. (1983). How are the physical and chemical properties of chrysotile asbestos altered by a 10-year residence in water and up to 5 days in simulated stomach acid? *Environmental Health Perspectives*, *53*, 143–148. https://doi.org/10.1289/ehp.8353143

Shedd, K. B. (1985). *Fiber dimensions of crocidolites from Western Australia, Bolivia, and the Cape and Transvaal provinces of South Africa* (RI-8998). U.S. Department of the Interior.

Somigliana, A. B. (2025). Validation of freeze-drier/plasma Asher method for analysis of asbestos in the lung tissue. *Frontiers in Chemistry*, *13*. https://doi.org/10.3389/fchem.2025.1581910

Sporn, T. A., & Roggli, V. L. (2013). Consideration of occupational lung disease and pneumoconiosis in forensic pathology. *Academic Forensic Pathology*, *3*(4), 370–385. https://doi.org/10.23907/2013.049

Stettler, L. E., Shaprnack, D. D., & Krieg, E. F. (2008). Chronic inhalation of short asbestos: Lung fiber burdens and histopathology for monkeys maintained for 11.5 years after exposure. *Inhalation Toxicology*, *20*(1), 63–73. https://doi.org/10.1080/08958370701665566

Suzuki, Y., & Kohyama, N. (1991). Translocation of inhaled asbestos fibers from the lung to other tissues. *American Journal of Industrial Medicine*, *19*(6), 701–704. https://doi.org/10.1002/ajim.4700190603

Suzuki, Y., & Yuen, S. R. (2002). Asbestos fibers contributing to the induction of human malignant mesothelioma. *Annals of the New York Academy of Sciences*, *982*(1), 160–176. https://doi.org/10.1111/j.1749-6632.2002.tb04931.x

Timbrell, V. (1982). Deposition and retention of fibres in the human lung. *Annals of Occupational Hygiene*, *26*(1–4), 347–369.

Tuomi, T. (1992). Fibrous minerals in the lungs of mesothelioma patients: Comparison between data on SEM, TEM, and personal interview information. *American Journal of Industrial Medicine*, *21*(2), 155–162. https://doi.org/10.1002/ajim.4700210205

Uibu, T., Vanhala, E., Sajantila, A., Lunetta, P., Mäkelä-Bengs, P., Goebeler, S., Jäntti, M., & Tossavainen, A. (2009). Asbestos fibers in para-aortic and mesenteric lymph nodes. *American Journal of Industrial Medicine*. https://doi.org/10.1002/ajim.20694

Utembe, W., Potgieter, K., Stefaniak, A. B., & Gulumian, M. (2015). Dissolution and biodurability: Important parameters needed for risk assessment of nanomaterials. *Particle and Fibre Toxicology*, *12*, 11–23. https://doi.org/10.1186/s12989-015-0088-2

Velasco-García, M. I., Cruz, M. J., Diego, C., Montero, M. A., Álvarez-Simón, D., & Ferrer, J. (2017). First identification of pulmonary asbestos fibres in a spanish population. *Lung*, *195*, 671–677. https://doi.org/10.1007/s00408-017-0042-1

Verkouteren, J. R., & Wylie, A. G. (2000). The tremolite-actinolite-ferro-actinolite series: Systematic relationships among cell parameters, composition, optical properties, and habit, and evidence of discontinuities. *American Mineralogist*, *85*(9), 1239–1254. https://doi.org/10.2138/am-2000-8-917

Vigliaturo, R., Jamnik, M., Drazic, G., Podobnik, M., Snidaric, M. T., Ventura, G., Redhammer, G., Znidarsic, N., Caserman, S., & Gieré, R. (2024). Localization and dimensional range of amphibole particles retrieved from human alveolar epithelial cells. *Minerals*, *14*, 101. https://doi.org/10.3390/min14010101

Visonà, S. D., Bertoglio, B., Capella, S., Belluso, E., Austoni, B., Colosio, C., Kurzhunbaeva, Z., Ivic-Pavlicic, T., & Taioli, E. (2023). Asbestos burden in lungs of mesothelioma patients with pleural plaques, lung fibrosis and/or ferruginous bodies at histology: A postmortem SEM-EDS study. *Carcinogenesis*, *45*(3), 131–139. https://doi.org/10.1093/carcin/bgad090

Vorwald, A. J., Dunkan, T. M., & Pratt, P. C. (1951). Experimental studies of asbestosis. *A.M.A. Archives of Industrial Hygiene and Occupational Medicine*, *3*(1), 1–43.

Wang, Q., Wang, Q., Zhao, Z., Alexander, D. B., Zhao, D., Xu, J., & Tsuda, H. (2020). Pleural translocation and lesions by pulmonary exposed multi-walled carbon nanotubes. *Journal of Toxicology & Pathology*, *33*(3), 145–151.

Warnock, M. L. (1989). Lung asbestos burden in shipyard and construction workers with mesothelioma: Comparison with burdens in subjects with asbestos or lung cancer. *Environmental Research*, *50*, 68–85. https://doi.org/10.1016/S0013-9351(89)80049-0

Watson, M. S. (1999). *Effects of intergrowths on the physical characteristics of fibrous anthophyllite* [MS thesis, University of Maryland].

World Health Organization (WHO). (1986). *Asbestos and other natural mineral fibres. international programme on chemical safety*. Environmental Health Criteria 53. https://www.inchem.org/documents/ehc/ehc/ehc53.htm

Wylie, A. G. (2016). Amphibole dusts: Fibers, fragments, and mesothelioma. *The Canadian Mineralogist*, *54*, 1403–1435. https://doi.org//10.3749/canmin.1500109

Wylie, A. G. (2024). Mineralogical characteristics and risk assessment of elongate mineral particles (EMP): Asbestos, fiber, and fragment. In A. Korchevskiy, J. Rasmuson, & E. Rasmuson (Eds.), *Health risk assessment for asbestos and other fibrous minerals*. John Wiley & Sons. ISBN: 978-1-119-43843-4. https://doi.org//10.1002/9781119438397

Wylie, A. G., & Korchevskiy, A. A. (2023). Dimensions of elongate mineral particles and cancer: A review. *Environmental Research*, *230*, 114688. https://doi.org/10.1016/j.envres.2022.114688

Wylie, A. G., & Korchevskiy, A. A. (2025). Critical values for dimensional parameters of mesotheliomagenic mineral fibers: Evidence from the dimensions and rigidity of MWCNT. *Frontiers in Toxicology*, *7*, 1568513. https://doi.org/10.3389/ftox.2025.1568513

Xu, J., Alexander, D. B., Futakuchi, M., Numano, T., Fukamachi, K., Suzui, M., Omori, T., Kanno, J., Hirose, A., & Tsuda, H. (2014). Size and shape- dependent pleural translocation, deposition, fibrogenesis and mesothelial proliferation by multiwalled carbon nanotubes. *Cancer Science*, *105*(7), 763–769. https://doi.org/10.1111/cas.12437

Zhu, W., von dem Bussche, A., Yi, X., Qiu, Y., Wang, Z., Weston, P., Hurt, R. H., Kane, A. B., & Gao, H. (2016). Nanomechanical mechanism for lipid bilayer damage induced by carbon nanotubes confined in intracellular vesicles. *Proceedings of the National Academies of Science United States of America*, *113*(44), 12374–12379. https://doi.org/10.1073/pnas.1605030113

7 Mechanical properties as a predictor of mesotheliomagenicity

A. Korchevskiy & A. Wylie

INTRODUCTION

The biological behavior of elongate particles, including toxicokinetics, how they spread in the body, and toxicodynamics, their interaction with cells, tissues, and organs, is determined by numerous factors. It is possible to determine the most important of these that correlate with mesothelioma mortality or other toxic effects.

Mesothelioma is one of the most significant and problematic health outcomes of asbestos exposure. There is still no adequate or even promising cure for this rare disease. This failure of our medical approach to mesothelioma seems to be related to a failure to understand the mode of action of elongate mineral particles (EMP), the prevailing, if not exclusive, factor increasing the baseline rate of mesothelial tumors in humans. The body seems to distinguish between spherical and elongate particles, with regular dust or even biologically active particles such as crystalline silica being unable to produce mesothelioma. Asbestos is very active in pleural mesothelioma, as well as in the development of other mesothelial tumors, like mesothelioma of the peritoneum, pericardium, or testes. The physical and chemical characteristics of fibers are very important in understanding why mesothelial tumors are so tightly related to "elongation," an elevated ratio of length to width.

In this chapter, we will specifically address the two mechanical properties most relevant to toxicity: tensile strength and rigidity, and we will demonstrate how these properties should be addressed for risk assessment purposes. The rigidity and tensile strength of fibers, as we will show, are functions of their dimensions. While rigidity and tensile strength are not expected to directly correlate with carcinogenic potency, they create important boundary conditions for toxicity that are often overlooked.

TENSILE STRENGTH

High tensile strength is a property frequently used to describe the unique mechanical property of asbestos. Tensile strength is a measure of the maximum extensional stress that can be applied to a fiber before it breaks. During mining and fabrication, the high tensile strength of asbestos results in aerosols that contain fibrils with extreme elongation. Tensile strength and the elongation of mineral particles are related.

 DOI: 10.1201/9781003424277-8

TABLE 7.1
Average tensile strength and fibril width among asbestiform fiber types from Aveston (1969)(a) (with standard deviation) and Zukowski and Gaze (1959)(b) (with average coefficient of variation) and EMPB, the percent of elongate mineral particles longer than 5 μm that have a width less than or equal to 0.25 μm (EMPB) from our database.

	Tensile Strength ($kg/cm^2 \times 10^4$)		EMPB
Asbestos type, source	**(a)**	**(b)**	**(%)**
Chrysotile, Thetford Mines, Quebec, Canada	3.86 (0.20)	4.99(36%)	69.2
Chrysotile, Arizona, U.S.A.		3.72(38%)	
Crocidolite, Cape, South Africa	2.26 (0.14)	7.27(26%)	64.7
Ferroactinolite (prieskite), Cape, South Africa	1.94 (0.31)		29.7[1]
Amosite, Penge Mine, Transvaal, South Africa	1.55 (0.13)	2.44(27%)	20.4
Anthophyllite, Finland	1.22(0.46)		26.6
Tremolite, Pakistan	0.42 (0.04)		5.0[2]

Measurements of the tensile strength of asbestos are high, but they are also variable among asbestos sources. For example, Hodgson (1965) reports tensile strengths of 3.5X 10^4 kg/cm^2 for crocidolite from South Africa and 0.5000 x 10^4 kg/cm^2 for fibrous tremolite from Pakistan. Average tensile strength measurements from Aveston (1969) and Zukowski and Gaze (1959) are shown in Table 7.1. All measurements of tensile strength in Table 7.1 are made on fiber bundles.

Different measurements for the same mineral type and source, for example, Cape crocidolite, will vary according to the length of the fiber being measured, with shorter fibers (measured in millimeters) demonstrating the highest tensile strength (Zukowski & Gaze, 1959).

While it is possible to measure the tensile strength of fibers with diameters as low as 10 to 20 μm by SEM or TEM, most published measurements were made on wider material. All measurements are of fiber bundles. Even an asbestos fiber 10 μm in width and thickness would be composed of $10^4 - 10^5$ fibrils.

The measurement process itself has significant uncertainty, and published measurements of tensile strength of the same type of asbestos vary. For example, Hodgson (1979) gives the tensile strength of anthophyllite asbestos exceeding that of chrysotile, while Aveston (1969) reports the reverse relationship.

Tensile strength might be influenced by chemical composition. For example, cations that form stronger bonds with oxygen in the silicate structure of amphiboles could enhance tensile strength. In general, the effect of common cations is Fe^{3+} > Fe^{2+}> Mg^{2+}. From a purely chemical approach, one would expect the tensile strength of crocidolite to be the highest and anthophyllite the lowest, consistent with observations (Hodgson, 1979).

It has been well established that tensile strength increases as the width of the EMP decreases, once EMPs are narrower than several micrometers. Griffith (1921) provided an expression that describes the relationship as

$$F = A \text{ and } B/D \tag{7.1}$$

where A and B are constants, F is the tensile strength, and D is the diameter (width).

Griffith recognized that atomic structure will also be a factor, and structural factors as a group are represented by A; defects or even the fibrillar structure itself can also affect tensile strength, which he considered as factor B.

For metal whiskers, the relationship given in Equation 7.1 has been experimentally demonstrated many times and discussed in detail by Zoltai (1986). To explain the increasing strength with decreasing width, A can be viewed as the internal strength while B/D is the surface strength. Zoltai argues that a strong surface theory to explain the high tensile strength of asbestos has been supported by direct observations from metal whiskers. High surface strength helps to explain the lack of cleavage surfaces and the presence of curved surfaces on fibrils. Strong surfaces could arise from fewer surface defects, although fewer surface defects on amphibole fibers than on fragments have not been verified.

Because amphiboles have a common structure and similar cell dimensions, they should have somewhat similar properties that contribute to tensile strength factor A in Griffith's equation (Eq. 7.1). This is consistent with the information in Table 7.3, which shows that Young's modulus is virtually the same for all the silicate minerals listed.

If tensile strength varies inversely with diameter, observed differences in tensile strength should correlate with differences in fibril diameter. Table 7.2 provides one measure of the abundance of narrow fibers derived from our database in terms of proportions with widths < 0.25 μm; these data are generally consistent with this inverse relationship.

It may be possible to generalize about the tensile strength or other physical and chemical characteristics by mining districts, for example, Cape crocidolite vs. Transvaal crocidolite, but it is not possible to generalize about all occurrences of a single mineral. Fibril diameters vary from one mine to another in both means and ranges; the tensile strength of fibers composed of fibrils will also vary.

The tensile strength of tremolite asbestos reported in the literature is lower than that of other amphibole asbestos, such as amosite and crocidolite, and most occurrences of tremolite asbestos in the database have fibrils, on average, wider than those of crocidolite. However, the fibril width of asbestiform tremolite varies widely among occurrences. For example, there is a high proportion of tremolite asbestos EMP-5s from Metsovo, Greece, with a width < 0.25 μm (EMPB = 68.8% (Wylie et al., 2020), and based on width alone, Metsovo tremolite asbestos would be expected to have higher tensile strength than the tremolite asbestos from Pakistan given in Table 7.2.

TABLE 7.2
Critical diameter based on Young's modulus (E)

Fiber type	Young's modulus (E)	Critical diameter
MWCNT	360 - 100 GPa	37 - 44 nm
Chrysotile	160 GPa	60 nm
Crocidolite	190 GPa	56 nm

TABLE 7.3
Young's modulus for various minerals

Mineral type, source	Young's modulus (GPa)	Reference source
Riebeckite (crocidolite), Cape, South Africa	181, 187, 196	Aveston (1969); Zukowski and Gaze (1959); Hodgson (1979)
Actinolite, Koegas, South Africa	150	Aveston (1969)
Grunerite (amosite), Transvaal, South Africa	180, 163, 170	Aveston (1969); Zukowski and Gaze (1959); Hodgson (1979)
Anthophyllite, Finland	158, 163	Aveston (1969); Hodgson (1979)
Tremolite, Pakistan	153	Aveston (1969)
Other amphiboles (glaucophane, fluoroedenite)	165 (estimate)	
Chrysotile, Thetford Mines, Quebec, Canada	174, 159, 156, 170	Aveston (1969); Zukowski and Gaze (1959); Golden (1968); Hodgson (1979)
Chrysotile, Arizona, U.S.A.	160	Zukowski and Gaze (1959)
Balangeroite	165 (estimate)	
Erionite	45	Bryukhanov et al. (2014)
Talc	16	Broz et al. (2006)
K-feldspar	101	Liu et al. (2024)
Illite	57	Húlan et al. (2020)
Kaolinite	40	Elhachemi et al. (2024)
Quartz	106.3	Broz et al. (2006)
Halloysite	130	Lu (2011)
Pyroxene (enstatite)	186	Gouriet et al. (2022)
Biotite (mica)	45	Liu et al. (2024)

On the other hand, chrysotile from many locations has almost the same tensile strength, despite slight differences in the chemical composition (Al, Fe) and in the manner in which the sheets of Si-O tetrahedra and Mg-OH octahedra are assembled into a tube (spiral vs. concentric circle construction). The constancy of tensile strength is attributed to the fact that the fibrils of chrysotile have essentially the same outer diameter, 0.010 to 0.08 μm (mode = 0.02–0.03[3]), and inner diameter, < 0.01 μm (mode = 0.005), among occurrences (Martin & Phillips, 1977; Chisholm, 1983).

Another interesting feature of amphibole asbestos is a significant loss of tensile strength on heating, beginning at about 200 C and reaching > 80% reduction by 500 C, well below the temperature at which structural changes evident by X-ray diffraction begin (Campbell et al., 1980). Hodgson (1979) reports that below 200 C, the tensile strength of crocidolite first increases slightly on heating, reaching a maximum of about 4.7 $Kg/cm^2 \times 10^4$ at about 150 C before decreasing significantly to less than 1 $Kg/cm^2 \times 10^4$ by about 550 C. The tensile strength of amosite is approximately constant at 2.6 $Kg/cm^2 \times 10^4$ until about 200C, after which, like crocidolite, it decreases rapidly to less than 0.3 $Kg/cm^2 \times 10^4$ at 550 C. Chrysotile, however, shows very little change in tensile strength until its tensile strength increases as it approaches its breakdown temperature, 500 C.

The changes observed in asbestos tensile strength following heating are generally thought to come about by alteration of the intrafibrillar bonds and are accompanied by a loss of adsorbed water. Adsorbed water forms weak hydrogen bonds between fibrils, and these bonds are broken as adsorbed water is driven off. Loss of tensile strength is also associated with the oxidation of iron. However, this explanation is inadequate to explain this behavior according to the Griffith equation because the loss of tensile strength does not correspond to any observable change in the internal atomic structure (A in the Griffith equation). Perhaps heating causes some annealing of individual fibrils already in close structural alignment, as observed in amosite (Cressey et al., 1982), thus increasing diameter and decreasing tensile strength.

Tensile strength will be affected by structural defects. According to Virta (2002), the inherent tensile strength of a single asbestos fiber, based on the strength of the Si-O-Si bonds, should be nearer 10 $Kg/cm^2 \times 10^4$ rather than 1. The fewer the defects in the structure, the greater the contribution of the A factor in Griffith's tensile strength equation will be. However, certain types of defects may actually enhance tensile strength. For example, if cracks propagating across a fibril encounter a planar defect resulting in slip parallel to the fiber axis rather than brittle failure across it, which can occur in both amphibole and chrysotile asbestos, tensile strength can be enhanced (Ahn & Busek, 1991; Martin & Phillips, 1977; Zussman, 1979). Planar defects are common in amphibole asbestos fibrils, but they are common in other non-fibrous forms as well (Dorling & Zussman, 1987). Because of defects, long fibers normally show lower tensile strength than shorter ones (Virta, 2002; Hodgson, 1979).

The tensile strength of single fibrils in most cases has not been measured directly. However, other characteristics of high tensile strength amphiboles, such as curved fibers, splaying of fibrils at the ends of bundles, and very narrow (< 0.2μm) high aspect ratio particles, can be observed by electron and optical microscopy and are indicative of elevated tensile strength.

TENSILE STRENGTH AND TOXICITY

The high tensile strength and narrow width of asbestos fibers make breakage perpendicular to the length very difficult, enabling very long, high aspect ratio fibers to penetrate and be deposited into the lung interstitium. While it has been shown that fiber bundles disaggregate in the rat lung following inhalation (Coffin et al., 1985), there is no evidence that biological processes can alter the length of narrow fibers due to their very high tensile strength. Tensile strength enhances elongation, with the narrowest fibers displaying the highest aspect ratios. While we generally try to understand the dimensional basis for mesothelioma and lung cancer in terms of length and width, it is the tensile strength resulting from the habit of growth that ultimately determines the relative magnitude of these two variables when respirable dust is created, and ultimately the length and width of particles in the lung.

STIFFNESS (RIGIDITY)

While the tensile strength of asbestos is integral to its use in building materials, its resistance to breakage, and in maintaining a fibrous shape, the mechanical property of stiffness is important in controlling the translocation of particles from the alveolar sacs to tumor sites in the lung interstitium, parietal pleura, peritoneum, and other organs of the body, in penetration of cell membranes, and in frustrated phagocytosis by macrophages. Rigidity regulates the integrity and function of physical and biological systems (Damavandi et al., 2022). Rigidity is referred to as the ability to withstand pressure, and in this way, this concept can be applied to objects, systems, or formations (Zhu & Hu, 2009).

CARBON NANOTUBES

The importance of stiffness in fiber toxicity is well illustrated through studies on carbon nanotubes (reviewed by Nel, 2023; Zhang et al., 2021; Murphy et al., 2022). Carbon nanotubes are nanomaterials that are characterized by a hollow, tube-shaped structure, which ranges in width from a few nanometers up to < 200 nm and in length from <1 μm to tens of micrometers. They are made by several different processes that affect their composition, size, and strength. They can be single- (SWCNT), double-(DWCNT), or multi-walled (MWCNT). Pristine carbon nanotubes, like amphibole asbestos fibers, carry a negative charge and are both biopersistent and hydrophobic.

Because carbon nanotubes are similar in width to the narrowest asbestos fibrils, they have been evaluated for their ability to cause inflammation and cancer, specifically mesothelioma. Animal inhalation and instillation studies show that some, but not all, MWCNT contribute to frustrated phagocytosis, inflammation, granuloma formation, and fibrosis, and are able to migrate to the pleura, where they initiate mesothelioma. However, there are many variables among the nanotubes whose rigidity has been studied, such as the presence of different lengths and widths, variations in composition, variations in the sample preparation process, as well as differences in strength and surface chemistry, making the identification of common factors for toxicity difficult (Barbarino & Giordano, 2021). Despite these uncertainties, a general picture of carcinogenic nanotubes has emerged.

In 2011, Nagai et al. proposed that it is the direct interaction between mesothelial cells and MWCNT that is the key for the initiation of mesothelial carcinogenesis. In studies of mesothelial cells, they showed an inverse correlation between diameter and toxicity for widths greater than about 30 nm. Below 30 nm in width, the tubes lack rigidity, and they are also on average quite short, often less than 1 μm. They also suggest that there is a maximum width of around 150 nm because fibers wider than this could be too wide to penetrate cells, although CNT samples with diameters greater than 150 nm and L > 5 μm have not been tested *in vivo*. Narrow tubes of essentially all widths are known to produce inflammation following inhalation or instillation (Jović et al., 2020). While the paradigm that inflammation in the pleura leads to mesothelioma is generally accepted, experiments on CNT have repeatedly shown that a high degree of inflammation does not necessarily lead to mesothelioma, or at least not in the lifetime of the exposed rats, and that stiffness of the fiber, width, and length are the important variables.

The first MWCNT identified as mesotheliomagenic is labeled MWCNT-7 or Mitsui–7. MWCNT-7 induced mesothelioma following intraperitoneal administration in rats (Takagi et al., 2012). Other MWCNTs with properties similar to MWCNT-7 have also produced mesothelioma, and it has been shown that less stiff, narrower single and multi-walled tubes do not (Kane et al., 2018; Nel, 2023; Fortini et al., 2020). More specifically, a proposal has been made by the Federal Institute for Occupational Safety and Health in Germany for a harmonized classification and labeling of multi-walled carbon nanotubes (MWCNT) as hazardous if they have a width ≥ 30 nm to 3μm and L ≥ 5 μm; below the 30 nm width, fibers lack the necessary stiffness to be a risk (BAuA, 2021), and short fibers are assumed to be less toxic. Due to their alignment with fluid flow, their effective aerodynamic diameter is closer to their actual width than that of more flexible or easily agglomerating fibers. Higher rigidity is associated with increased crystallinity, surface charge, and conductivity along the tube's length.

Rigid fibers present a challenge for macrophages to engulf (Fortini et al., 2020). It is often assumed that frustrated phagocytosis is associated only with long fibers and specifically with those longer than 10–15 μm, but there is some evidence that shorter MWCNTs can also produce the type of inflammation associated with frustrated phagocytosis. Murphy et al. (2021) point out that frustrated phagocytosis is not a well-defined phenomenon that can be readily measured and that even short fibers that are engulfed by macrophages can cause lysosomal disruption within the cell and stimulate pro-inflammatory responses. In their review of the literature, they argue that it is not possible to define a threshold whereby high aspect ratio nanotubes can be identified as causing frustrated phagocytosis. Both L > 10 μm and L = 5–10 μm are associated with a pro-inflammatory state in the pleura (Schinwald & Donaldson, 2012).

Lee et al. (2018) reported experiments with intrapleural injection in rats, showing that rigidity is strongly correlated with inflammogenic potential and proposed that only MWCNT that are highly rigid can pierce macrophages and induce frustrated phagocytosis. In a recent review, Fortini et al. (2020) concluded that the property of flexural rigidity is associated with cell lesions, incomplete phagocytosis, and mesothelioma. Fortini et al. suggested substituting rigidity for diameter, such that a general statement about the carcinogenicity of EMPs is that they are respirable (aerodynamic diameter < 4 μm), long (> 5 μm), rigid, and biodurable.

Quantifying rigidity

Biological rigidity might be defined as the stiffness necessary for a fiber to pierce a macrophage's cell membrane during engulfment. Rigidity can be mathematically defined based on factors such as width, length, and crystal structural strength (Young's modulus).

We proposed the following framework for the quantitative estimation of rigidity for elongate particles (Wylie & Korchevskiy, 2025). Our model is based on the quantitative evaluation of the stiffness for elongate particles from the data on their dimensions and elasticity. Stiffness, defined as the resistance to bending, can be described through Euler's buckling theory, which models the critical force needed to buckle a long, elastic particle under an end-applied force.

The critical buckling force, F_{crit}, is calculated by the formula

$$F_{crit} = \pi^2 EI_A / L_{eff}^{\ 2}, \tag{7.2}$$

where E is Young's modulus and IA is the area moment of inertia. The product EI_A represents bending stiffness or **flexural rigidity**, which is independent of the particle's length. As discussed later in the chapter, flexural rigidity has been used as a measure of biological rigidity as well.

Euler buckling theory describes four modes of buckling. In the first mode, with one fiber end fixed and the other free, Leff=2L, and Equation 7.2 becomes Equation 7.3:

$$F_{crit1} = \pi^2 EI_A / 4L^2. \tag{7.3}$$

For the second buckling mode, where both ends of the fiber are fixed, Equation 7.2 becomes Equation 7.4:

$$F_{crit2} = \pi^2 EI_A / L^2. \tag{7.4}$$

In examining fiber stiffness and lysosomal disruption, Zhu et al. (2016) assumed the second buckling mode. However, the first mode could also apply in cases where a fiber pierces a cell wall. Given uncertainties in the buckling mode, among other factors, a Rigidity Index (RI) is calculated as follows:

$$\textbf{Rigidity Index (RI)} = \pi^2 EI_A / 4L^2 \text{x } 10000. \tag{7.5}$$

With length and width data for particles, the RI can be computed for each particle and averaged to represent a population's characteristics.

The cross-sectional shape (IA) affects RI:

- For a circular cross-section: $I_A = \pi\, r^4/4$ where r = 1/2 W; (7.6)
- For a square cross-section: $I_A = W^4/12$; (7.7)
- For a rectangular cross-section: $I_A = (T^3)(W)/12$ where T = thickness; and (7.8)
- For a hollow tube (with outer diameter W_o and inner diameter W_i): $I_A = \pi\left(W_o^{\ 4} - W_i^{\ 4}\right)/64$. (7.9)

Broßell et al. (2020) used Euler's buckling theory to study fiber bending by macrophages. They found that, assuming conditions of Equation 7.3, fibers with an RI around 10^{-19} N ×m^2 could bend under a 10 nN force applied by a macrophage, facilitating removal. In Table 7.2, we list critical diameters when fibers lose biological rigidity; this diameter depends on Young's modulus (E). In our studies, we assumed 160 Gpa for CNT produced by chemical vapor deposition, 5125 Gpa for Mitsui 7, and 1200 Gpa for all others:

Chrysotile fibrils are cylindrical tubes with varying outer and inner diameters. Chisholm (1983) measured outer diameters from 10 to 85 nm (mean range 13 to 38 nm) and inner diameters from 0 to 10 nm. The small inner diameter can be disregarded in RI calculations, as it minimally reduces the index. Fibril lengths vary, and widths above 40 nm indicate composite fibers. According to Atkinson et al. (1970), average lengths range from 2 to 4 μm, though some fibrils reach several millimeters.

Broßell et al. (2020) noted that a 60 nm threshold for biological rigidity would exclude most single chrysotile fibrils. Population rigidity measurements often involve composite fibers, thus increasing calculated rigidity; however, inhalation could disaggregate chrysotile into weak single fibrils, with disaggregation depending on interfibrillar adhesion.

Fiber thickness (see Chapter 3 of this book for a description of this important metric) significantly affects IA for rectangular cross-sections, as seen in Equation 7.7. Wylie et al. (1982) related log-thickness to log-width for crocidolite and amosite as

$$\text{Log thickness} = 0.692\,\text{logwidth} - 0.493 \tag{7.10}$$

This relationship was used in this study for asbestiform amphiboles, while non-asbestiform amphiboles (cleaving into rhombuses with an ideal width-to-thickness ratio of 1.88) and other silicates used approximations for width-to-thickness ratios:

- Erionite: 1:1
- Balangeroite: 1.1:1
- Talc: 3:1

These estimates of width to thickness are derived from best estimates for other minerals that fall into the same silicate structural group as discussed in Wylie and Korchevskiy (2025). Going forward, more precise measurements of the thickness are needed before it will be possible to understand cell-EMP interactions fully, especially for the phyllosilicates, the group most likely to have the highest ratio of width to thickness and the greatest potential for lacking biological rigidity. The phyllosilicates include antigorite, mica, talc, chlorite, palygorskite, and sepiolite.

Young's modulus, a measure of lattice strength, remains constant regardless of habit, although it varies by lattice direction. Since Young's modulus is a characteristic that derives primarily from the atomic structure rather than particle size, the moduli of amphiboles and chrysotile parallel to elongation are very similar. Both the double chains of amphibole and the axis of the rolled sheets of Si-O tetrahedra in chrysotile are parallel to the elongation axis. The fact that Young's modulus is similar across asbestos types means that the primary contributor to differences in the stiffness of asbestos is fiber width.

Table 7.3 shows values of Young's modulus parallel to elongation of common minerals relevant to lung pathology:

We also applied the rigidity index approach to the dimensional database of elongate mineral particles to compare with carbon nanotubes. Groups 0–3 designate carbon nanotube populations that are not reported to produce lung cancer, fibrosis, or mesothelioma, respectively (Wylie & Korchevskiy, 2025) (see Table 7.4). We determined

TABLE 7.4
Estimated rigidity index for categories of elongate particles

Category of particles	Average rigidity index (standard deviation) ($\mu m^2 GPa \times 10^4$)	Fraction of particles with rigidity index < $0.05\ \mu m^2 GPa \times 10^4$
Mesothelioma reported MWCNTs (Group 1)	51.86 (81.23)	0*
No mesothelioma reported MWCNTs (Group 0)	7.5 (26.25)	44.4*
Lung cancer reported (Group 2)	15.64 (27.08)	66.7*
Fibrosis reported (no cancer) (Group 3)	7.93 (13.41)	23.1*
Elongate asbestiform particles (L >5 μm, L/W ≥3, W ≥0.05 μm, W ≤3 μm) (All EMP, asbestiform)	509.35 (5887.6)	2.2
Elongate non-asbestiform particles (L >5 μm, L/W ≥3, W ≥0.05 μm, W ≤3 μm) (All EMP non-asbestiform)	20033 (29759)	0
EMPA particles (L >5 μm, L/W ≥3, W ≥0.05 μm, W≤0.15 μm) (Group 4)	0.98 (1.48)	11.6
Non-EMPA particles (L >5 μm, L/W ≥3, W >0.15 μm, W ≤3 μm) (Group 5)	6448 (19976)	0.2
Particles from datasets with EMPA fraction ≥ 1%	1074 (7869)	2.1
Particles from datasets with EMPA fraction < 1%	16996 (27873)	0

* For carbon nanotubes, the fraction is calculated from average rigidity index values, and not from the distribution of individual particles.

the rigidity index for each particle in the database for asbestiform EMPs, non-asbestiform EMPs, and from two groups designated as Groups 4–5 and averaged them. Group 4 contains the so-called EMPA particles (with length >5µm, width ≤0.15 µm) that were determined as "signature mesotheliomagenic" particles in our previous studies (Wylie et al., 2020; Wylie & Korchevskiy, 2023). Group 5 results from removing "signature mesotheliomagenic" fibers from consideration. We have assumed Group 5 to be non-mesotheliomagenic (with length >5 µm, width >0.15 µm) because of the removal of EMPA, Group 4. This assumption is supported by the fact that there are no reported occurrences of excess mesothelioma from inhalation of mineral dust (environmental or occupational) where the dust does not contain Group 4 (EMPA) fibers.

When direct measurements were unavailable, the following assumptions were made: data for erionite were extrapolated from zeolites, and for balangeroite, the amphibole average was used because the published Young's moduli for other single-chain silicates were very similar to the amphiboles as a group.

Table 7.4 contains estimates of the rigidity index for several categories of elongate particles. The index value of 0.05 μm^2GPa x 10^4 was suggested by Wylie and Korchevskiy (2025) as a convenient dividing line between mesotheliomagenic and non-mesotheliomagenic carbon nanotubes.

Figure 7.1 demonstrates the relationship between average width and average rigidity index of particle populations in the four groups in our CNT study.

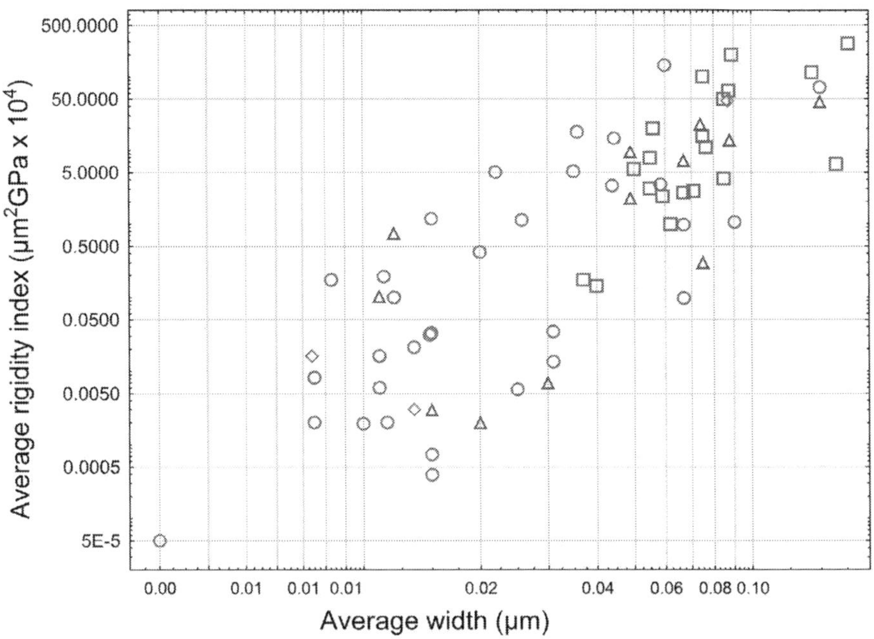

FIGURE 7.1 Relationship between width and rigidity index for categories of carbon nanotubes. Green circles denote no mesothelioma reported, red squares denote mesothelioma reported, magenta rhombuses denote lung cancer reported but not mesothelioma, and blue triangles denote fibrosis reported but no mesothelioma or lung cancer.

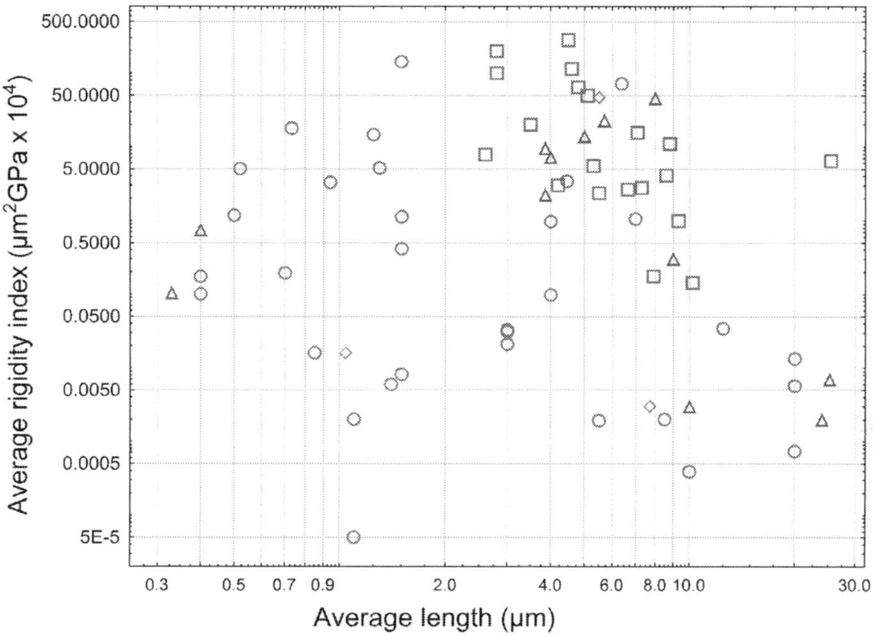

FIGURE 7.2 Relationship between average length and average rigidity index for categories of carbon nanotube populations. Green circles denote no mesothelioma reported, red squares denote mesothelioma reported, magenta rhombuses denote lung cancer reported but not mesothelioma, and blue triangles denote fibrosis reported but no mesothelioma or lung cancer.

Similarly, Figure 7.2 demonstrates the relationship between average length and average rigidity index of populations of CNT.

Several observations can be made from Figures 7.1 and 7.2. In particular, no mesotheliomagenic CNT population had an average rigidity index less than about 0.05 – 0.1 $\mu m^2 GPa \times 10^4$ and/or an average width less than 0.03 μm and/or an average length less than 2 μm. Therefore, at least some carbon nanotubes should have a level of sufficient rigidity to produce mesothelioma (RI > 0.05).

Recently, we introduced a new metric for the mesotheliomagenic potential of particles with various sizes (Korchevskiy & Wylie, 2025a, 2025b). This metric is called the dimensional coefficient of carcinogenicity (DCC), and it is described in more detail in Chapter 6 of this book. DCC can be calculated by the following formula:

$$DCC = 1 - \exp(-0.11SA/(1000\ Width^3 + 1)),$$

where SA is the surface area of the particle (μm^2) and Width is the particle width (μm).

DCC has a conditional probabilistic meaning, with no units, and changes from 0 to 1 for particles with various levels of carcinogenic potential. It was suggested that most mesotheliomagenic particle populations have an average DCC ≥0.05; and no mesotheliomagenic particle populations, by our observations, have an average DCC <0.02.

As we can see from the plot, the majority of mesotheliomagenic CNTs and EMPA have both average DCC ≥0.05 and RI ≥0.05 μm^{2}GPa x 10^4. There are no sets among these groups with DCC <0.05 and RI <0.05 μm^{2}GPa x 10^4. There is only 8.7% of datasets with RI <0.05 μm^{2}GPa x 10^4 and DCC >0.05. It can also be seen that with average DCC <0.05, the majority of datasets do not have mesothelioma potency, irrespective of their rigidity.

Therefore, we hypothesized that the rigidity index for particles with DCC ≥0.05 should reflect the true characterization of the biological behavior of particles with high or low propensity to buckle or penetrate cell walls when interacting with cells and tissues.

Figure 7.3 shows the relationship between rigidity index and DCC for the four groups of particles in our study: Group 0 (no mesothelioma reported CNTs), Group 1 (mesothelioma reported CNTs), Group 4 (EMPA), and Group 5 (non-EMPA EMPs). All datapoints are average values for various datasets or sources of information.

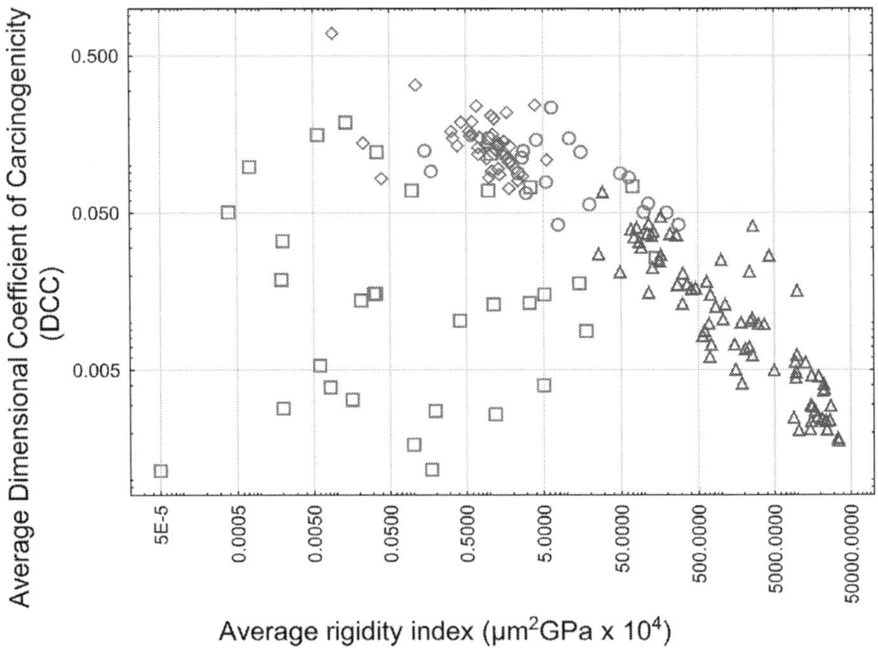

FIGURE 7.3 Relationship between average rigidity index and average DCC for four categories of particles. Green squares denote no mesothelioma or lung cancer CNTs, magenta circles denote mesothelioma reported CNTs (Group 1), red rhombuses denote EMPA mineral particles (Group 4), and blue triangles denote all EMPs excluding EMPA (Group 5).

Table 7.5 contains average rigidity indices for major mineral types of EMP-5 particles. Specifically, the average rigidity index for particles with DCC ≥0.05 is demonstrated, along with the fraction of particles with rigidity index ≥0.05 $\mu m^2 GPa \times 10^4$ and DCC ≥0.05.

We can demonstrate that the mesothelioma potency of elongate mineral particles depends on their biosolubility (as in Gualtieri et al., 2018), along with the average rigidity index for particles with DCC ≥0.05 and the fraction of particles with DCC ≥0.05 and RI ≥0.05 $\mu m^2 GPa \times 10^4$.

TABLE 7.5

Dimensional and rigidity characteristics for major types of elongate mineral particles (particles with length ≥5 μm, length/width ≥3 μm, width ≥0.05 μm, width ≤3 μm).

Mineral type Habit	Average Rigidity Index for sets with DCC ≥0.05 ($\mu m^2 GPa \times 10^4$)	Fraction of individual particles with Rigidity Index ≥0.05 and DCC ≥0.05 (%) in each set
Chrysotile, fibers Asbestiform	5.38	51
Chrysotile fibrils (width 0.02 μm) Asbestiform	0.002	0
Crocidolite Asbestiform	1.75	49
Riebeckite Non-asbestiform	4.7	0.2
Amosite Asbestiform	1.99	41
Grunerite Non-asbestiform	3.16	0.07
Anthophyllite Asbestiform	2.13	10.5
Anthophyllite Non-asbestiform	2.94	0.5
Libby amphiboles Mixed	3.15	11.4
Glaucophane Mixed	3.4	6.2
Balangeroite Asbestiform	25.8	16
Fibrous talc Mixed	0.04	7.5
Wooly erionite Asbestiform	5.5	37.4

The following regression model can be developed for estimation of the mesothelioma potency factor R_M:

$$Log_{10}R_M = -5.65 + 2.09*\log_{10}(RigidityIndex) + 0.04Fraction + 1.43\log_{10}(Biopersistence)),$$

where Rigidity Index is the average rigidity index for particles with DCC ≥0.05 (μm²GPa x 10⁴),

Fraction is the fraction of particles with Rigidity Index ≥0.05 μm²GPa x 10⁴, and

Biopersistence is the biosolubility of particles in Gamble's solution as described in Gualtieri et al. (2018) (lifetime of fibers in years)

$$(R = 0.99, R^2 = 0.97, p < 0.04).$$

Table 7.6 contains the assumed values of particle biopersistence along with published and modeled mesothelioma potency factors.

The proposed model yields reasonable estimations for the majority of EMP types. The model for R_M estimations included rigidity index and dimensionality parameters, along with the biosolubility of particles. As we can see, non-asbestiform varieties of EMPs yielded significantly lower values of potency. The only exception is anthophyllite, which showed lower but close values of potency for the non-asbestiform and asbestiform varieties. In general, it is possible that the biopersistence value published by Gualtieri is too high (a possible outlier), obscuring the true difference between habits of anthophyllite.

For chrysotile fibrils and fibrous talc, the model demonstrated negligible estimations of potency.

Figure 7.4 demonstrates the relationship between observed and published values of mesothelioma potency R_M for various mineral types.

We also determined that the threshold for minimal rigidity necessary to produce biological effects in the human body can be supported by different biological observations.

Earlier, we mentioned flexural rigidity as a different metric of the biological stiffness of elongate mineral particles. According to Fortini et al. (2020), for a potentially toxic action of a chemically inert fiber inside the lung tissue, high flexural rigidity can be assumed to negatively affect macrophages' phagocytosis and other lung clearance mechanisms. Fortini suggested that the flexural rigidity threshold for a macrophage to be able to perform the complete phagocytosis of a biopersistent nanofiber is 10^{-19} N x m². This means that fibers presenting a flexural rigidity lower than 10^{-19} N x m² are classified as flexible and harmless; fibers with rigidity in the order of 10^{-19} N x m² could be either flexible or rigid; and fibers with rigidity above 10^{-19} N x m² are rigid and pose a hazard to macrophages.

It is easy to see that flexural rigidity for cylindrical particles is equal to 491 x Young's Modulus x Width⁴, and for tetrahedral particles, 833 x Young's Modulus x Thickness³ x Width.

Based on the data from the dimensional database, we demonstrated that for particles longer than 5 μm, with length/width ≥3, width ≥0.05 μm, width ≤3 μm, Rigidity

TABLE 7.6
Assumed biopersistence of elongate particles and estimations of their mesothelioma potency R_M (%)

Mineral type Habit	Biopersistence (Years)	R_M, published (%)	R_M, modeled (%)
Chrysotile, fibers Asbestiform	0.3[*]	0.0014[***]	0.0015
Chrysotile fibrils (width 0.02 μm) Asbestiform	0.3[*]	N/A	9.15×10^{-13}[******]
Crocidolite Asbestiform	66[*]	0.52[***]	0.26
Riebeckite Non-asbestiform	66[*]	N/A	0.02
Amosite	74[*]	0.11[***]	0.19
Grunerite Non-asbestiform	74[*]	N/A	0.01
Anthophyllite Asbestiform	245[*]	0.056[****]	0.07
Anthophyllite Non asbestiform	245[*]	N/A	0.05
Libby amphiboles Asbestiform and non-asbestiform	49[*]	0.03[***]	0.02
Glaucophane Asbestiform and non-asbestiform	N/A	0.0085[****]	N/A
Balangeroite Asbestiform	N/A	0.045[*****]	N/A
Fibrous talc Asbestiform	4.1[**]	N/A	4.02×10^{-8}
Wooly erionite Asbestiform	181[*]	4.67[****]	4.19

[*] Gualtieri et al. (2018)
[**] Jurinski and Rimstidt (2001)
[***] Darnton (2023)
[****] Korchevskiy et al. (2019)
[*****] Korchevskiy and Wylie (2023)
[******] The fraction of particles with DCC ≥ 0.05 and RI ≥ 0.05 μm^{2}GPa x 10^4 is zero for chrysotile fibrils. This parameter was replaced by a very low value (0.01%) to get the estimation of potency that seems to be negligible independent of assumptions on this parameter.

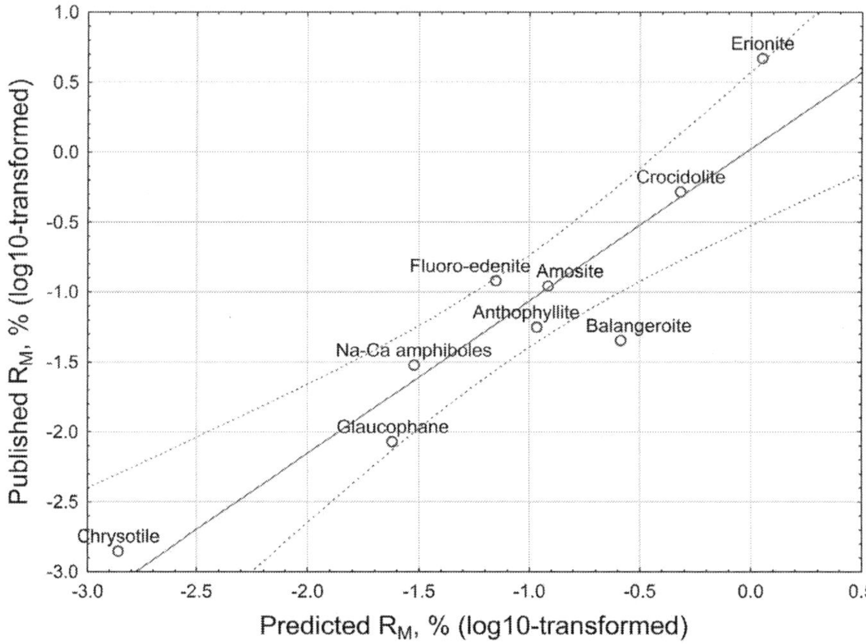

FIGURE 7.4 Observed and published values of mesothelioma potency R_M for various mineral types.

Index (RI) can be approximated by flexural rigidity by the following regression equation:

$$\text{Log}_{10}\,(\text{Rigidity Index}) = -1.04 + 1.02\log_{10}\,(\text{Flexural Rigidity}*10^{19}),$$
$$R = 0.95,\ R^2 = 0.89,\ F(1,\ 94677) = 836400,\ p < 0.00001,$$

where Rigidity Index is inμm^2GPa x 10^4,

Flexural Rigidity is in N x m^2.

In this case, the threshold of 10^{-19} N x m^2 corresponds to a value of Rigidity Index at 0.1 μm^2GPa x 10^4. It is quite consistent with the value of 0.05 μm^2GPa x 10^4 that we determined as a possible rigidity-related threshold for mesotheliomagenic CNTs and EMPs.

NOTES

1 W ≤ 0.27 μm.
2 Sample from India of similar texture.
3 Modal values for chrysotile from Deer et al. (2009).

REFERENCE LIST

Ahn, J. H., & Buseck, P. R. (1991). Microstructures and fiber-formation mechanisms of crocidolite asbestos. *American Mineralogist*, *76*(9–10), 1467–1478.

Atkinson, A. W., Gettins, R. B., & Rickards, A. L. (1970). Estimation of fibril lengths in chrysotile asbestos fibre. *Nature, 226*, 937–938. https://doi.org/10.1038/226937a0

Aveston, J. (1969). The mechanical properties of asbestos. *Journal of Materials Science, 4*, 625–633. https://doi.org/10.1007/BF00550118

Barbarino, M., & Giordano, A. (2021). Assessment of the carcinogenicity of carbon nanotubes in the respiratory system. *Cancers (Basel)*, *13*(6), 1318. https://doi.org/10.3390/cancers13061318

BAuA. (2021). *Proposal for harmonised classification and labelling of multi-walled carbon tubes to European chemical agency (2.0)* (pp. 1–111). BAuA.

Broßell, D., Meyer-Plath, A. A., Kaempf, K., Plitzko, S., Wohlleben, W., Stahlmecke, B., Wiemann, M., & Haase, A. (2020). A human risk banding scheme for high aspect-ratio materials. In R. M. Wagtervelci, J. C. M. Marynissen, L. Gradon, & A. Moskai (Eds.), *Synthetic nano-and microfibers*. Westim European Center of Excellence for Sustainable Water Technology. https://www.researchgate.net/publication/344190022_A_human_risk_banding_scheme_for_high_aspect-ratio_materials

Broz, M. E., Cook, R. F., & Whitney, D. L. (2006). Microhardness, toughness and modulus of Mohs scale minerals. *American Mineralogist*, *91*(1), 135–142. https://doi.org/10.2138/am.2006.1844

Bryukhanov, I. A., Rybakov, A. A., Kovalev, V. L., & Larin, A. V. (2014). Influence of carbonate species on elastic properties of NaX and NAKX zeolites. *Microporous and Mesoporous Materials, 195*, 276–283. https://doi.org/10.1016/j.micromeso.2014.04.036

Campbell, W. J., Huggins, C. W., & Wylie, A. G. (1980). *Chemical and physical characterization of amosite, chrysotile, crocidolite, and nonfibrous tremolite for oral ingestion studies*. National Institute of Environmental Health Sciences.

Chisholm, J. E. (1983). Transmission electron microscopy of asbestos. In S. S. Chissick & R. Derricott (Eds.), *Asbestos: Properties, applications and hazards* (Vol. 2, pp. 85–168). John Wiley and Sons.

Coffin, D. L., Palekar, L. D., & Cook, P. M. (1985). Correlation of in vitro and in vivo methods by means of mass dose and fiber distribution for amosite and fibrous ferroactinolite. *Environmental Health Perspectives*, *51*, 49–53. https://doi.org/10.1289/ehp.835149

Cressey, B. A., Whittaker, E. J. W., & Hutchison, J. L. (1982). Morphology and alteration of asbestiform grunerite and anthophyllite. *Mineralogical Magazine*, *46*(338), 77–87. https://doi.org/10.1180/minmag.1982.046.338.13

Damavandi, O. K., Hagh, V. F., Santangelo, C. D., & Manning, M. L. (2022). Energetic rigidity. I: A unifying theory of mechanical stability. *Physical Review E*, *105*, 025003. https://doi.org/10.1103/PhysRevE.105.025003

Darnton, L. (2023). Quantitative assessment of mesothelioma and lung cancer risk based on phase contrast microscopy (PCM) estimates of fibre exposure: An update of 2000 asbestos cohort data. *Environmental Research*, *230*, 114753. https://doi.org/10.1016/j.envres.2022.114753

Deer, W. A., Howie, R. A., & Zussman, J. (2009). *Rock forming minerals 3B: Layered silicates excluding micas and clay minerals* (2nd ed., Serpentine, p. 157). Published by the Geological Society of London.

Dorling, M., & Zussman, J. (1987). Characteristics of asbestiform and non-asbestiform calcic amphiboles. *Lithos*, *20*(6), 469–489. https://doi.org/10.1016/0024-4937(87)90030-2

Elhachemi, K., Khellafi, H., Bendouba, M., & Djebli, A. (2024). Quantification of Young's modulus of kaolin, sodalite and nanocomposite based on polycaprolactone/sodalite using atomic force microscopy. *Materials Research Express*, *11*(7), 075008. https://doi.org/10.1088/2053-1591/ad6236

Fortini, R., Meyer-Plath, A., Kehren, D., Gernert, U., Jácome, L. A., & Sturm, H. (2020). Measurement of flexural rigidity of multi-walled carbon nanotubes by dynamic scanning electron microscopy. *Fibers, 8*(5), 31. https://doi.org/10.3390/fib8050031

Golden, J. (1968). Whisker-like fibers from chrysotile asbestos. *Nature, 220*, 64–65. https://doi.org/10.1038/220064a0

Gouriet, K., Roussel, P., Carrez, P., & Cordier, P. (2022). Ultimate mechanical properties of enstatite. *Physics and Chemistry of Minerals, 49*(30). https://doi.org/10.1007/s00269-022-01206-5

Griffith, A. A. (1921). VI: The phenomena of rupture and flow in solids. *Philosophical Transactions of the Royal Society of London. Series A, Containing Papers of a Mathematical or Physical Character*, *221*, 163–198. https://doi.org/10.1098/rsta.1921.0006

Gualtieri, A. F., Pollastri, S., Gandolfi, N. B., & Gualtieri, M. L. (2018). *In vitro* acellular dissolution of mineral fibres: A comparative study. *Scientific Reports, 8*, 7071. https://doi.org/10.1038/s41598-018-25531-4

Hodgson, A. A. (1965). The thermal decomposition of miscellaneous crocidolites. *Mineralogical Magazine and Journal of the Mineralogical Society*, *35*(270), 291–305. https://doi.org/10.1180/minmag.1965.035.270.04

Hodgson, A. A. (1979). Chemistry and physics of asbestos. In L. Michaels & S. S. Chissick (Eds.), *Asbestos, properties, applications, and hazards* (pp. 65–115). John Wiley & Sons.

Húlan, T., Štubňa, I., Ondruška, J., Csáki, S., Lukáč, F., Mánik, M., Vozár, L., Ozolins, J., Kaljuvee, T., & Trnik, A. (2020). Young's modulus of different illitic clays during heating and cooling stage of firing. *Materials, 13*(21), 4968. http://dx.doi.org/10.3390/ma13214968

Jović, D., Jaćević, V., Kuča, K., Borišev, I., Mrdjanovic, J., Petrovic, D., Seke, M., & Djordjevic, A. (2020). The puzzling potential of carbon nanomaterials: General properties, application, and toxicity. *Nanomaterials (Basel)*, *10*(8), 1508. https://doi.org/10.3390/nano10081508

Jurinski, J., & Rimstidt, J. (2001). Biodurability of talc. *American Mineralogist*, *86*, 392–399. https://doi.org/10.2138/am-2001-0402

Kane, A. B., Hurt, R. H., & Gao, H. (2018). The asbestos-carbon nanotube analogy: An update. *Toxicology and Applied Pharmacology*, *361*, 68–80. https://doi.org/10.1016/j.taap.2018.06.027

Korchevskiy, A. A., Rasmuson, J. O., & Rasmuson, E. J. (2019). Empirical model of mesothelioma potency factors for different mineral fibers based on their chemical composition and dimensionality. *Inhalation Toxicology*, *31*(5), 180–191. https://doi.org/10.1080/08958378.2019.1640320

Korchevskiy, A. A., & Wylie, A. G. (2023). Toxicological and epidemiological approaches to carcinogenic potency modeling for mixed mineral fiber exposure: The case of fibrous balangeroite and chrysotile. *Inhalation Toxicology*, *35*(7–8), 185–200. https://doi.org/10.1080/08958378.2023.2213720

Korchevskiy, A. A., & Wylie, A. G. (2025a). Habit of elongate amphibole particles as a predictor of mesothelial carcinogenicity. *Toxicology Reports*, *14*, 101908. https://doi.org/10.1016/j.toxrep.2025.101908

Korchevskiy, A. A., & Wylie, A. G. (2025b, April 24). The empirical metric of mesothelial carcinogenicity for carbon nanotubes and elongate mineral particles. *Inhalation Toxicology* (online). https://doi.org/10.1080/08958378.2025.2486087

Lee, D.-K., Jeon, S., Han, Y., Kim, S.-H., Lee, S., Yu, J. Y., Song, K. S., Kang, A., Yun, W. S., Kang, S.-M., Huh, Y. S., & Cho, W.-S. (2018). Threshold rigidity values for the asbestos-like pathogenicity of high aspect ratio carbon nanotubes in a mouse pleural inflammation model. *ACS Nano, 12*(11), 10867–10879. https://doi.org/10.1021/acsnano.8b03604

Liu, C., He, H., Zhu, Y., Xu, W., & Yang, S. (2024). The utilization of 1-Dodecyl-3-methylimidazolium bromine ionic liquid in the reverse flotation separation of feldspar from apatite. *Advanced Powder Technology, 35*(6), 104499. https://doi.org/10.1016/j.apt.2024.104499

Lu, D. (2011). Direct measurement of the Young's modulus of a single halloysite nanotube using a transmission electron microscope with a bending stage. *Journal of Nanoscience and Nanotechnology, 11*, 7789–7793. https://doi.org/10.1166/jnn.2011.4720

Martin, C. J., & Phillips, V. A. (1977). The texture of chrysotile asbestos in relationship to mechanical properties. *Materials Science and Engineering, 30*(1), 81–87. https://doi.org/10.1016/0025-5416(77)90082-9

Murphy, F., Dekkers, S., Braakhuis, H., Ma-Hock, L., Johnston, H., Janer, G., de Cristo, L., Sabella, S., Jacobsen, N. R., Oomen, A. G., Haase, A., Fernandes, T., & Stone, V. (2021). An integrated approach to testing and assessment of high aspect ratio nanomaterials and its application for grouping based on a common mesothelioma hazard. *NanoImpact, 22*, 100314. https://doi.org/10.1016/j.impact.2021.100314

Murphy, F., Jacobsen, N. R., Di Ianni, E., Johnston, H., Braakhuis, H., Peijnenburg, W., Oomen, A., Fernandes, T., & Stone, V. (2022). Grouping MWCNTs based on their similar potential to cause pulmonary hazard after inhalation: A case-study. *Particle and Fibre Toxicology, 19*(1), 50. https://doi.org/10.1186/s12989-022-00487-6

Nagai, H., Okazaki, Y., Chew, S. H., Misawa, N., Yamashita, Y., Akatsuka, S., Ishihara, T., Yamashita, K., Yoshikawa, Y., Yasui, H., Jiang, L., Ohara, H., Takahashi, T., Ichihara, G., Kostarelos, K., Yasumitsu, M., Shinohara, H., & Toyokuni, S. (2011). Diameter and rigidity of multiwalled carbon nanotubes are critical factors in mesothelial injury and carcinogenesis. *Proceedings of the National Academy of Sciences-USA, 108*(49), E1330–E1338. https://doi.org/10.1073/pnas.1110013108

Nel, A. (2023). Carbon nanotube pathogenicity conforms to a unified theory for mesothelioma causation by elongate materials and fibers. *Environmental Research, 230*, 114580. https://doi.org/10.1016/j.envres.2022.114580

Schinwald, A., & Donaldson, K. (2012). Use of back-scatter electron signals to visualize cell/nanowires interactions in vitro and in vivo; frustrated phagocytosis of long fibers in macrophages and compartmentalization in mesothelial cells in vivo. *Particle and Fibre Toxicology, 9*(1), 34. https://doi.org/10.1186/1743-8977-9-34

Takagi, A., Hirose, A., Futakuchi, M., Tsuda, H., & Kanno, J. (2012). Dose-dependent mesothelioma induction by intraperitoneal administration of multi-wall carbon nanotubes in p53 heterozygous mice. *Cancer Science, 103*(8), 1440–1444. https://doi.org/10.1111/j.1349-7006.2012.02318.x

Virta, R. L. (2002). *Asbestos: Geology, mineralogy, mining, and uses* (Open File Report 02-149). U.S. Department of the Interior, U.S. Geological Survey, John Wiley & Sons, Inc.

Wylie, A. G., & Korchevskiy, A. A. (2023). Dimensions of elongate mineral particles and cancer: A review. *Environmental Research, 230*, 114688. https://doi.org/10.1016/j.envres.2022.114688

Wylie, A. G., & Korchevskiy, A. A. (2025). Critical values for dimensional parameters of mesotheliomagenic mineral fibers: Evidence from the dimensions and rigidity of MWCNT. *Frontiers in Toxicology, 7*, 1568513. https://doi.org/10.3389/ftox.2025.1568513

Wylie, A. G., Korchevskiy, A. A., Segrave, A. M., & Duane, A. (2020). Modeling mesothelioma risk factors from amphibole fiber dimensionality: Mineralogical and epidemiological perspective. *Journal of Applied Toxicology, 40*(4), 515–524. https://doi.org/10.1002/jat.39230

Wylie, A. G., Shedd, K. B., & Taylor, M. E. (1982, August 9–13). Measurement of the thickness of amphibole asbestos fibers with scanning electron microscope and transmission electron microscope. In K. F. J. Heinrich (Ed.), *Microbeam analysis: Proceedings of the annual 17th annual conference of the microbeam analysis society*. https://archive.org/details/1982-mas-proc-washington-dc/page/n1/mode/2up

Zhang, C., Wu, L., de Perrot, M., & Zhao, Z. (2021). Carbon nanotubes: A summary of beneficial and dangerous aspects of an increasingly popular group of nanomaterials. *Frontiers in Oncology, 11*. https://doi.org/10.3389/fonc.2021.693814

Zhu, G., & Hu, J. (2009). Stiffness matrix and quantitative measure of formation rigidity. In *Proceedings of the IEEE conference on decision and control (CDC)* (pp. 3057–3062). IEEE. https://doi.org/10.1109/CDC.2009.5400387

Zhu, W., von dem Bussche, A., Yi, X., Qiu, Y., Wang, Z., Weston, P., Hurt, R. H., Kane, A. B., & Gao, H. (2016). Nanomechanical mechanism for lipid bilayer damage induced by carbon nanotubes confined in intracellular vesicles. *Proceedings of the National Academy of Science USA, 113*(44), 12374–12379. https://doi.org/10.1073/pnas.1605030113

Zoltai, T. (1986). Asbestos, strength and surfaces. In *Proceedings of the 13th general meeting of the IMA, 1982 in physics of minerals and ore microscopy*. Bulgarian Academy of Sciences.

Zukowski, R., & Gaze, R. (1959). Tensile strength of asbestos. *Nature, 183*, 35–37. https://doi.org/10.1038/183035b0

Zussman, J. (1979). The mineralogy of asbestos. In L. Michaels & S. S. Chissick (Eds.), *Asbestos: Properties, applications, and hazards* (Vol. 1, pp. 45–65). John Wiley and Sons.

8 Characteristics of elongate mineral particles relevant for carcinogenic risk assessment

A. Korchevskiy & A. Wylie

INTRODUCTION

Various quantitative characteristics can be used to estimate the toxicological behavior of elongate mineral particles. All dimensional parameters for elongate mineral particles, as a rule, can be derived from their length, width, and thickness, as well as the interrelationship of these three metrics in a sample.

In 2022, we used a series of dimensional characteristics for various mineral types of elongate amphibole particles to determine which of them would most closely correlate with mesothelioma potency factors (Korchevskiy & Wylie, 2022). In this chapter, we will expand our study by using dimensional parameters that we previously tested, as well as new parameters, along with an expanded list of mineral particle types. We utilized the dimensional database described elsewhere in this book. For each mineral type in consideration, we calculated averages of each of the continuous characteristics, along with averages of logged values. For fractional characteristics, we only calculated averages. Then, all parameters in the study were correlated with each other and with mesothelioma potency factors and biopersistence, as reported below. Only amphiboles and single-chain silicate mineral types were used first, assuming that they may have similar chemical compositions with respect to biopersistence and potency. Then, we used the "best subset" linear regression method to detect the best combination of dimensional characteristics.

DIMENSIONAL PARAMETERS

The following dimensional parameters will be used for the analysis:

Length, width, and aspect ratio

Length, width, and aspect ratio are the most important and most described parameters of elongate mineral particles. In general, length is the measurement of the longest dimension, and width is the measurement of the longest dimension perpendicular to length of the two-dimensional particles observed under a microscope. Most fibers and cleavage fragments have parallel sides, but in the event that this is not the case, most analysts approximate an average. The aspect ratio is defined as the ratio of length to width of elongate particles.

DOI: 10.1201/9781003424277-9

Thickness

The thickness of particles (Th) was determined by the following empirical algorithm:

for erionite, Th = W,

for asbestiform and mixed amphiboles, $\log_{10}(Th) = 0.692\log_{10}(W) - 0.493$ (based on measurements reported by Wylie et al., 1982),

for non-asbestiform amphibole particles,
Th = W/1.9,

for balangeroite and other single-chain silicates,
Th = W/1.1, and

for talc (and other nontubular sheet silicates),
Th = W/3 (Wylie & Korchevskiy, 2025).

Fibrosity index

Wylie's fibrosity index is useful for discriminating asbestos from cleavage fragment populations. It was calculated as the F coefficient in Equation 8.1:

$$\text{Log W} = \text{F log L} + \text{Cq} \quad (8.1),$$

where W is the width, L is the length of the particles (Siegrist & Wylie, 1980; Wylie & Schweitzer, 1982), and F and C are derived from the linear regression relationship. The fibrosity index is calculated for particles longer than 2 μm, with width ≥0.05 μm, width ≤3 μm, and length/width ≥3.

Pearson index

For Equation 8.1, a linear Pearson correlation was also calculated as another metric of the relationship between logged length and logged width (referred to as the "Pearson index"). The Pearson index is a modification of the fibrosity index, allowing evaluation of the statistical independence of length and width. Independence between these parameters has been observed for populations of asbestiform fibers, but not for mineral fragments. The Pearson index is calculated for particles longer than 2 μm, with width ≥0.05 μm, width ≤3 μm, and length/width ≥3.

EMPA and EMPB

Parameters EMPA and EMPB were calculated as in Wylie et al. (2020), who showed a close correlation between these parameters and mesothelioma risk factors. The EMPA index is defined as the fraction of EMPs with aspect ratio ≥3, length >5 μm, and width ≤0.15 μm to total EMPs with aspect ratio ≥3 and length >5 μm. The EMPB index is the fraction of EMPs with aspect ratio ≥3, length >5 μm, and width ≤0.25 μm to all EMPs with aspect ratio ≥3, and length >5 μm.

Lippmann lung cancer index

As in Korchevskiy and Wylie (2022), the term Lippmann lung cancer (or just Lippmann) index refers to a fraction of particles with an aspect ratio ≥3:1, length >10 μm, and width >0.15 μm. It should be noted that Lippmann (1988) also suggested that the mesothelioma potency of fibers is most highly dependent on exposure to particles with width <0.15 μm (the Lippmann mesothelioma index). Because it is almost the same as the EMPA parameter, it was not considered independently.

Stanton index

Stanton et al. (1981) showed that the highest correlation between logit tumor probability and the abundance of particles per microgram of material implanted on the pleura of rats occurred with particles of length >8 μm and width ≤0.25 μm. The Stanton Index is the proportion of all elongate particles (aspect ratio or L:W ≥3:1) that are >8 μm long and ≤0.25 μm wide.

Surface area

The surface area (SA) of each of the non-serpentine particles was estimated from Equation 8.2:

$$SA = 2LW + 2LTh + 2WTh \quad (8.2),$$

where L = length, W = width, and Th = thickness.

For chrysotile fibers, the surface area was found as

$$S = \pi \times W^2 / 2 + \pi \times W \times L \cdot$$

Specific surface area

The specific surface area (ratio of surface area to volume) (SSA) was found as

SSA = S/V, where volume was determined as

$V = WTL$ for non-chrysotile particles, and

$V = \pi \times (W/2)^2 \times L$ for chrysotile particles.

This parameter is closely related to the often-published specific surface area per weight that can be found as SA/V/ρp, where ρp is the density of particles (in gm/cm^3). Specific surface area per unit of fiber mass was mentioned by Oberdörster et al. (2005) as a strong predictor of the biological reactivity of particles.

Aerodynamic diameter

Two models for the calculation of aerodynamic diameter (AD) of elongate mineral particles were used.

The first model is based on Timbrell (1965):

$$AD(Timb) = 66W \left(AR/(2{+}4\,AR)\right)^{2.2} x \left(\rho p/\rho_0\right)^{0.5} \quad (8.3),$$

where AD is the aerodynamic diameter, W is the measured width of the EMP, AR is the length/width, ρp is the density in gm/cm^3, and ρ0 is 1.0 gm/cm^3. The density of minerals is provided as basic information in descriptive mineral texts. The influence of small density variations (second decimal place) on AD is minor, so the use of literature values for mineral compositions is reasonable even if the exact composition can only be approximated from a qualitative chemical analysis or precise determination of the indices of refraction.

The second version of the AD calculation was derived from Gonda and Khalik (1985). The following formula was used:

$$\mathrm{AD}(\mathrm{New}) = W\sqrt{\frac{\rho}{\rho_0}\frac{1}{\frac{2}{9}\left(\frac{1}{Ln(2AR)-0.5}\right)+\frac{8}{9}\left(\frac{1}{Ln(2AR)+0.5}\right)}}$$

Dimensional Coefficient of Carcinogenicity (DCC)

DCC, introduced by Korchevskiy and Wylie (2025a, 2025b), was found by the formula

$$\mathrm{DCC} = 1 - \exp(-0.11\mathrm{SA}/(1000\mathrm{W}^3 + 1)).$$

The fraction of particles with DCC ≥0.05 was also determined for each mineral type.

Rigidity Index and Flexural Rigidity

The rigidity index (RI), as determined in Wylie and Korchevskiy (2025), was calculated as follows:

$$\text{Rigidity Index (RI)} = \pi^2 \mathrm{EI}_A / 4\mathrm{L}^2 \times 10000,$$

where E is Young's modulus for the material, and

I_A is determined as

- For a circular cross-section, $I_A = \pi r^4/4$ where r = ‰W (chrysotile); (8.4)
- For a rectangular cross-section, $I_A = (\mathrm{Th}^3)(\mathrm{W})/12$ where Th = thickness (amphiboles, zeolites, single-chain silicates). (8.5)

The fraction of particles with RI ≥0.05 was also calculated.
Flexural Rigidity (FR) of particles was calculated as

$$\mathrm{FR} = \pi \times \mathrm{W}^4 \times \mathrm{E} \times 10^4/64 \text{ for chrysotile particles, and}$$

$$\mathrm{FR} = \mathrm{Th}^3 \times \mathrm{W} \times \mathrm{E} \times 10^4/12 \text{ for non-serpentines.}$$

Shape factor

The shape factor for a particle is a ratio of the surface area of a sphere with the same volume as the particle to the surface area of the particle.

The shape factor can be closely approximated as
Shape Factor = $3.3\ \pi^{1/3}\ V^{2/3}/SA$.

Chatfield index

The Chatfield index is a proportion of elongate mineral particles longer than 5 μm adhering to Chatfield criteria. Based on Chatfield (2023), EMPs with width greater than 1.5 μm are considered non-asbestiform.

From the remaining particles,

Among particles with 5 μm ≤Length ≤10 μm, asbestiform have aspect ratio greater or equal to 35:1,

Among particles with 10 μm <Length ≤20 μm, asbestiform have aspect ratio greater or equal to 30:1, and

Among particles with Length >20 μm, asbestiform have an aspect ratio greater than or equal to 20:1.

Berman criteria

In Berman and Crump (2008), the "long thin" particle index is equal to the proportion of particles with an aspect ratio of more than 3:1, longer than 10 μm, and width < 0.40 μm. The "long, all width" index includes particles longer than 10 μm and narrower than 3 μm.

PCME index

The PCME index refers to the fraction of the particle category with W > 0.25 μm among all particles with AR ≥ 3:1 and L > 5 μm. This category was extensively used by NIOSH in their attempt to reconcile electron microscopy methods with the historical PCM technique. NIOSH now recognizes that amphibole fibers as narrow as 0.05 μm and chrysotile fibers as narrow as 0.15 μm are visible by PCM (Rooker et al., 1982; Kenny et al., 1987). Though the PCME index was used for different reasons in various publications (in particular, Berman, 2011 attempted to reconcile PCME criteria with other dimensional protocols), the complete exclusion of fibers narrower than 0.25 μm from counting cannot be considered a useful approach.

Corrected aspect ratio

Based on Korchevskiy and Wylie (2021), we used the corrected aspect ratio as the median of the value $Length^{1.19}/Width^{2.97}$.

In this paper, we used the geometric mean of the same value to account for the log-normal distribution of continuous variables used for size characterization of EMPs.

Mesothelioma potency (R_M) and biopersistence

As metrics for the carcinogenic potency of various mineral exposures, Hodgson and Darnton (2000) slope factors were utilized. We used the mesothelioma potency factor $R_{M,}$ defined by Hodgson and Darnton as a percent of expected mortality from all causes (adjusted to the age of first exposure of 30) per unit of cumulative exposure:

$$R_M = 100\frac{O_M}{\left(E_{Adj} \times X\right)} \tag{8.6},$$

where O_M is the number of mesothelioma deaths, E_{Adj} is the total expected deaths from all causes adjusted to the age of first exposure of 30, and X is the mean cumulative exposure in PCME fibers/cubic centimeter-years (f/cc-years).

Biopersistence for various mineral types of particles was estimated in terms of the predicted lifetime of mineral particles of a certain diameter (0.25 μm) during acellular dissolution, as described by Gualtieri et al. (2018).

Table 8.1 contains values of mesothelioma potency factors, biopersistence, and sources of the most recent information on fiber potency.

Table 8.2 contains average values of all parameters included to this study for mineral types listed in Table 8.1.

We performed correlation analysis to determine characteristics of EMPs that would be most efficiently predictive of the mesothelioma potency R_M. The results of the correlation analysis are provided in Table 8.3.

TABLE 8.1
The values of mesothelioma potency factors and biopersistence of major mineral types

Mineral type, Source	Mesothelioma potency factor R_M (%)	Biopersistence (years)*
Chrysotile, Quebec	0.0014**	0.3
Amosite, South Africa	0.11**	74
Crocidolite, South Africa and Australia	0.52**	66
Anthophyllite, Russia and Finland	0.056***	245
Libby amphiboles, Montana, U.S.A.	0.03**	49
Balangeroite, Italy	0.045****	N/A
Fluoro-edenite, Italy	0.12*****	N/A
Glaucophane, California, U.S.A.	0.0085*****	N/A
Erionite, Turkey	4.67*****	181

* Gualtieri et al. (2018)
** Darnton (2023, 2024)
*** Korchevskiy et al. (2013)
**** Korchevskiy and Wylie (2023)
***** Korchevskiy et al. (2019)

TABLE 8.2

Average values for major characteristics of selected mineral types of particles

Mineral type, source	Length, μm	Length, μm (Log)	Width, μm	Width, μm (Log)	Aspect Ratio	Aspect Ratio (Log)	AD, Timbrell, μm	AD, Timbrell, μm (Log)	AD, new, μm	AD, new, μm (Log)	Surface Area, μm^2	Surface Area, μm^2 (Log)
Chrysotile, Quebec	14.345	1.043	0.379	−0.571	70.033	1.613	1.770	0.109	1.151	−0.062	21.493	0.977
Amosite, South Africa	10.149	0.937	0.476	−0.397	29.595	1.334	2.184	0.272	1.380	0.080	14.480	1.003
Crocidolite, South Africa and Australia	15.212	1.030	0.313	−0.642	87.944	1.672	1.689	0.103	1.106	−0.064	13.475	0.874
Anthophyllite, Russia	10.368	0.943	0.830	−0.174	19.309	1.117	4.057	0.529	2.492	0.323	25.083	1.217
Glaucophane, California	9.059	0.919	0.859	−0.187	16.758	1.106	4.038	0.505	2.467	0.299	23.149	1.182
Libby amphiboles, Montana	10.798	0.976	0.663	−0.276	23.216	1.253	3.270	0.428	2.037	0.230	21.977	1.154
Fluoro-edenite, Italy	17.937	1.172	0.482	−0.390	46.067	1.563	2.523	0.333	1.657	0.158	25.845	1.242
Erionite, Turkey	12.998	0.979	0.452	−0.514	60.363	1.493	1.853	0.118	1.177	−0.061	24.945	1.078
Balangeroite, Italy	13.140	1.010	0.650	−0.274	28.261	1.284	3.204	0.428	2.022	0.233	39.364	1.332

Mineral type, source	SSA, 1/μm	SSA, 1/μm (Log)	AR, corrected	AR, corrected (Log)	Shape Factor	Shape Factor (Log)	RI, μm^2 x GPAx10000	RI, μm^2 x GPAx10000 (Log)	FR, nN	FR, nN (Log)	DCC	DCC (Log)
Chrysotile, Quebec	20.100	1.180	9320.750	2.935	0.390	−0.428	2393.052	1.548	58386.509	2.639	0.085	−1.393
Amosite, South Africa	19.237	1.232	1440.816	2.294	0.344	−0.471	182.184	1.597	1239.598	2.476	0.031	−1.803
Crocidolite, South Africa and Australia	31.008	1.423	10695.812	3.133	0.289	−0.556	110.971	0.656	1128.877	1.722	0.109	−1.308
Anthophyllite, Russia	13.318	1.062	744.377	1.640	0.379	−0.429	853.283	2.212	7045.797	3.105	0.016	−2.235
Glaucophane, California	13.884	1.072	300.358	1.648	0.381	−0.424	1201.786	2.241	10301.330	3.085	0.014	−2.231

(Continued)

TABLE 8.2 *(Continued)*
Average values for major characteristics of selected mineral types of particles

Mineral type, source	SSA, 1/μm	SSA, 1/μm (Log)	AR, corrected	AR, corrected (Log)	Shape Factor	Shape Factor (Log)	RI, μm² x GPAx10000	RI, μm² x GPAx10000 (Log)	FR, nN	FR, nN (Log)	DCC	DCC (Log)
Libby amphiboles, Montana	15.680	1.138	515.356	1.983	0.352	−0.459	398.148	1.850	4621.654	2.809	0.021	−1.995
Fluoro-edenite, Italy	18.396	1.223	953.435	2.554	0.291	−0.545	65.614	1.108	1411.837	2.459	0.044	−1.575
Erionite, Turkey	18.927	1.127	8484.616	2.691	0.394	−0.426	4551.031	1.554	46782.790	2.519	0.083	−1.460
Balangeroite, Italy	9.963	0.911	895.740	2.015	0.442	−0.367	13825.393	2.893	112367.170	3.918	0.033	−1.828

Mineral type, source	Fraction of DCC>0.05	EMPA	EMPB	Chatfield Index	Stanton Index	Lippmann Index	Berman, long thin	Berman, all width	PCME	Fibrosity Index	Pearson Index	Number of datapoints
Chrysotile, Quebec	0.443	0.261	0.452	0.526	0.281	0.334	0.320	0.493	0.548	0.287	0.324	3060
Amosite, South Africa	0.181	0.067	0.237	0.270	0.091	0.271	0.106	0.289	0.763	0.184	0.272	3455
Crocidolite, South Africa and Australia	0.559	0.357	0.579	0.619	0.312	0.234	0.300	0.410	0.421	0.273	0.394	12840
Anthophyllite, Russia	0.059	0.025	0.071	0.133	0.024	0.296	0.056	0.304	0.929	0.531	0.500	1038
Glaucophane, California	0.062	0.021	0.128	0.106	0.023	0.309	0.049	0.314	0.872	1.049	0.684	6255
Libby amphiboles, Montana	0.113	0.026	0.188	0.225	0.038	0.379	0.093	0.417	0.812	0.507	0.547	3059
Fluoro-edenite, Italy	0.339	0.046	0.211	0.587	0.165	0.697	0.294	0.725	0.789	0.257	0.285	109
Erionite, Turkey	0.456	0.221	0.405	0.445	0.175	0.205	0.138	0.240	0.595	0.192	0.233	1891
Balangeroite, Italy	0.161	0.054	0.089	0.321	0.054	0.464	0.125	0.482	0.911	0.354	0.472	56

TABLE 8.3
Correlation matrix for various characteristics of fibers

	R_M	R_M (Log)	Biopersistence	Biopersistence (Log)	Length, µm	Length, µm (Log)	Width, µm	Width, µm (Log)	Aspect Ratio	Aspect Ratio (Log)
R_M	1.00	**0.85**	−0.32	−0.26	0.51	0.29	**−0.79**	**−0.92**	**0.97**	**0.81**
R_M (Log)	**0.85**	1.00	−0.24	−0.15	0.65	0.48	**−0.89**	**−0.88**	**0.86**	**0.86**
Biopersistence	−0.32	−0.24	1.00	**0.99**	−0.34	−0.45	0.71	0.61	−0.40	−0.60
Biopersistence (Log)	−0.26	−0.15	**0.99**	1.00	−0.31	−0.47	0.63	0.53	−0.34	−0.54
Length, µm	0.51	0.65	−0.34	−0.31	1.00	**0.95**	**−0.68**	−0.61	**0.68**	**0.83**
Length, µm (Log)	0.29	0.48	−0.46	−0.47	**0.95**	1.00	−0.52	−0.41	0.47	**0.69**
Width, µm	**−0.79**	**−0.89**	0.71	0.63	**−0.68**	−0.52	1.00	**0.96**	**−0.89**	**−0.95**
Width, µm (Log)	**−0.92**	**−0.88**	0.61	0.53	−0.61	−0.41	**0.96**	1.00	**−0.96**	**−0.94**
Aspect Ratio	**0.97**	**0.86**	−0.40	−0.34	**0.68**	0.47	**−0.89**	**−0.96**	1.00	**0.94**
Aspect ratio (Log)	**0.81**	**0.86**	−0.60	−0.54	**0.83**	**0.69**	**−0.95**	**−0.94**	**0.94**	1.00
AD, Timbrell, µm	**−0.76**	**−0.86**	0.72	0.63	−0.59	−0.42	**0.98**	**0.96**	**−0.87**	**−0.92**
AD, Timbrell, µm (Log)	**−0.89**	**−0.87**	0.64	0.56	−0.53	−0.32	**0.94**	**0.98**	**−0.92**	**−0.90**
AD, new, µm	**−0.77**	**−0.86**	0.72	0.63	−0.56	−0.38	**0.98**	**0.96**	**−0.86**	**−0.90**
AD, new, µm (Log)	**−0.88**	**−0.86**	0.65	0.56	−0.50	−0.29	**0.93**	**0.98**	**−0.91**	**−0.88**
Surface area, µm2	−0.55	−0.43	0.67	0.57	0.09	0.15	0.42	0.47	−0.39	−0.32
Surface area, µm2 (Log)	**−0.79**	−0.62	0.61	0.52	−0.11	0.07	**0.70**	**0.80**	**−0.73**	−0.61
SSA, 1/µm	**0.94**	**0.80**	−0.51	−0.44	0.45	0.28	**−0.79**	**−0.85**	**0.85**	**0.78**
SSA, 1/µm (Log)	**0.82**	0.74	−0.60	−0.53	0.41	0.31	**−0.70**	**−0.72**	**0.69**	**0.68**
AR, corrected	**0.99**	**0.77**	−0.32	−0.27	0.43	0.19	**−0.77**	**−0.91**	**0.94**	**0.79**
AR, corrected (Log)	**0.89**	**0.89**	−0.61	−0.54	**0.72**	0.55	**−0.97**	**−0.99**	**0.96**	**0.98**
Shape Factor	−0.64	−0.65	0.64	0.58	−0.45	−0.47	0.43	0.38	−0.38	−0.47

(Continued)

TABLE 8.3 *(Continued)*
Correlation matrix for various characteristics of fibers

	R_M	R_M (Log)	Biopersistence	Biopersistence (Log)	Length, µm	Length, µm (Log)	Width, µm	Width, µm (Log)	Aspect Ratio	Aspect Ratio (Log)
Shape factor (Log)	−0.71	−0.71	0.58	0.52	−0.55	−0.54	0.52	0.48	−0.49	−0.57
RI, µm2 x GPAx10000	−0.25	−0.19	0.89	0.82	0.05	−0.01	0.11	0.14	−0.11	−0.11
RI, µm2 x GPAx10000 (Log)	**−0.77**	−0.75	0.60	0.53	−0.57	−0.48	**0.76**	**0.77**	**−0.76**	**−0.79**
FR, nN	−0.25	−0.19	0.76	0.67	0.13	0.05	−0.04	−0.03	0.05	0.05
FR, nN (Log)	**−0.77**	−0.70	0.60	0.53	−0.39	−0.27	**0.70**	**0.74**	**−0.71**	**−0.69**
DCC	**0.98**	**0.85**	−0.40	−0.35	0.61	0.37	**−0.87**	**−0.96**	**0.99**	**0.90**
DCC (Log)	**0.82**	**0.87**	−0.63	−0.57	**0.77**	0.59	**−0.97**	**−0.96**	**0.94**	**0.98**
Fraction of DCC>0.05	**0.92**	**0.87**	−0.46	−0.40	**0.73**	0.53	**−0.91**	**−0.97**	**0.98**	**0.96**
EMPA	**0.99**	**0.78**	−0.36	−0.30	0.46	0.21	**−0.80**	**−0.93**	**0.96**	**0.81**
EMPB	**0.96**	**0.78**	−0.57	−0.52	0.48	0.27	**−0.87**	**−0.96**	**0.96**	**0.86**
Chatfield Index	0.75	**0.82**	−0.53	−0.47	**0.92**	**0.79**	**−0.90**	**−0.87**	**0.89**	**0.98**
Stanton Index	**0.95**	**0.87**	−0.42	−0.35	**0.70**	0.52	**−0.90**	**−0.96**	**0.98**	**0.95**
Lippmann Index	−0.29	−0.03	−0.09	−0.20	0.56	**0.76**	0.06	0.23	−0.19	0.09
Berman, long thin	0.75	**0.79**	−0.48	−0.43	**0.88**	**0.81**	**−0.82**	**−0.81**	**0.85**	**0.93**
Berman, all width	0.08	0.27	−0.57	−0.64	**0.78**	**0.92**	−0.27	−0.13	0.19	0.44
PCME	**−0.96**	**−0.78**	0.57	0.52	−0.48	−0.27	**0.87**	**0.96**	**−0.96**	**−0.86**
Fibrosity Index	−0.44	**−0.83**	0.52	0.40	−0.59	−0.47	**0.81**	**0.68**	−0.57	**−0.71**
Pearson Index	−0.39	**−0.78**	0.29	0.16	−0.58	−0.47	**0.80**	**0.70**	−0.58	**−0.72**

TABLE 8.3 ***(Continued)***
Correlation matrix for various characteristics of fibers

	AD, Timbrell, μm	AD, Timbrell, μm (Log)	AD, new, μm	AD, new, μm (Log)	Surface Area, μm2	Surface Area, μm2 (Log)	SSA, 1/μm	SSA, 1/μm (Log)	AR, corrected	AR, corrected (Log)
R_M	**−0.76**	**−0.89**	**−0.77**	**−0.88**	−0.55	**−0.79**	**0.94**	**0.82**	**0.99**	**0.89**
R_M (Log)	**−0.86**	**−0.87**	**−0.86**	**−0.86**	−0.43	−0.62	**0.80**	0.74	**0.77**	**0.89**
Biopersistence	0.72	0.64	0.72	0.65	0.67	0.61	−0.51	−0.60	−0.32	−0.61
Biopersistence (Log)	0.63	0.56	0.63	0.56	0.57	0.52	−0.44	−0.53	−0.27	−0.54
Length, μm	−0.59	−0.53	−0.56	−0.50	0.09	−0.11	0.45	0.41	0.43	**0.72**
Length, μm (Log)	−0.42	−0.32	−0.38	−0.29	0.15	0.07	0.28	0.31	0.19	0.55
Width, μm	**0.98**	**0.94**	**0.98**	**0.93**	0.42	**0.70**	**−0.79**	**−0.70**	**−0.77**	**−0.97**
Width, μm (Log)	**0.96**	**0.98**	**0.96**	**0.98**	0.47	**0.80**	**−0.85**	**−0.72**	**−0.91**	**−0.99**
Aspect ratio	**−0.87**	**−0.92**	**−0.86**	**−0.91**	−0.39	**−0.73**	**0.85**	**0.69**	**0.94**	**0.96**
Aspect ratio (Log)	**−0.92**	**−0.90**	**−0.90**	**−0.88**	−0.32	−0.61	**0.78**	**0.68**	**0.79**	**0.98**
AD, Timbrell, μm	1.00	**0.97**	**1.00**	**0.97**	0.42	**0.72**	**−0.75**	−0.65	**−0.80**	**−0.95**
AD, Timbrell, μm (Log)	**0.97**	1.00	**0.98**	**1.00**	0.44	**0.79**	**−0.78**	−0.64	**−0.91**	**−0.96**
AD, new, μm	**1.00**	**0.98**	1.00	**0.98**	0.44	**0.75**	**−0.75**	−0.65	**−0.81**	**−0.95**
AD, new, μm (Log)	**0.97**	**1.00**	**0.98**	1.00	0.45	**0.79**	**−0.77**	−0.63	**−0.91**	**−0.94**
Surface area, μm2	0.42	0.44	0.44	0.45	1.00	**0.85**	**−0.76**	**−0.86**	−0.39	−0.41
Surface area, μm2 (Log)	**0.72**	**0.79**	**0.75**	**0.79**	**0.85**	1.00	**−0.88**	**−0.82**	**−0.78**	**−0.72**
SSA, 1/μm	**−0.75**	**−0.78**	**−0.75**	**−0.77**	**−0.76**	**−0.88**	1.00	**0.95**	**0.77**	**0.83**
SSA, 1/μm (Log)	−0.65	−0.64	−0.65	−0.63	**−0.86**	**−0.82**	**0.95**	1.00	0.57	**0.71**
AR, corrected	**−0.80**	**−0.91**	**−0.81**	**−0.91**	−0.39	**−0.78**	**0.77**	0.57	1.00	**0.87**
AR, corrected (Log)	**−0.95**	**−0.96**	**−0.95**	**−0.94**	−0.41	**−0.72**	**0.83**	**0.71**	**0.87**	1.00
Shape factor	0.34	0.27	0.32	0.24	**0.68**	0.44	**−0.71**	**−0.87**	−0.16	−0.43
Shape factor (Log)	0.43	0.36	0.41	0.34	0.65	0.47	**−0.77**	**−0.89**	−0.26	−0.53
RI, μm2 x GPAx10000	0.09	0.10	0.09	0.10	**0.84**	0.50	−0.50	**−0.70**	−0.07	−0.13

(Continued)

TABLE 8.3 *(Continued)*
Correlation matrix for various characteristics of fibers

	AD, Timbrell, μm	AD, Timbrell, μm (Log)	AD, new, μm	AD, new, μm (Log)	Surface Area, μm2	Surface Area, μm2 (Log)	SSA, 1/μm	SSA, 1/μm (Log)	AR, corrected	AR, corrected (Log)
RI, μm2 x GPAx10000 (Log)	**0.72**	**0.71**	**0.71**	**0.69**	**0.75**	**0.73**	**−0.92**	**−0.96**	−0.61	**−0.79**
FR, nN	−0.07	−0.09	−0.07	−0.09	**0.76**	0.34	−0.42	−0.64	0.12	0.04
FR, nN (Log)	**0.68**	**0.69**	**0.69**	**0.69**	**0.86**	**0.83**	**−0.94**	**−0.97**	−0.62	**−0.73**
DCC	**−0.87**	**−0.94**	**−0.87**	**−0.93**	−0.35	**−0.73**	**0.81**	0.63	**0.97**	**0.94**
DCC (Log)	**−0.95**	**−0.94**	**−0.94**	**−0.93**	−0.25	−0.61	**0.73**	0.60	**0.83**	**0.98**
Fraction of DCC>0.05	**−0.90**	**−0.94**	**−0.90**	**−0.93**	−0.33	−0.67	**0.81**	0.66	**0.91**	**0.98**
EMPA	**−0.81**	**−0.90**	**−0.81**	**−0.90**	−0.43	**−0.80**	**0.83**	0.63	**0.99**	**0.89**
EMPB	**−0.87**	**−0.94**	**−0.88**	**−0.94**	−0.58	**−0.87**	**0.90**	**0.77**	**0.95**	**0.93**
Chatfield Index	**−0.84**	**−0.81**	**−0.82**	**−0.79**	−0.19	−0.46	**0.71**	0.62	**0.71**	**0.94**
Stanton Index	**−0.87**	**−0.91**	**−0.87**	**−0.90**	−0.43	**−0.74**	**0.84**	**0.72**	**0.90**	**0.97**
Lippmann Index	0.16	0.31	0.20	0.34	0.47	0.60	−0.31	−0.17	−0.47	−0.08
Berman, long thin	**−0.75**	**−0.72**	**−0.72**	**−0.70**	−0.23	−0.47	**0.67**	0.62	0.66	**0.88**
Berman, all width	−0.14	−0.02	−0.10	0.01	0.27	0.27	0.04	0.12	−0.10	0.28
PCME	**0.87**	**0.94**	**0.88**	**0.94**	0.58	**0.87**	**−0.90**	**−0.77**	**−0.95**	**−0.93**
Fibrosity Index	**0.80**	**0.69**	**0.78**	**0.68**	0.12	0.35	−0.43	−0.37	−0.47	**−0.70**
Pearson Index	**0.83**	**0.75**	**0.82**	**0.74**	0.21	0.39	−0.44	−0.41	−0.49	**−0.72**

TABLE 8.3 *(Continued)*
Correlation matrix for various characteristics of fibers

	Shape Factor	Shape Factor (Log)	RI, µm2 x GPAx10000	RI, µm2 x GPAx10000 (Log)	FR, nN	FR, nN (Log)	DCC	DCC (Log)	Fraction of DCC>0.05	EMPA
R_M	−0.64	−0.71	−0.25	**−0.77**	−0.25	**−0.77**	**0.98**	**0.82**	**0.92**	**0.99**
R_M (Log)	−0.65	−0.71	−0.19	−0.75	−0.19	−0.70	**0.85**	**0.87**	**0.87**	**0.78**
Biopersistence	0.64	0.58	0.89	0.60	0.76	0.60	−0.40	−0.63	−0.46	−0.36
Biopersistence (Log)	0.58	0.52	0.82	0.53	0.67	0.53	−0.35	−0.57	−0.40	−0.30
Length, µm	−0.45	−0.55	0.05	−0.57	0.13	−0.39	0.61	**0.77**	**0.73**	0.46
Length, µm (Log)	−0.47	−0.54	−0.01	−0.48	0.05	−0.27	0.37	0.59	0.53	0.21
Width, µm	0.43	0.52	0.11	**0.76**	−0.04	**0.70**	**−0.87**	**−0.97**	**−0.91**	**−0.80**
Width, µm (Log)	0.38	0.48	0.14	**0.77**	−0.03	**0.74**	**−0.96**	**−0.96**	**−0.97**	**−0.93**
Aspect ratio	−0.38	−0.49	−0.11	**−0.76**	0.05	**−0.71**	**0.99**	**0.94**	**0.98**	**0.96**
Aspect ratio (Log)	−0.47	−0.57	−0.11	**−0.79**	0.05	**−0.69**	**0.90**	**0.98**	**0.96**	**0.81**
AD, Timbrell, µm	0.34	0.43	0.09	**0.72**	−0.07	**0.68**	**−0.87**	**−0.95**	**−0.90**	**−0.81**
AD, Timbrell, µm (Log)	0.27	0.36	0.10	**0.71**	−0.09	**0.69**	**−0.94**	**−0.94**	**−0.94**	**−0.90**
AD, new, µm	0.32	0.41	0.09	**0.71**	−0.07	**0.69**	**−0.87**	**−0.94**	**−0.90**	**−0.81**
AD, new, µm (Log)	0.24	0.34	0.10	**0.69**	−0.09	**0.69**	**−0.93**	**−0.93**	**−0.93**	**−0.90**
Surface Area, µm2	**0.68**	0.65	**0.84**	**0.75**	**0.76**	**0.86**	−0.35	−0.25	−0.33	−0.43
Surface Area, µm2 (Log)	0.44	0.47	0.50	**0.73**	0.34	**0.83**	**−0.73**	−0.61	−0.67	**−0.80**
SSA, 1/µm	**−0.71**	**−0.77**	−0.50	**−0.92**	−0.42	**−0.94**	**0.81**	**0.73**	**0.81**	**0.83**
SSA, 1/µm (Log)	**−0.87**	**−0.89**	**−0.70**	**−0.96**	−0.64	**−0.97**	0.63	0.60	0.66	0.63
AR, corrected	−0.16	−0.26	−0.07	−0.61	0.12	−0.62	**0.97**	**0.83**	**0.91**	**0.99**
AR, corrected (Log)	−0.43	−0.53	−0.13	**−0.79**	0.04	**−0.73**	**0.94**	**0.98**	**0.98**	**0.89**
Shape factor	1.00	**0.99**	**0.75**	**0.86**	**0.79**	**0.82**	−0.28	−0.33	−0.38	−0.24
Shape factor (Log)	**0.99**	1.00	**0.68**	**0.89**	**0.71**	**0.85**	−0.39	−0.44	−0.49	−0.34
RI, µm2 x GPAx10000	**0.75**	**0.68**	1.00	0.66	**0.94**	**0.72**	−0.04	0.02	−0.09	−0.08

(Continued)

TABLE 8.3 *(Continued)*
Correlation matrix for various characteristics of fibers

	Shape Factor	Shape Factor (Log)	RI, µm2 x GPAx10000	RI, µm2 x GPAx10000 (Log)	FR, nN	FR, nN (Log)	DCC	DCC (Log)	Fraction of DCC>0.05	EMPA
RI, µm2 x GPAx10000 (Log)	**0.86**	**0.89**	0.66	1.00	0.57	**0.97**	**−0.69**	**−0.70**	**−0.76**	−0.65
FR, nN	**0.79**	**0.71**	**0.94**	0.57	1.00	0.64	0.12	0.18	0.07	0.09
FR, nN (Log)	**0.82**	**0.85**	**0.72**	**0.97**	0.64	1.00	−0.66	−0.62	**−0.70**	−0.66
DCC	−0.28	−0.39	−0.04	**−0.69**	0.12	−0.66	1.00	**0.93**	**0.98**	**0.98**
DCC (Log)	−0.33	−0.44	0.02	**−0.70**	0.18	−0.62	**0.93**	1.00	**0.97**	**0.84**
Fraction of DCC>0.05	−0.38	−0.49	−0.09	**−0.76**	0.07	**−0.70**	**0.98**	**0.97**	1.00	**0.92**
EMPA	−0.24	−0.34	−0.08	−0.65	0.09	−0.66	**0.98**	**0.84**	**0.92**	1.00
EMPB	−0.40	−0.49	−0.26	**−0.79**	−0.08	**−0.80**	**0.96**	**0.87**	**0.93**	**0.96**
Chatfield Index	−0.48	−0.59	−0.04	**−0.74**	0.09	−0.61	**0.85**	**0.95**	**0.93**	**0.74**
Stanton Index	−0.42	−0.52	−0.18	**−0.78**	0.01	**−0.72**	**0.95**	**0.93**	**0.96**	**0.92**
Lippmann Index	−0.22	−0.22	0.13	0.05	0.08	0.25	−0.29	−0.01	−0.13	−0.44
Berman, long thin	−0.49	−0.58	−0.14	**−0.71**	0.04	−0.57	**0.77**	**0.86**	**0.84**	**0.69**
Berman, all width	−0.36	−0.40	0.05	−0.23	0.09	−0.02	0.08	0.32	0.22	−0.05
PCME	0.40	0.49	0.26	**0.79**	0.08	**0.80**	**−0.96**	**−0.87**	**−0.93**	**−0.96**
Fibrosity Index	0.22	0.30	−0.11	0.46	−0.18	0.39	−0.57	**−0.75**	−0.63	−0.47
Pearson Index	0.25	0.32	0.04	0.55	−0.07	0.48	−0.58	**−0.76**	**−0.68**	−0.46

TABLE 8.3 *(Continued)*
Correlation matrix for various characteristics of fibers

	EMPB	Chatfield Index	Stanton Index	Lippmann Index	Berman, long thin	Berman, all width	PCME	Fibrosity Index	Pearson Index
R_M	**0.96**	0.75	**0.95**	−0.29	0.75	0.08	**−0.96**	−0.44	−0.39
R_M (Log)	**0.78**	**0.82**	**0.87**	−0.03	**0.79**	0.27	**−0.78**	**−0.83**	**−0.78**
Biopersistence	−0.57	−0.53	−0.42	−0.09	−0.48	−0.57	0.57	0.52	0.29
Biopersistence (Log)	−0.52	−0.47	−0.35	−0.20	−0.43	−0.64	0.52	0.40	0.16
Length, µm	0.48	**0.92**	**0.70**	0.56	**0.88**	**0.78**	−0.48	−0.59	−0.58
Length, µm (Log)	0.27	**0.79**	0.52	**0.76**	**0.81**	**0.92**	−0.27	−0.47	−0.47
Width, µm	**−0.87**	**−0.90**	**−0.90**	0.06	**−0.82**	−0.27	**0.87**	**0.81**	**0.80**
Width, µm (Log)	**−0.96**	**−0.87**	**−0.96**	0.23	**−0.81**	−0.13	**0.96**	**0.68**	**0.70**
Aspect ratio	**0.96**	**0.89**	**0.98**	−0.19	**0.85**	0.19	**−0.96**	−0.57	−0.58
Aspect ratio (Log)	**0.86**	**0.98**	**0.95**	0.09	**0.93**	0.44	**−0.86**	**−0.71**	**−0.72**
AD, Timbrell, µm	**−0.87**	**−0.84**	**−0.87**	0.16	**−0.75**	−0.14	**0.87**	**0.80**	**0.83**
AD, Timbrell, µm (Log)	**−0.94**	**−0.81**	**−0.91**	0.31	**−0.72**	−0.02	**0.94**	**0.69**	**0.75**
AD, new, µm	**−0.88**	**−0.82**	**−0.87**	0.20	**−0.72**	−0.10	**0.88**	**0.78**	**0.82**
AD, new, µm (Log)	**−0.94**	**−0.79**	**−0.90**	0.34	**−0.70**	0.01	**0.94**	**0.68**	**0.74**
Surface area, µm2	−0.58	−0.19	−0.43	0.47	−0.23	0.27	0.58	0.12	0.21
Surface area, µm2 (Log)	**−0.87**	−0.46	**−0.74**	0.60	−0.47	0.27	**0.87**	0.35	0.39
SSA, 1/µm	**0.90**	**0.71**	**0.84**	−0.31	**0.67**	0.04	**−0.90**	−0.43	−0.44
SSA, 1/µm (Log)	**0.77**	0.62	**0.72**	−0.17	0.62	0.12	**−0.77**	−0.37	−0.41
AR, corrected	**0.95**	**0.71**	**0.90**	−0.47	0.66	[illegible]	**−0.95**	−0.47	−0.49
AR, corrected (Log)	**0.93**	**0.94**	**0.97**	−0.08	**0.88**	0.28	**−0.93**	**−0.70**	**−0.72**
Shape factor	−0.40	−0.48	−0.42	−0.22	−0.49	−0.36	0.40	0.22	0.25
Shape factor (Log)	−0.49	−0.59	−0.52	−0.22	−0.58	−0.40	0.49	0.30	0.32
RI, µm2 x GPAx10000	−0.26	−0.04	−0.18	0.13	−0.14	0.05	0.26	−0.11	0.04
RI, µm2 x GPAx10000 (Log)	**−0.79**	**−0.74**	**−0.78**	0.05	**−0.71**	−0.23	**0.79**	0.46	0.55

(Continued)

TABLE 8.3 *(Continued)*
Correlation matrix for various characteristics of fibers

	EMPB	Chatfield Index	Stanton Index	Lippmann Index	Berman, long thin	Berman, all width	PCME	Fibrosity Index	Pearson Index
FR, nN	−0.08	0.09	0.01	0.08	0.04	0.09	0.08	−0.18	−0.07
FR, nN (Log)	**−0.80**	−0.61	**−0.72**	0.25	−0.57	−0.02	**0.80**	0.39	0.48
DCC	**0.96**	**0.85**	**0.95**	−0.29	**0.77**	0.08	**−0.96**	−0.57	−0.58
DCC (Log)	**0.87**	**0.95**	**0.93**	−0.01	**0.86**	0.32	**−0.87**	**−0.75**	**−0.76**
Fraction of DCC>0.05	**0.93**	**0.93**	**0.96**	−0.13	**0.84**	0.22	**−0.93**	−0.63	**−0.68**
EMPA	**0.96**	**0.74**	**0.92**	−0.44	**0.69**	−0.05	**−0.96**	−0.47	−0.46
EMPB	1.00	**0.77**	**0.94**	−0.39	**0.73**	−0.01	−1.00	−0.50	−0.53
Chatfield Index	**0.77**	1.00	**0.90**	0.24	**0.94**	0.55	**−0.77**	**−0.69**	**−0.70**
Stanton Index	**0.94**	**0.90**	1.00	−0.12	**0.91**	0.28	**−0.94**	−0.56	−0.60
Lippmann Index	−0.39	0.24	−0.12	1.00	0.30	**0.90**	0.39	−0.07	−0.05
Berman, long thin	**0.73**	**0.94**	**0.91**	0.30	1.00	0.65	**−0.73**	−0.55	−0.56
Berman, all width	−0.01	0.55	0.28	**0.90**	0.65	1.00	0.01	−0.22	−0.17
PCME	−1.00	**−0.77**	**−0.94**	0.39	**−0.73**	0.01	1.00	0.50	0.53
Fibrosity Index	−0.50	**−0.69**	−0.56	−0.07	−0.55	−0.22	0.50	1.00	**0.91**
Pearson Index	−0.53	**−0.70**	−0.60	−0.05	−0.56	−0.17	0.53	**0.91**	1.00

The following parameters yield the maximum correlation coefficients with R_M and logged R_M values:

For R_M

AR, corrected	0.99
EMPA	0.99
DCC	0.98
Aspect ratio	0.97
EMPB	0.96
Stanton Index	0.95
SSA, 1/μm	0.94
Fraction of DCC>0.05	0.92
AR, corrected (Log)	0.89
SSA, 1/μm (Log)	0.82
DCC (Log)	0.82
Aspect ratio (Log)	0.81

For $Log(R_M)$

AR, corrected (Log)	0.89
Stanton Index	0.87
Fraction of DCC>0.05	0.87
DCC (Log)	0.87
Aspect ratio	0.86
Aspect ratio (Log)	0.86
DCC	0.85
Chatfield Index	0.82
SSA, 1/μm	0.80
Berman, long thin	0.79
EMPA	0.78
EMPB	0.78
AR, corrected	0.77

We also performed principal component (factor) analysis, projecting all parameters in our study on a two-dimensional plane. The results are demonstrated in Figure 8.1.

We also expanded our analysis by including erionite and chrysotile in the modeling process. We used the logged mesothelioma potency factor and utilized best subset regression analysis, as described earlier (Korchevskiy et al., 2019, 2024). We also assumed that biopersistence should be included as a mandatory factor, along with at least one of the dimensional parameters.

The best five models derived from the analysis are included in Table 8.4.

We averaged the predictions for the five listed models and compared the predicted and observed values of mesothelioma potency, as demonstrated in Figure 8.2.

We can therefore conclude that dimensional parameters are highly predictive for mesothelioma potency for various classes of minerals. For amphiboles and single-chain silicates, the corrected aspect ratio (median of $length^{1.19}/width^{2.97}$) is

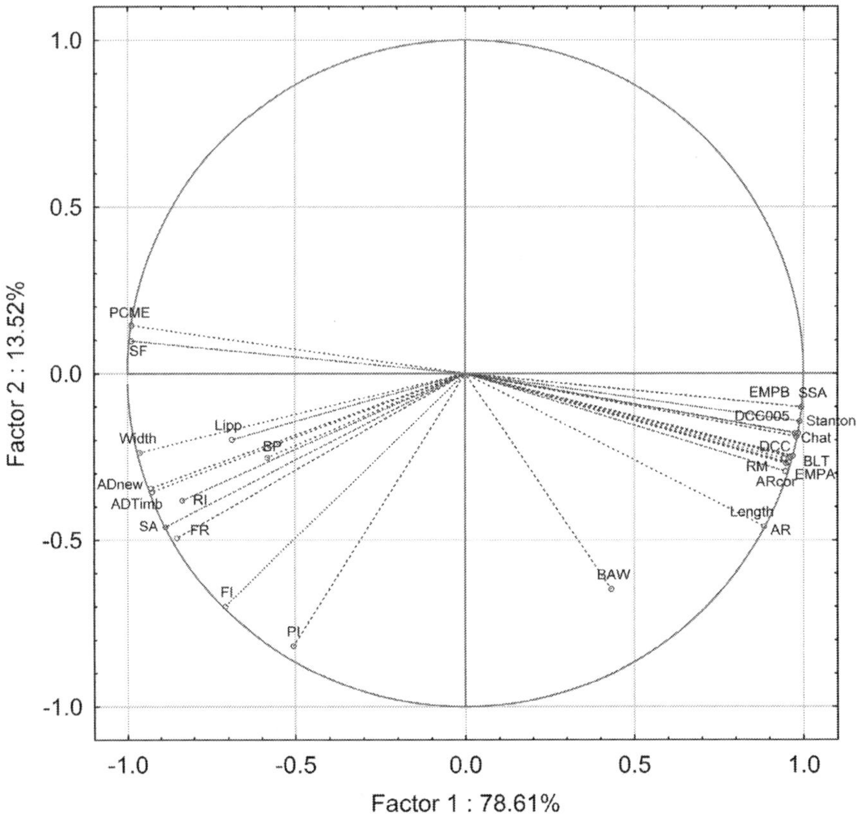

FIGURE 8.1 Projection of various parameters on the two-dimensional plane. R_M – mesothelioma potency factor, BP – biopersistence, AR – aspect ratio, ADTimb – aerodynamic diameter by Timbrell, ADnew – aerodynamic diameter by Gonda, SA – surface area, SSA – specific surface area, ARcorr – corrected aspect ratio, SF – shape factor, RI – rigidity index, FR – flexural rigidity, DCC – dimensional coefficient of carcinogenicity, EMPA – EMPA parameter, EMPB – EMPB parameter, Chat – Chatfield index, Stanton – Stanton index, Lipp – Lippmann index, BLT – Berman "long thin" index, BAW – Berman "all, width" index, PCME – PCME parameter, FI – fibrosity index, PI – Pearson index, DCC005 – fraction of particles with DCC ≥0.05.

TABLE 8.4
The "best subset" models selected for the analysis

Model	Statistical characteristics
$Log_{10}(RM) = -2.56+1.19*Log_{10}(Bioper) -4.7Log_{10}(ADNew)$	$R = 0.987, R^2 = 0.978, p < 0.0039$
$Log_{10}(RM) = -1.796+1.19*Log_{10}(Bioper) -4.34Log_{10}(ADTimb)$	$R = 0.986, R^2 = 0.974, p < 0.0043$
$Log_{10}(RM) = 0.66+1.198Log_{10}(Bioper) + 2.11*Log_{10}(DCC)$	$R = 0.979, R^2 = 0.959, p < 0.008$
$Log_{10}(RM) = -0.84+1.15Log_{10}(Bioper) - 1.30*ADNew$	$R = 0.968, R^2 = 0.937, p < 0.016$
$Log_{10}(RM) = -3.82+1.10Log_{10}(Biope)r + 3.46(DCC \geq 0.05 \text{ fraction})$	$R = 0.967, R^2 = 0.937, p < 0.016$

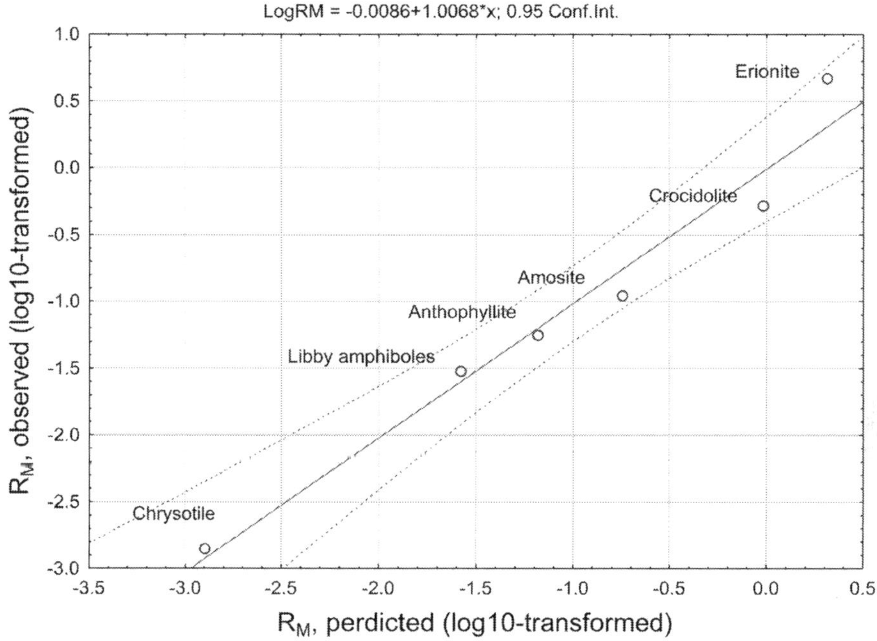

FIGURE 8.2 Relationship between observed and predicted mesothelioma potency (log_{10}-transformed)

confirmed as having the highest correlation coefficient, along with the EMPA fraction and dimensional coefficient of carcinogenicity (DCC). If serpentine, amphiboles, zeolites, and single-chain silicates are combined, and logged biopersistence is included as one of the independent variables, the aerodynamic diameter of the fibers, along with DCC (and the fraction of DCC ≥0.05) would be the strongest predictors of mesothelioma potency.

This analysis supports the idea that there is a true toxicological difference between asbestiform and non-asbestiform varieties of elongate particles. The corrected aspect ratio serves as a good discrimination function between asbestiform particles and cleavage fragments and, at the same time, correlates with the mesothelioma potency of amphiboles because non-asbestiform particles are not mesotheliomagenic, while asbestiform particles can cause mesothelioma (though not every asbestiform particle is mesotheliomagenic).

The modeling confirms that there are objective differences among types of mineral fibers regarding their propensity to produce mesothelioma. Canadian chrysotile has the lowest potency among commercial asbestos varieties. Libby amphiboles and California glaucophane represent the low tail of amphibole potency, while crocidolite (SA and Australia) is the most potent mesothelial amphibole carcinogen. Turkish erionite appears to be a type of fiber with the highest mesothelioma potency, though other types of erionite (and other zeolites) may have lower potency values.

The fibrous form of the mineral talc (without intergrown amphibole) is another example of a mineral with absent epidemiological data on mesothelioma mortality. Based on Jurinski and Rimstidt (2001), we can estimate the biopersistence of a fibrous talc particle with diameter of 0.25 μm as approximately 4.1 years (in terms of Gualtieri's biosolubility estimation). The average $\log_{10}$-transformed aerodynamic diameter (μm) of fibrous talc, based on the database information, is 0.08. The mesothelioma potency factor for fibrous talc, according to the first of the "best subset" models in our analysis, would be predicted as 0.006%, significantly lower than for all types of amphibole fibers. It should be noted that the potency of fibrous talc would be even lower (and most probably negligible), considering its low rigidity index (see Chapter 7).

It is noteworthy that parameters predictive of mesothelioma potency R_M also allow us to distinguish asbestiform from non-asbestiform particles.

For example, corrected AR ($\text{length}^{1.17}/\text{width}^{2.97}$) demonstrates the best predictive power for mesothelioma potency.

We can demonstrate that log-transformed corrected AR also allows for the distinction between asbestiform and non-asbestiform particles following the equation:

$\text{Log}_{10}(\text{ARcorrected}) \geq 1.87$ for asbestiform variety.

This statement is illustrated in Figure 8.3.

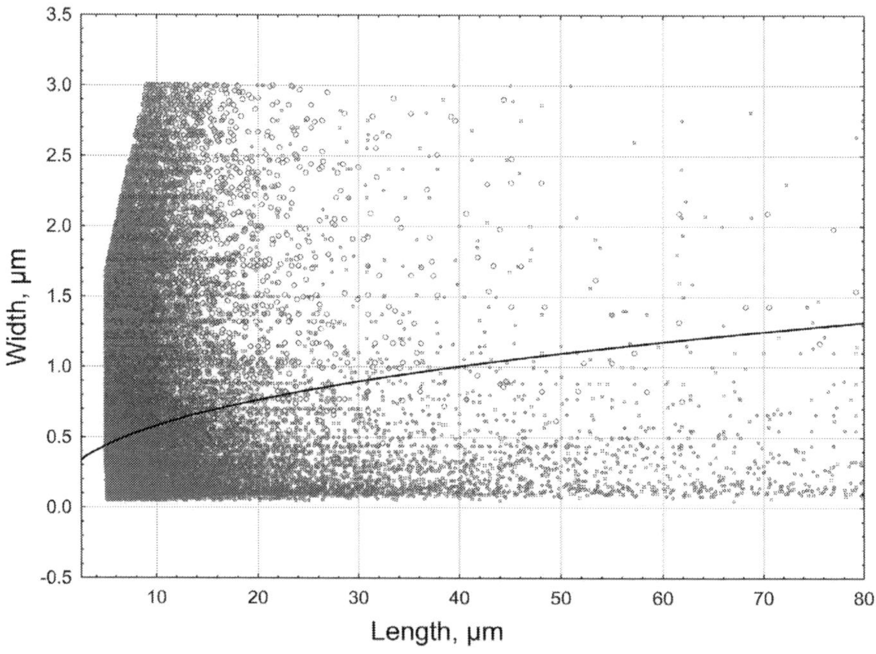

FIGURE 8.3 Distinguishing between asbestiform and non-asbestiform particles (amphiboles, zeolites, single-chain silicates) with log-transformed corrected aspect ratio. Green circles denotes non-asbestiform particles, red dots denotes asbestiform particles, the black line shows the value of the decision boundary $\log_{10}(\text{ARcorrected})=1.87$.

The quality of the prediction method is as follows:

Accuracy: 84%
True positive rate (recall): 80.9%
False positive rate: 9.7%
Precision: 93.9%

See other effective discrimination methods for asbestiform and non-asbestiform particles in Chapter 9.

Also, we can use the developed models to estimate the average mesothelioma potency factor for particles with a non-asbestiform habit (cleavage fragments). For example, we can assume as a worse-scenario case that the biopersistence of non-fibrous riebeckite would be comparable to the biopersistence of crocidolite, which is 66 years. For this type of riebeckite, log-transformed aerodynamic diameter has a level of 0.42. The conservative estimation of non-fibrous riebeckite potency would be 0.004%, which is 130 times lower than that for asbestiform crocidolite.

The modeled potency factors can be recalculated to lifetime mesothelioma risk estimations. For example, if a worker were exposed to 0.1 f/cc of non-asbestiform riebeckite for 10 years, 8 hours per day, 5 days per week, starting at the age of 30, his total lifetime excess mesothelioma risk would be
Risk = 0.004/100 x 0.1 f/cc x 10 years x 10,000 = 0.4 (cases per 10,000).

This excess risk is within the range of acceptable levels set by NIOSH or the U.S. EPA (see Korchevskiy et al., 2024). It is also lower than the baseline level of mesothelioma risk in the general population (Price & Ware, 2009).

If the person were exposed to asbestiform crocidolite, the excess risk would be estimated as

Risk = 0.52/100 x 0.1 f/cc x 10 years x 10,000 = 52 (cases per 10,000).

The comparison shows that the mesothelioma excess mortality rate in workers exposed to non-asbestiform varieties of amphiboles is negligible compared to the asbestiform counterpart. Refer to Chapter 9 for more information on the difference in habit as a predictor of potency. Exposure to asbestiform amphibole asbestos, especially the commercial types, can, to the contrary, cause significant health concerns.

REFERENCE LIST

Berman, D. W. (2011). Apples to apples: The origin and magnitude of differences in asbestos cancer risk estimates derived using varying protocols. *Risk Analysis*, *31*(10), 1308–1326. https://doi.org/10.1111/j.1539-6924.2010.01581.x

Berman, D. W., & Crump, K. S. (2008). A meta-analysis of asbestos-related cancer risk that addresses fiber size and mineral type. *Critical Reviews in Toxicology*, *38*(Suppl 1), 49–73. https://doi.org/10.1080/10408440802273156

Chatfield, E. J. (2023). Asbestiform fibers and cleavage fragments: Conceptual approaches for differentiation in laboratory practice and data analysis. *Environmental Research*, *230*, 114529. https://doi.org/10.1016/j.envres.2022.114529

Darnton, L. (2023). Quantitative assessment of mesothelioma and lung cancer risk based on phase contrast microscopy (PCM) estimates of fibre exposure: An update of 2000 asbestos cohort data. *Environmental Research, 230*, 114753. https://doi.org/10.1016/j.envres.2022.114753

Darnton, L. (2024). The Hodgson and Darnton approach to quantifying the risks of mesothelioma and lung cancer in relation to asbestos exposure. In A. Korchevskiy, J. Rasmuson, & E. Rasmuson (Eds.), *Health risk assessment for asbestos and other fibrous minerals* (pp. 233–269). John Wiley & Sons, Inc. ISBN: 978-1-119-43843-4. https://doi.org/10.1002/9781119438397

Gonda, I., & Abd El Khalik, A. F. (1985). On the calculation of aerodynamic diameters of fibers. *Aerosol Science and Technology*, *4*(2), 233–238. https://doi.org/10.1080/02786828508959051

Gualtieri, A. F., Pollastri, S., Gandolfi, N. B., & Gualtieri, M. L. (2018). In vitro acellular dissolution of mineral fibres: A comparative study. *Scientific Reports, 8*, 7071. https://doi.org/10.1038/s41598-018-25531-4

Hodgson, J. T., & Darnton, A. (2000). The quantitative risks of mesothelioma and lung cancer in relation to asbestos exposure. *Annals of Occupational Hygiene, 44*(8), 565–601.

Jurinski, J. B., & Rimstidt, J. (2001). Biodurability of talc. *American Mineralogist*, *86*(4), 392–399. https://doi.org/10.2138/am-2001-0402

Kenny, L., Rood, A. P., & Blight, B. J. (1987). A direct measurement of the visibility of amosite asbestos fibres by phase contrast optical microscopy. *Annals of Occupational Hygiene*, *31*, 261–264. https://doi.org/10.1093/ANNHYG/31.2.261

Korchevskiy, A. A., Rasmuson, E. J., Rasmuson, J. O., & Strode, R. D. (2013, February 24–27). *Asbestos mining in Russia: Approaches to public health risk assessment* (Preprint 13–117). Mining: It's All About People. Pre-Prints of the Society for Mining, Metallurgy & Exploration Annual Meeting, Denver, CO.

Korchevskiy, A. A., Rasmuson, J. O., & Rasmuson, E. J. (2019). Empirical model of mesothelioma potency factors for different mineral fibers based on their chemical composition and dimensionality. *Inhalation Toxicology*, *31*(5), 180–191. https://doi.org/10.1080/08958378.2019.1640320

Korchevskiy, A. A., Rasmuson, J. O., & Rasmuson, E. J. (2024). Mathematical modeling of cancer potency for various fibrous minerals. In A. Korchevskiy, J. Rasmuson, & E. Rasmuson (Eds.), *Health risk assessment for asbestos and other fibrous minerals* (pp. 396). John Wiley & Sons. https://doi.org/10.1002/9781119438397

Korchevskiy, A. A., & Wylie, A. G. (2021). Dimensional determinants for the carcinogenic potency of elongate amphibole particles. *Inhalation Toxicology*, *33*(6–8), 244–259. https://doi.org/10.1080/08958378.2021.1971340

Korchevskiy, A. A., & Wylie, A. G. (2022). Asbestos exposure, lung fiber burden, and mesothelioma rates: Mechanistic modelling for risk assessment. *Computational Toxicology*, *24*, 100249. https://doi.org/10.1016/j.comtox.2022.100249

Korchevskiy, A. A., & Wylie, A. G. (2023). Toxicological and epidemiological approaches to carcinogenic potency modeling for mixed mineral fiber exposure: The case of fibrous balangeroite and chrysotile. *Inhalation Toxicology*, *35*(7–8), 185–200. https://doi.org/10.1080/08958378.2023.2213720

Korchevskiy, A. A., & Wylie, A. G. (2025a). Habit of elongate amphibole particles as a predictor of mesothelial carcinogenicity. *Toxicology Report*, *14*, 101908. https://doi.org/10.1016/j.toxrep.2025.101908

Korchevskiy, A. A., & Wylie, A. G. (2025b, April 24). The empirical metric of mesothelial carcinogenicity for carbon nanotubes and elongate mineral particles. *Inhalation Toxicology* (online). https://doi.org/10.1080/08958378.2025.2486087

Lippmann, M. (1988). Asbestos exposure indices. *Environmental Research*, *46*(1), 86–106. https://doi.org/10.1016/s0013-9351(88)80061-6

Oberdörster, G., Oberdörster, E., & Oberdörster, J. (2005). Nanotoxicology: An emerging discipline evolving from studies of ultrafine particles. *Environmental Health Perspectives, 113*(7), 823–839. https://doi.org/10.1289/ehp.7339

Price, B., & Ware, A. (2009). Time trend of mesothelioma incidence in the United States and projection of future cases: An update based on SEER data for 1973 through 2005. *Critical Reviews in Toxicology, 39*(7), 576–588. https://doi.org/10.1080/10408440903044928

Rooker, S. J., Vaughan, N. P., & Le Guen, J. M. (1982). On the visibility of fibers by phase contrast microscopy. *American Industrial Hygiene Association Journal, 43*(7), 505–515. https://doi.org/10.1080/15298668291410125

Siegrist, H. G., & Wylie, A. G. (1980). Characterizing and discriminating the shape of asbestos particles. *Environmental Research, 23*, 348–361. https://doi.org/10.1016/0013-9351(80)90070-5

Stanton, M. F., Layard, M., Tegeris, A., Miller, E., May, M., Morgan, E., & Smith, A. (1981). Relation of particle dimension to carcinogenicity in amphibole asbestoses and other fibrous minerals. *Journal of the National Cancer Institute, 67*(5), 965–975.

Timbrell, V. (1965). Human exposure to asbestos: Dust controls and standards. The inhalation of fibrous dusts. *Annals of the New York Academy of Sciences, 132*(1), 255–273. https://dx.doi.org/10.1111/j.1749-6632.1965.tb41107.x

Wylie, A. G., & Korchevskiy, A. A. (2025). Critical values for dimensional parameters of mesotheliomagenic mineral fibers: Evidence from the dimensions and rigidity of MWCNT. *Frontiers in Toxicology, 7*. https://doi.org/10.3389/ftox.2025.1568513

Wylie, A. G., Korchevskiy, A. A., Segrave, A. M., & Duane, A. (2020). Modeling mesothelioma risk factors from amphibole fiber dimensionality: Mineralogical and epidemiological perspective. *Journal of Applied Toxicology, 40*(4), 515–524. https://doi.org/10.1002/jat.3923

Wylie, A. G., & Schweitzer, P. (1982). The effects of sample preparation and measuring techniques on the shape and shape characterization of mineral particles: The case of wollastonite. *Environmental Research, 27*(1), 52–73. https://doi.org/10.1016/0013-9351(82)90057-3

Wylie, A. G., Shedd, K. B., & Taylor, M. E. (1982, August 9–13). Measurement of the thickness of amphibole asbestos fibers with scanning electron microscope and transmission electron microscope. In K. F. J. Heinrich (Ed.), *Microbeam analysis: Proceedings of the annual 17th annual conference of the microbeam analysis society*. https://archive.org/details/1982-mas-proc-washington-dc/page/n1/mode/2up

9 Classification of elongate mineral particles by habit

A. Korchevskiy & A. Wylie

THE NEED FOR HABIT CLASSIFICATION

Asbestos and its analogues, asbestiform minerals, continue to be an issue of concern in many countries. The unique characteristics of asbestos made it an important industrial commodity. Virtually the same characteristics (flexibility in combination with persistence) made commercial asbestos a primary hazard in many occupational environments. However, commercial asbestos is not unique in nature because many other minerals express the asbestiform habit (Libby amphiboles or wooly erionite are good examples).

At the same time, various minerals, when mechanically affected, can produce non-asbestiform elongate mineral particles, with the majority being categorized as so-called cleavage fragments. As Belardi et al. (2018) stated,

> [N]on-asbestos crystals can break, during crushing or grinding, along preferred cleavage planes leading to splinter-like cleavage that may be mistaken for asbestos fibres. Therefore, any exploiting of rock and mineral deposits hosting nonasbestos particles may result in an exposure to airborne particles with morphology resembling asbestos. Notably, the classification of a particle as either a real asbestiform mineral or a cleavage fragment (non-asbestos) has a key role in assessing a reliable asbestos hazard scenario.

Distinguishing between asbestiform and non-asbestiform elongate mineral particles is an important and complex process. Many attempts have been made to determine the characteristics of asbestiform fibers that can be definitively detected during laboratory analysis; however, the results of individual classifications of elongate particles as cleavage fragments or asbestiform fibers under a microscope have been demonstrated to be quite subjective (Aust et al., 2011; Case, 1991; Meeker et al., 2006).

Therefore, it appears to be important to find easily measurable parameters that would distinguish biologically active asbestiform fibers from benign cleavage fragments. Dimensions of elongate particles appear to be an obvious choice. The U.S. Occupational Safety and Health Administration (OSHA, 1994) stated that "[m]ost cleavage fragments of the minerals are easily distinguishable from true asbestos fibers. This is because cleavage fragments usually have larger diameters than 1 μm." The issue with this statement is the choice of the dimensional cutpoint. Based on our data, 40% of non-asbestiform elongate amphibole particles with length >5 μm and an aspect ratio greater than 3:1 would have width ≤1 μm; 9.9% would have width ≤0.5 μm.

More elaborate methods are needed to discriminate between asbestiform fibers and cleavage fragments based on dimensional characteristics. The major question is

 DOI: 10.1201/9781003424277-10

as follows: are the dimensions of elongate particles sufficiently distinctive to evaluate their habit with some reasonable limits of error?

CLASSIFICATION OF PARTICLES BASED ON RELATIVE FREQUENCY OF HABITS

One of the straightforward new methods that can be used for this purpose is the relative frequency model. In our database on the dimensions of elongate mineral particles, we can measure the density of asbestiform fibers and cleavage fragments for short increments of length and width. For this method, we used rectangles for various values of length L (μm) and width W (μm), as shown in Figure 9.1.

For each combination of L and W in the database, we found parameters DensAsb and DensNonAsb equal to the numbers of asbestiform and non-asbestiform elongate particles, respectively, with dimensions that fall within the rectangle, as demonstrated in Figure 9.1.

The relative density of asbestiform particles in each size category is demonstrated in Figure 9.2.

We proposed the following empirical algorithm to classify particles with length > 5 μm, AR ≥3:1, width ≥0.05 μm, and width ≤3 μm (we call this category EMP-5).

1. If DensAsb<DensNonAsb/5, then the first classification variable is assigned a value of 0, otherwise 1.
2. If DensNonAsb<DensAsb/5, then the second classification variable is assigned a value of 1, otherwise 0.
3. If the classification variables yield equal values, then the combination of L and W is assumed to belong to the asbestiform habit if the variables are equal to 1 and to the non-asbestiform habit if equal to 0.

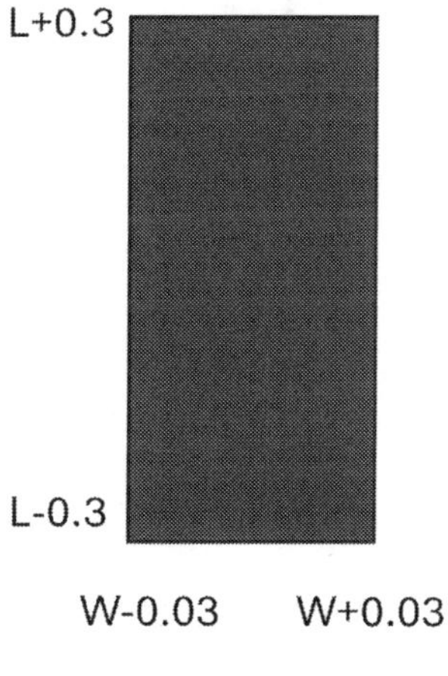

FIGURE 9.1 Dimensional rectangles to determine the density of asbestiform fibers and cleavage fragments

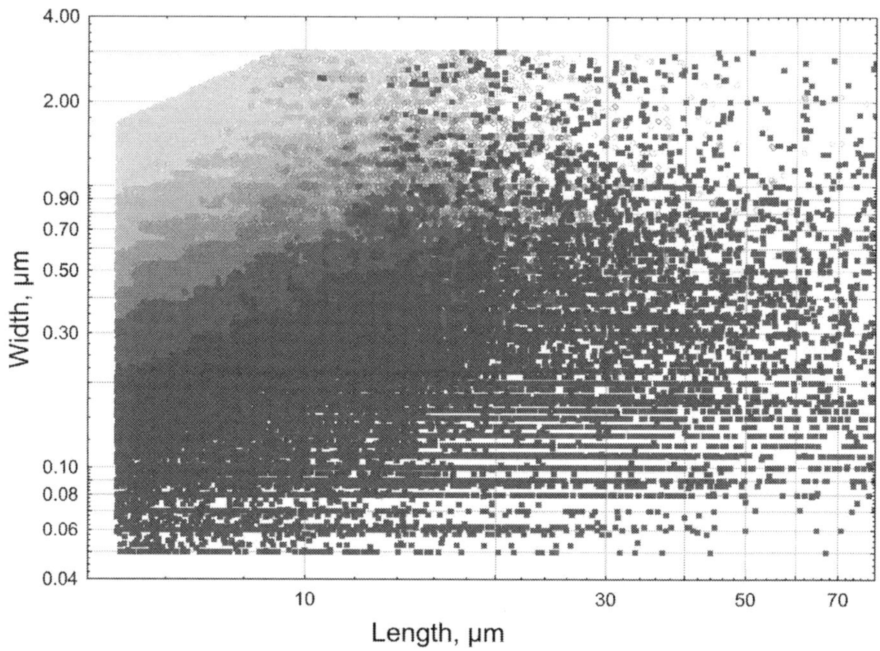

FIGURE 9.2 Relative density of asbestiform particles in each length and width category. Darker tone shows higher density.

4. If the classification variables yield non-equal values and DensAbs< DenNonAsb, then the combination of L and W is assumed to be non-asbestiform, otherwise asbestiform.

The classification using this algorithm (where the database plays the role of a training set) yields the correct assignment of habits for 87.8% of the records (a total of 53,750 records following the selection criteria).

Table 9.1 contains the estimation of correct identification of a series of various types of elongate mineral particles.

The relative frequencies of asbestiform and non-asbestiform particles around the dimensions of interest demonstrate that these dimensions are quite sufficient for predicting the habit of most individual particles. This method, however, produces higher errors for particles of several mineral types and habits, such as non-asbestiform riebeckite, asbestiform anthophyllite, asbestiform tremolite, and non-asbestiform fluoro-edenite. Also, the method requires complex calculations with a large database to determine the frequency of asbestiform and non-asbestiform particles in proximity to certain length and width values.

UTILIZATION OF LINEAR DISCRIMINANT FUNCTION

The alternative approach is the utilization of linear discriminant analysis for the classification of elongate particles with various habits.

TABLE 9.1
Fraction of correctly identified habit by probability frequency method (by location?)

Mineral type and habit	Correctly identified (%)
Cummingtonite-grunerite (asbestiform) (SA)	90.8
Cummingtonite-grunerite (non-asbestiform) (various locations)	89.8
Riebeckite (asbestiform) (SA and Australia)	94.4
Riebeckite (non-asbestiform) (various locations)	68.1
Anthophyllite (asbestiform) (Russia and Finland)	61.4
Anthophyllite (non-asbestiform) (various locations)	76.5
Tremolite (asbestiform) (various locations)	77.1
Tremolite (non-asbestiform) (various locations)	82.8
Actinolite (asbestiform) (various locations)	83.8
Actinolite (non-asbestiform) (various locations)	81.9
Fluoro-edenite (asbestiform) (Italy)	95.2
Fluoro-edenite (non-asbestiform) (Italy)	59.4
Erionite (Turkey)	85.5
Fibrous talc (NY state)	83.9
Total	87.8

Several landmark works have been published to evaluate the utilization of discriminant analysis for the purposes of EMP classification. In particular, Siegrist and Wylie (1980) utilized discriminant analysis to separate asbestiform particles from cleavage fragments on the basis of length and width. The procedure was applied to four populations of asbestos and three populations of cleavage fragments. For both, all measurements were made by scanning electron microscopy (SEM). In their original analyses, Siegrist and Wylie used data with lengths as short as 0.5 μm. The discriminant function (Equation 9.1) they derived was

$$Y = 2.17 \log_{10} \mathit{Length} - 1.26 \log_{10} \mathit{Aspect\ Ratio} + 2.75 \tag{9.1}$$

The value of Y>0 should predict the non-asbestiform, and Y<0 the asbestiform variety. As a result, 87.9% of the amphibole cleavage fragment population and 97.8% of the asbestos populations were correctly classified.

In 1985, Wylie, Virta, and Russek applied discriminant analysis to two populations of airborne amosite (a mixture of asbestiform grunerite and actinolite) and two populations of airborne amphibole cleavage fragments (one grunerite and the other actinolite). All particles met the 3:1 criterion and were longer than 2 μm, as measured by SEM. The discriminant model (Equation 9.2) they derived to separate the populations as asbestiform vs. non-asbestiform was

$$Y = 5.9 \log_{10} \mathit{Length} - 9.2 \log_{10} \mathit{Width} - 6.63 \tag{9.2}$$

The classification efficiency of Equation 9.2 was 81% for asbestiform fibers and 91% for non-asbestiform particles.

In 2022, Wylie et al. presented a study where discriminant analysis was utilized on a large multi-dimensional database. The analysis included over 300,000 measurements of amphibole. The datasets were pre-classified as "asbestiform," "non-asbestiform," and "inhomogeneous," and these classifications were used to develop models characterizing the habits of individual particles. The study analyzed the correct classification rates and misclassification rates, as well as identifying particle characteristics that impact their classification.

The database contains 56 independent aggregated datasets from bulk and air samples of asbestiform amphiboles, totaling 67,876 particle measurements. These datasets include samples used as asbestos reference materials by the National Institute of Standards and Technology (NIST), the National Institute of Environmental Health Sciences (NIEHS), and the Health and Safety Executive (HSE), as well as samples used in animal and cellular experiments on asbestos toxicity. The datasets include asbestos from major mines worldwide. Specifically, there are nine datasets for grunerite asbestos from the Transvaal region of South Africa (marketed as amosite or brown asbestos), known for mesothelioma excess in epidemiological studies, and 16 datasets for riebeckite asbestos, known as blue asbestos or crocidolite (also linked to mesothelioma excess). Nine crocidolite datasets are from various mines in South Africa's Cape Province, and three are from Hamersley, Australia – two of the world's primary crocidolite suppliers. Additionally, there are two crocidolite datasets from Cochabamba, Bolivia, where the material is used locally for roofing tiles. The world's anthophyllite asbestos, predominantly from Finland (associated with mesothelioma excess), is represented by three samples. Other sources include anthophyllite asbestos from mines in Georgia, in Sysert, Russia (mesothelioma excess), and India (two datasets). There are 20 samples of asbestiform particles with tremolite or actinolite composition from mines worldwide, including the United States (California and Virginia), Italy, Korea, Greece (mesothelioma excess), South Africa, India, Japan, and Scotland. A rare asbestiform Al-rich amphibole of edenite composition from Australia is also included.

The lengths and widths of non-asbestiform amphibole particles formed by crushing rock are found in 37 datasets, totaling 235,247 measurements. These datasets, from 29 different locations with varied chemical compositions, include amphiboles from some of the oldest rocks on Earth, such as banded iron formations and crystalline basement rocks, to younger volcanic rocks in Italy and Japan. The database includes samples from young mountain ranges in California, the Rockies, the Appalachian Blue Ridge, the Himalayas, and the Alps. It also represents volcanic and hydrothermal environments, regionally metamorphosed marbles, and amphibolites. Data from a gold mine, iron mine, marble quarries, and crushed stone mines are included. The compositions of these fragmented amphiboles vary as much as the asbestos samples, broadly reflecting common fragmented amphibole, except for Ca-Al-rich amphiboles common in granite (hornblende), which rarely form fibers or high-aspect-ratio fragments.

The inhomogeneous and anomalous category includes 12 samples of mixed amphibole cleavage fragments, asbestos fibers, and other brittle glassy, non-asbestiform fibers (35,277 measurements). These include air samples from El Dorado County, California; Boulder City, Nevada; and Rockhill Quarry, Pennsylvania, where both asbestos and non-asbestos forms of tremolitic and actinolitic compositions can occur in excavated rock or disturbed soil. Air samples from the Calaveras Dam excavation, constructed from rock producing anomalous amphibole glaucophane particles, are also included, as well as amphiboles from Libby, Montana. Libby amphiboles, known for excess mesothelioma mortality among workers, include a fraction of non-asbestiform particles referred to as prismatic amphibole (Meeker et al., 2003). The non-asbestiform component in the Libby aerosol is also described as byssolite fibers (Verkouteren & Wylie, 2000, 2002). Glaucophane excavated for the Calaveras Dam in California displayed an anomalous growth form, resulting in long, thin particles resembling asbestos but that were actually cleavage fragments (similar to reports for glaucophane from Italy by Vigliaturo et al., 2021).

Throughout the study, the populations were treated as either "asbestiform" or "non-asbestiform" based on the primary habit of the amphibole source. In many cases, this is unlikely to be entirely accurate. Amphibole fibers typically occur within massive rock composed of the same amphibole in a non-asbestiform habit, detectable in raw asbestos. Different EMP habits can be intergrown. Misclassification in a category labeled asbestiform may occur because some particles are not asbestiform; similarly, some particles in a non-asbestiform set could be asbestiform. However, asbestos in samples labeled non-asbestiform is uncommon in our non-asbestiform datasets because most materials were crushed laboratory samples chosen for their lack of asbestiform characteristics. Asbestos forms in discrete, normally planar zones, making it unlikely to be overlooked in a hand sample. The "inhomogeneous and anomalous" category designates populations with known asbestiform and non-asbestiform components, including cleavage fragments and, in some cases, brittle byssolite fibers.

General discriminant analysis was used on various dataset combinations to develop and cross-validate functions distinguishing elongate particles as asbestiform or non-asbestiform. The "best subset" approach selected the shape of the discriminant function for efficient discrimination between particle habits. Discriminant analysis then identified the specific discriminant function minimizing the overall misclassification rate.

Equation 9.3 is the universal discriminant function developed for all datasets, with particles L>5 μm, W≤3 μm, AR≥3:1:

$$Y = 2.99\log_{10} L - 5.82\log_{10} W - 3.80. \tag{9.3}$$

The particles with $Y \geq 0$ were classified as "criteria particles" and those with $Y < 0$ as "non-criteria particles."

The discriminant function yielded the correct overall classification rate of 84.66%, 82.8% for non-asbestiform particles, and 85.74% for asbestiform particles. Therefore, criteria particles approximate the group of asbestiform fibers, and non-criteria particles represent the group of non-asbestiform particles.

Table 9.2 demonstrates a fraction of correctly identified habits of individual particles according to Equation 9.3 in this chapter.

TABLE 9.2
Fraction of correctly identified habit by discriminant function method (Equation 9.3) (by mineral type and location)

Mineral type, habit, and source	Correctly identified (%)
Cummingtonite-grunerite (asbestiform) (South Africa)	74.1
Cummingtonite-grunerite (non-asbestiform) (various locations)	99.4
Crocidolite (asbestiform) (Australia and South Africa)	84.3
Riebeckite (non-asbestiform) (various locations)	87.3
Anthophyllite (asbestiform) (Russia)	54.1
Anthophyllite (non-asbestiform) (various locations)	90.2
Tremolite (asbestiform) (various locations)	58.9
Tremolite (non-asbestiform) (various locations)	75.4
Actinolite (asbestiform) (various locations)	70.1
Actinolite (non-asbestiform) (various locations)	86.1
Fluoro-edenite (asbestiform) (Italy)	90.4
Fluoro-edenite (non-asbestiform) (Italy)	48.1
Erionite (asbestiform) (Turkey)	71.5
Fibrous talc (mixed) (NY state)	77.0
Total	84.7

It can be shown that the discriminant function in terms of length and width can also be developed for the length and aspect ratio of particles.

The corresponding discriminant function is

$$Y = -3.14*\log_{10}L + 6.13\log_{10}AR - 4.40 \tag{9.4}$$

The negative coefficient by length in this function reflects the fact that the second variable (aspect ratio) is a function of length, μm and width. The corresponding coefficients in Equations 9.3 and 9.4 are slightly different because of the deviation of statistical estimations.

Figure 9.3 illustrates the discriminant function in a space of length and aspect ratio of particles.

For every length value, an increasing cutpoint of aspect ratio exists, differentiating asbestiform and non-asbestiform particles.

The cutpoint can be found in Equation 9.5:

$$\text{Aspect Ratio} \geq 5.22 \times \text{Length}^{0.51} \tag{9.5}$$

For example, for a length of 15 μm, the minimal aspect ratio for asbestiform fibers would be 20.77. For a length of 5 μm, the minimal aspect ratio for asbestiform fibers would be 12.

To the contrary, the cutpoint for aspect ratio in the so-called Chatfield yellow box method (Chatfield, 2023) decreases with increasing length. In one of our recent

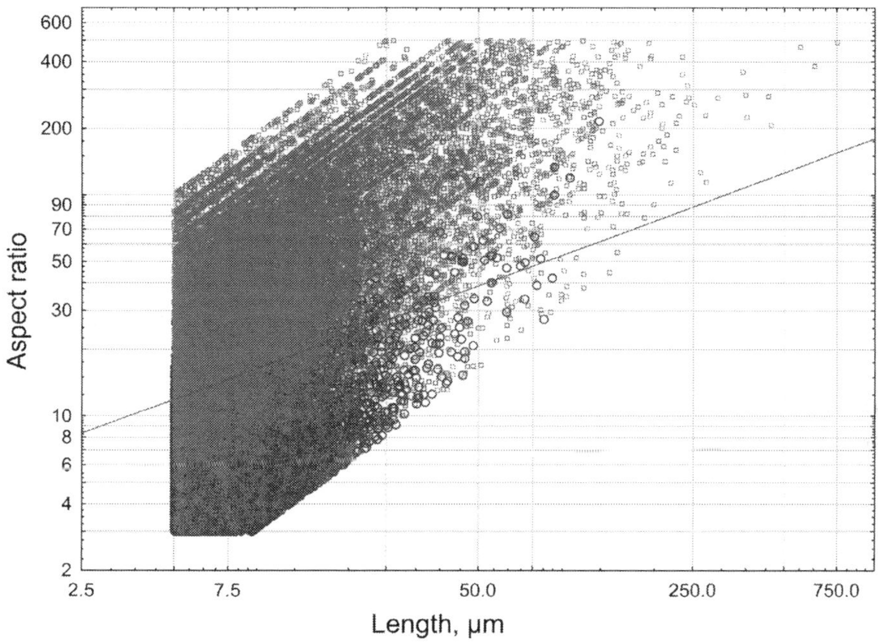

FIGURE 9.3 Discriminant function demonstrated in relationship to length and aspect ratio of particles. Red circles are from asbestiform and blue are from non-asbestiform populations.

publications, we demonstrated that our discriminant function method produces significantly lower misclassification error than the Chatfield method (Wylie & Korchevskiy, 2023).

Figure 9.4 illustrates a conceptual model developed in this study to distinguish between asbestiform and non-asbestiform particles. Particles that fall above the Discriminant Function (1) line are categorized as non-asbestiform, while those below are classified as asbestiform. Some particles in both regions are misclassified because they originate from the opposite group, appearing as "contaminants" (though they may naturally occur). This means that cleavage fragments and prismatic crystals can be found in asbestiform-labeled samples (although some of these particles may be fiber bundles). Conversely, most non-asbestiform samples are prepared from materials without asbestiform characteristics, so non-asbestiform particles mistakenly classified as asbestos are likely misclassified cleavage fragments or similar structures. The Discriminant Function Equation (9.3) effectively separates the populations, correctly predicting the source label approximately 85% of the time, leaving only 15% of each population as "misclassified" (ambiguous origin).

Areas 1 and 2 in Figure 9.4 contain EMPs identified by the discriminant function (Equation 9.3) as non-asbestiform, with the majority in Area 1. As mentioned earlier, only 14% of asbestiform EMPs are found in Areas 1 and 2, and many of these are likely actual non-asbestiform particle contamination in the asbestiform sets. The number of non-asbestiform particles decreases for those longer than 20 μm, marking the division between Area 1 and Area 2.

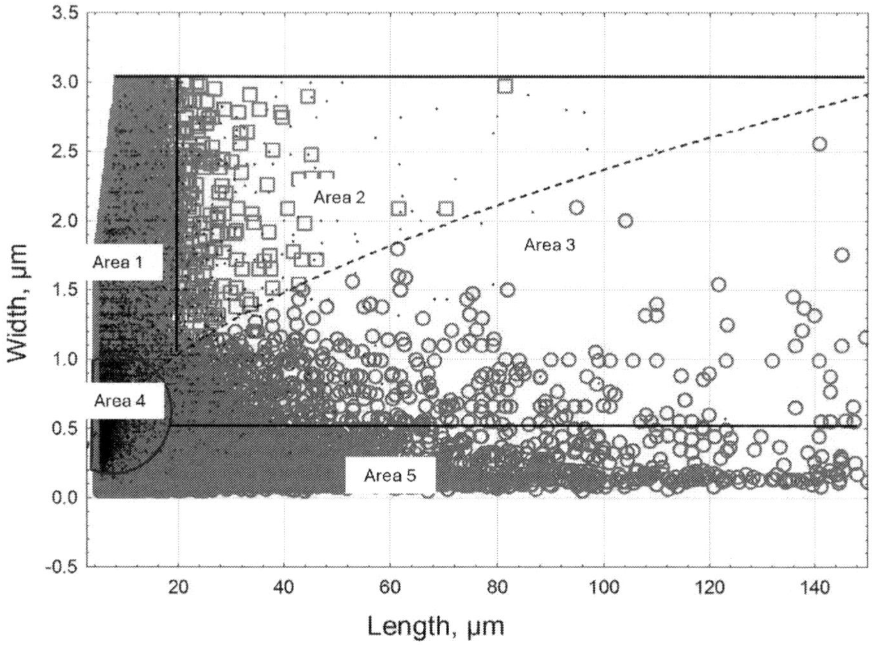

FIGURE 9.4 A schematic depiction of the discrimination process between asbestiform and non-asbestiform particles. Red circles represent correctly classified asbestiform particles, green squares represent correctly classified non-asbestiform particles, the dotted line shows the Discriminant Function (Equation 9.3), and black dots represent misclassified particles. Area 1: Particles designated as non-asbestiform with lengths less than 20 μm (excluding particles from Area 4). Area 2: Particles designated as non-asbestiform with lengths greater than 20 μm. Area 3: Particles designated as asbestiform with widths greater than 0.5 μm (excluding particles from Area 4). Area 4: Short fibrils, bundles of fibrils, prismatic crystals, and cleavage fragments that can belong to either asbestiform or non-asbestiform populations. Area 5: Particles designated as asbestiform with widths less than 0.5 μm (excluding particles from Area 4).

Areas 3 and 5 contain particles classified as asbestiform. Area 5 includes most of these particles, mainly composed of asbestos fibrils and small bundles of fibrils, each ranging in width from about 0.5 down to < 0.04 μm. Cleavage fragments are uncommon in this width range, especially for widths < 0.2 μm and are unknown below 0.1 μm. In Area 3, there are very few, if any, single asbestos fibrils above 0.5 μm. Here, composite asbestos particles of wider widths occur, which can be distinguished from cleavage fragments by their morphology in SEM, composite fibrillar structure in TEM, or by their unique optical properties under polarized light microscopy (PLM).

Area 4 has the highest proportions of misclassified particles, containing particles from both population types, including short fibrils, bundles of fibrils, prismatic crystals, and cleavage fragments. Particles in Area 4 cannot be readily distinguished as asbestiform or non-asbestiform based only on dimensions.

Cleavage fragments often accompany asbestiform material. To the extent that cleavage fragments contaminate asbestiform particle populations, they could be found in Area 4, mostly with W > 0.5 μm. Morphology can help determine whether a particle > 0.5 μm in width is composite. However, there are cleavage fragments as narrow as 0.2 μm, and for those with widths less than 0.5 μm, there are few tools available for discrimination (Figure 9.4). In Figure 9.4, the area below the 0.5 μm line with lengths less than about 8 μm remains a region where discrimination by length and width is unreliable. Therefore, considering the potency of "misclassified" or ambiguous EMPs based solely on dimensions may be useful in assessing risk.

The conceptual model can also be interpreted toxicologically. Most particles in Areas 1 and 2 are not expected to be carcinogenic. However, Area 5 corresponds to the asbestiform habit with the highest carcinogenic potential. The fraction of particles above the discriminant function (Equation 9.3) curve in Area 4 that are potentially carcinogenic and misclassified as non-asbestiform is small.

THE "BLIND" CLUSTER MODEL FOR PARTICLE CLASSIFICATION

Cluster analysis was performed to analyze possible "blind" classification of elongate mineral particles by length and width, without preliminary information about the habit or other characteristics of the particles.

Figure 9.5 illustrates the distribution of particles by length and width. Three clusters were determined. Cluster I corresponds to asbestiform EMPs, and Cluster II

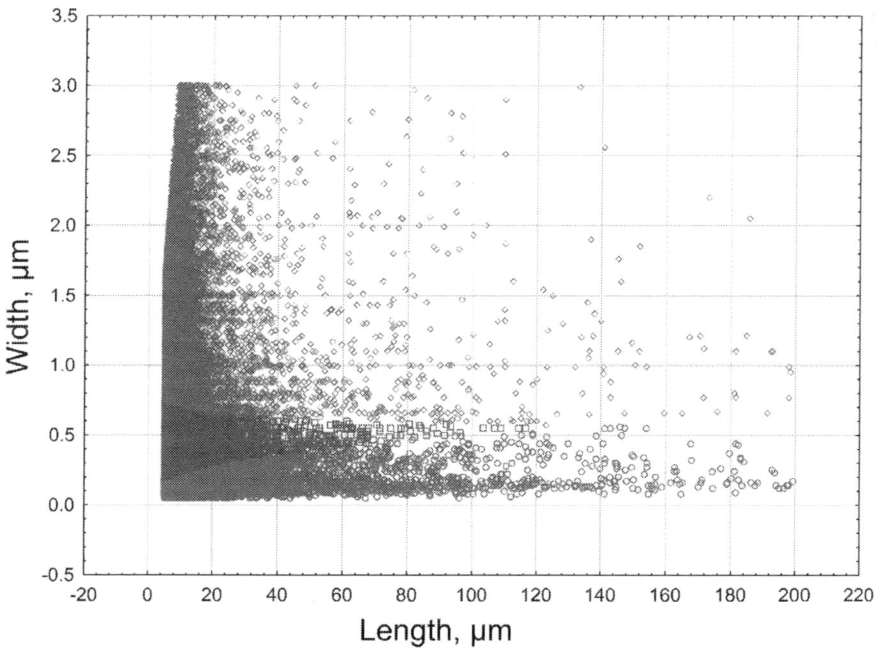

FIGURE 9.5 Cluster analysis of the dimensional data. Red circles represent Cluster I, blue rhombuses – represent Cluster II, and green squares represent Cluster III.

corresponds to non-asbestiform particles. Cluster III is a transitional category, with comparatively thin fibers but without sufficient aspect ratio and/or biological activity. Cluster III may partly correspond to Area 4 in Figure 9.4.

FIBROSITY INDEX AND CLASSIFICATION OF ASBESTIFORM AND NON-ASBESTIFORM PARTICLES

An additional tool to distinguish between the true habits of elongate particles is a fibrosity index that can be found by the following regression equation (Equation 9.6):

$$\text{Log10}(\text{Width}) = \text{A} + \text{B}\ \text{log10}(\text{Length}) \qquad (9.6),$$

where length >2 μm, width ≥0.05 μm, width ≤3 μm, length/width ≥3, and B is the fibrosity index (slope factor).

Table 9.3 contains the estimation of fibrosity index for several categories of fibers derived from our database.

The fibrosity index can provide valuable insights for the classification of asbestiform and non-asbestiform particles. For example, the fibrosity index for asbestiform tremolite is 0.22, while it is 0.66 for the non-asbestiform variety.

Table 9.4 demonstrates the fibrosity index in application to the classification of particles based on the discriminant function (Equation 9.3).

We can conclude that non-criteria particles found in asbestiform datasets have characteristics of cleavage fragments (higher fibrosity index), indicating the possible presence of fragments produced by mechanical forces in the sets.

Any particles in non-asbestiform datasets with length and width resembling asbestiform fibers still have a non-asbestiform nature (high fibrosity index) and are expected to have similar toxicological characteristics.

The following combined method is proposed to determine the habit based on the dimensional data for a sample of elongate particles.

1. Explore the fibrosity index. If high, the source is most probably non-asbestiform, and if low, asbestiform.

TABLE 9.3
Fibrosity index for various categories of elongate mineral particles (length>5 μm, width ≥0.05 μm, width ≤3 μm, length/width ≥3)

Category of EMPs	Fibrosity index
Asbestiform	0.19
Non-asbestiform	0.54
Mixed	0.55

TABLE 9.4
Fibrosity index for particles classified by Equation 9.3 (length>5 μm, length/width ≥3, width ≥0.05 μm, width ≤3 μm).

Category of EMPs	Fibrosity index
Asbestiform	
Identified as asbestiform by Equation 9.3	0.22
Identified as non-asbestiform by Equation 9.3	0.51
Non-asbestiform	
Identified as asbestiform by Equation 9.3	0.45
Identified as non-asbestiform by Equation 9.3	0.57

2. In asbestiform populations, the fraction of "non-criteria" particles (by Equation 9.3) indicates a possible presence of cleavage fragments. Rigid particles with a width less than or equal to 0.15 μm are mesothelioma carcinogens (see Chapter 3).

   In non-asbestiform populations, there are no known mesothelioma carcinogenic particles. The fraction of criteria particles (according to Equation 9.3) indicates rare occasions of long, thin cleavage fragments that are misclassified as asbestiform.
3. Mixed populations can have a high fibrosity index coupled with a high fraction of asbestiform criteria particles (by Equation 9.3), or a low fibrosity index and a low fraction of asbestiform criteria particles (by Equation 9.3).

PEARSON INDEX AND DECISION BOUNDARY CLASSIFICATION METHODOLOGY

The decision boundary classification methodology was proposed in one of our recent publications (Korchevskiy & Wylie, 2025a).

The methodology is based on the Pearson Index for sets of particles. The Pearson Index is a modification of the Fibrosity Index and is calculated as a linear correlation coefficient corresponding to Equation 9.6 above.

The following formula for the boundary was found:

Asbestiform Criteria Particles Fraction ≥0.34Pearson Index +0.35, (Equation 9.7),

where Asbestiform Criteria Particles Fraction is the fraction of asbestiform particles based on Equation 9.3.

Equation 9.7 allows us to distinguish asbestiform and non-asbestiform samples with an error rate of 5.7%.

We also explored modifications of this method, assuming that mixed populations of particles may be present in a sample, making it difficult to determine the combined habit or fraction of particles for each habit in the sample. It was suggested that if the fraction of asbestiform criteria particles (by Equation 9.3) is in the range from 0.2 to 0.4, but the Pearson index is between 0.1 and 0.4, the samples can be misclassified. Additional resampling may be required to resolve the controversy. This approach reduces the error rate of the method to about 3% (meaning that only 3% of samples would be misidentified as asbestiform or non-asbestiform based on initial mineralogical characterization).

CANCER POTENCY OF ASBESTIFORM AND NON-ASBESTIFORM ELONGATE PARTICLES

Figure 9.6 illustrates the relationship between the habit of EMPs, as predicted by the Discriminant Function (Equation 9.3), and particles in the so-called EMPA category which includes elongate mineral particles longer than 5 μm having a width less than or equal to 0.15 μm.

As we can see, no "non-criteria" particles (with Y<0) belong to the carcinogenic EMPA category.

Among all non-asbestiform EMP5 particles out of 15,234 total particles, only 9 particles, or 0.06%, would be EMPA, clearly demonstrating that EMP-5 fragments with very narrow widths are extremely rare. It is also possible that they are accidental

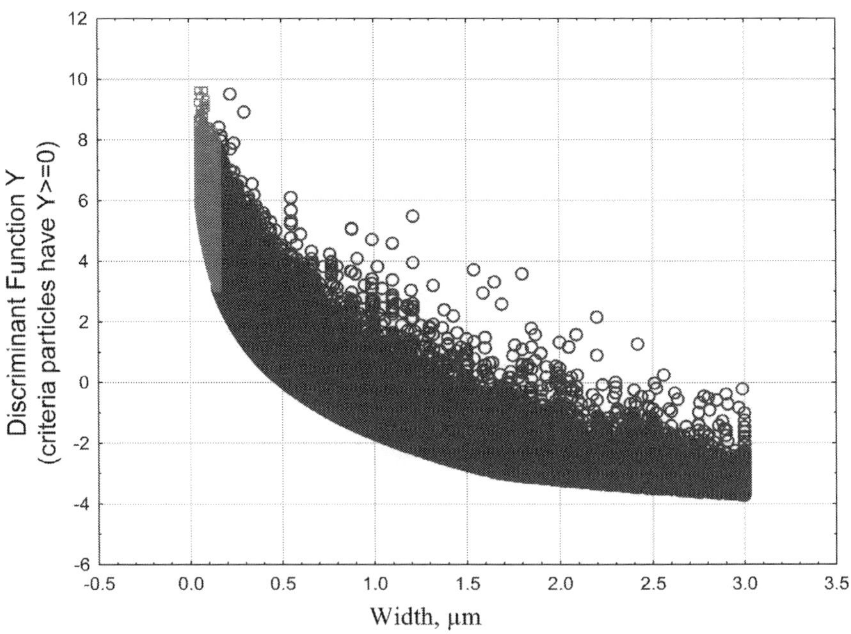

FIGURE 9.6 Relationship between the width of particles and discriminant function Y (Equation 9.3). Red squares represent EMPA particles and blue dots represent non-EMPA particles (Length >5 μm, length/width ≥3, width ≥0.05 μm, width ≤3 μm).

contamination, not corresponding to a specific habit of the samples, or that they are particles that were measured incorrectly.

Based on Wylie et al. (2020), the fraction of 0.06% of EMPA particles would yield a mesothelioma risk estimation of 0% for the linear model, or 0.00076% for the non-linear model (10 times lower than for Quebec chrysotile, and most probably below the level of statistical significance).

For asbestiform particles in our database longer than 5 μm (a total of 39,075 particles), 8,894 or 22.8% are EMPA, corresponding to a mesothelioma potency of 0.21% by the non-linear model, or 0.24% for the linear model. This is a value between the mesothelioma potency of amosite (about 0.11%) and crocidolite (0.52%).

The dimensional coefficient of carcinogenicity (DCC), described in Chapters 4 and 8, provides a good framework for estimations of mesothelioma potency for non-asbestiform particles. Korchevskiy and Wylie (2025a, 2025b) demonstrated, based on both DCC and EMPA parameters, that non-asbestiform tremolite particles have negligible mesothelioma potency.

Figure 9.7 shows the values of DCC for particles classified as non-asbestiform and asbestiform, based on Equation 9.3 (so-called criteria and non-criteria particles).

As can be seen, all particles classified as non-asbestiform by Equation 9.3 have DCC < 0.05, which enables their classification as non-mesotheliomagenic. Some fraction of particles classified as asbestiform by Equation 9.3 have DCC > 0.05, but

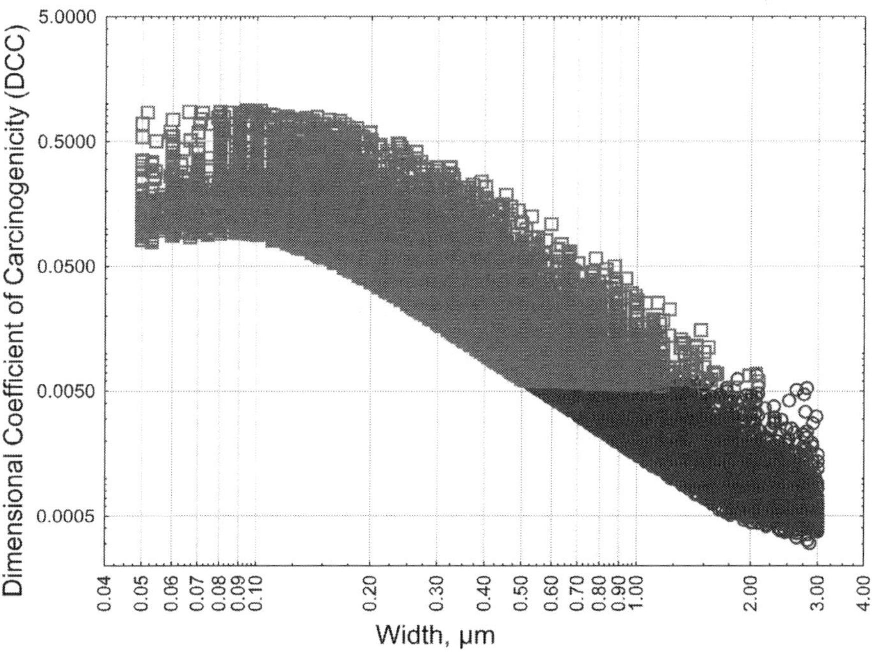

FIGURE 9.7 Dimensional coefficient of carcinogenicity (DCC) and width of criteria (red squares) and non-criteria (blue circles) EMPs based on Equation 9.3.

a significant portion also have DCC < 0.05, emphasizing the fact that not all asbestiform particles are carcinogenic.

The application of DCC demonstrates and explains that non-asbestiform particles would not produce an elevated level of mesothelioma in exposed humans. It is possible to distinguish non-asbestiform populations of elongate mineral particles from asbestiform based on dimensional characteristics. Asbestiform populations by themselves often have a mixed nature, with some fraction of thicker particles that can belong to a non-asbestiform variety. It is necessary to explore the dimensional characteristics of potential exposure in detail to determine the mineralogical source of the elongate particles. A single asbestiform sample that does not contain the mesotheliomagenic fraction EMPA can still be suspected to be potentially carcinogenic, given the inhomogeneous nature of fiber dimensions in some occurrences. However, the non-asbestiform (cleavage fragments) nature of the source (massive, prismatic) makes carcinogenic effects improbable.

REFERENCE LIST

Aust, A. E., Cook, P. M., & Dodson, R. F. (2011). Morphological and chemical mechanisms of elongated mineral particle toxicities. *Journal of Toxicology and Environmental Health, Part B, Critical Reviews*, *14*(1–4), 40–75. https://doi.org/10.1080/10937404.2011.556046

Belardi, G., Vignaroli, G., Trapasso, F., Pacella, A., & Passeri, D. (2018). Detecting asbestos fibres and cleavage fragments produced after mechanical tests on ophiolite rocks: Clues for the asbestos hazard evaluation. *Journal of Mediterranean Earth Sciences*, *10*, 63–78. https://doi.org/10.3304/JMES.2018.016

Case, B. W. (1991). On talc, tremolite, and tergiversation. Ter-gi-ver-sate: 2: To use subterfuges. *British Journal of Industrial Medicine*, *48*, 357–360. https://doi.org/10.1136%2Foem.48.5.357

Chatfield, E. J. (2023). Asbestiform fibers and cleavage fragments: Conceptual approaches for differentiation in laboratory practice and data analysis. *Environmental Research*, *230*, 114529. https://doi.org/10.1016/j.envres.2022.114529

Korchevskiy, A. A., & Wylie, A. G. (2025a). Habit of elongate amphibole particles as a predictor of mesothelial carcinogenicity. *Toxicology Reports*, *14*, 101908. https://doi.org/10.1016/j.toxrep.2025.101908

Korchevskiy, A. A., & Wylie, A. G. (2025b, April 24). The empirical metric of mesothelial carcinogenicity for carbon nanotubes and elongate mineral particles. *Inhalation Toxicology* (online). https://doi.org/10.1080/08958378.2025.2486087

Meeker, G. P., Bern, A. M., Brownfield, I. K., Lowers, H. A., Sutley, S. J., & Hoefen, T. M. (2003). The composition and morphology of amphiboles from the Rainy Creek Complex, near Libby, Montana. *American Mineralogist*, *88*, 1955–1969. https://doi.org/10.2138/am-2003-11-1239

Meeker, G. P., Lowers, H. A., Swayze, G. A., Van Gosen, B. S., Sutley, S. J., & Brownfield, I. K. (2006). *Mineralogy and morphology of amphiboles observed in soils and rocks in El Dorado Hills, California* (U.S. Geological Survey Open-File Report 06-1362). https://pubs.usgs.gov/of/2006/1362/

Occupational Safety and Health Administration (OSHA). (1994). *Rules and regulations, department of labor: 29 CFR parts 1910, 1915 and 1926, 59 FR 40964, RIN: 1218-AB25; occupational exposure to asbestos; August 1994-final rule; appendix B of 1910.1001; 1. Introduction*. OSHA.

Siegrist, H. G., & Wylie, A. G. (1980). Characterizing and discriminating the shape of asbestos particles. *Environmental Research*, *23*, 348–361. https://doi.org/10.1016/0013-9351(80)90070-5

Verkouteren, J. R., & Wylie, A. G. (2000). The tremolite-actinolite-ferro-actinolite series: Systematic relationships among cell parameters, composition, optical properties, and habit, and evidence of discontinuities. *American Mineralogist*, *85*(9), 1239–1254. https://doi.org/10.2138/am-2000-8-917

Verkouteren, J., & Wylie, A. (2002). Anomalous optical properties of fibrous tremolite, actinolite, and ferro-actinolite. *American Mineralogist*, *87*(8–9), 1090–1095. https://doi.org/10.2138/am-2002-8-905

Vigliaturo, R., Elkassas, S. M., Ventura, G. D., Redhammer, G. J., Ruiz-Zepeda, F., O'Shea, M. J., Dražić, G., & Gieré, R. (2021). Multi-scale characterization of glaucophane from Chiavolino (Biella, Italy): Implications for international regulations on elongate mineral particles. *European Journal of Mineralogy*, *33*(1), 77112. https://doi.org/10.5194/ejm-33-77-2021

Wylie, A. G., & Korchevskiy, A. A. (2023). Dimensions of elongate mineral particles and cancer: A review. *Environmental Research*, *230*, 114688. https://doi.org/10.1016/j.envres.2022.114688

Wylie, A. G., Korchevskiy, A. A., Segrave, A. M., & Duane, A. (2020). Modeling mesothelioma risk factors from amphibole fiber dimensionality: Mineralogical and epidemiological perspective. *Journal of Applied Toxicology*, *40*(4), 515–524. https://doi.org/10.1002/jat.3923

Wylie, A. G., Korchevskiy, A. A., Van Orden, D. R., & Chatfield, E. J. (2022). Discriminant analysis of asbestiform and non-asbestiform amphibole particles and its implications for toxicological studies. *Computational Toxicology*, *23*, 100233. https://doi.org/10.1016/j.comtox.2022.100233

Wylie, A. G., Virta, R. L., & Russek, E. (1985). Characterizing and discriminating airborne amphibole cleavage fragments and amosite fibers: Implications for the NIOSH method. *American Industrial Hygiene Association Journal*, *46*(4), 197–201. https://www.webofscience.com/wos/WOSCC/full-record/A1985AFY1000005

10 Toxicological assessment for a mixture of fibrous dusts

The case of the Boulder City Bypass Project

Kelly Bailey, Andrey Korchevskiy, and Ann Wylie

INTRODUCTION

In large construction projects, it is important to understand the mineralogical nature of the project area that is to be disturbed. Sometimes, when Mother Earth is dug into, she will bite back! This is because some mineralogical assemblages contain substances that can be hazardous if excessive exposures to workers occur. The most common particulate substance likely to be encountered in construction is respirable crystalline silica, which is strictly regulated by the Occupational Safety and Health Administration (OSHA, 2016). Another group of substances that can be encountered, which is the subject of this book, is naturally occurring asbestos (NOA). This is especially possible in areas that contain igneous and/or metamorphic rock (Kuryvial et al., 1974; Van Gosen, 2005, 2006, 2007, 2008, 2010; Van Gosen & Clinkenbeard, 2011). OSHA's asbestos standard for the construction industry is the primary regulation governing NOA exposures (OSHA, 1995).

The project engineer, with the assistance of a geologist knowledgeable about NOA, should know the mineralogical makeup of the construction project before the first shovel is driven into the ground. This typically involves an examination of relevant literature dealing with the local mineralogy (i.e., federal and state geological surveys and maps, local university geology department papers on the local area, and U.S. Geological Survey publications). Secondly, a field examination to look at and sample outcrops and road cuts in and near the construction site is an important element of due diligence prior to construction activity. If these activities reveal the presence of NOA, then more extensive and intensive mineralogical examinations would be necessary to understand the potential for exposure to the hazardous minerals identified. This further examination would most likely involve surface and subsurface soil sampling, core drilling, and geological/mineralogical mapping of the construction site as it pertains to NOA. After the identification of NOA-containing areas within the construction project site, industrial hygiene monitoring of potentially exposed

DOI: 10.1201/9781003424277-11

workers needs to be planned and conducted, along with protective measures to keep workers and nearby communities from being overexposed for the duration of the construction project.

When NOA is encountered, it will almost always be accompanied by the non-asbestiform growth habit of the same mineral. Because of this fact of nature, it is critical to have samples analyzed by transmission electron microscopy (TEM) so that all widths of countable fibers or particles are recorded. This is critical to assist in distinguishing the asbestos fibers from the non-asbestiform particles or the hazardous exposure from the nonhazardous exposure.

The purpose of this chapter is to show that by relying on TEM determinations of the dimensions of asbestiform and non-asbestiform elongate particles of actinolite that occur in an excavation-related mineral aerosol, it is possible to use particle dimensions to predict both their potency and, if exposure concentration is known, to predict risk based on the principles described earlier in this book (see Chapter 3). This chapter is included in hopes that it will guide approaches to assessing risk in similar circumstances in the future.

This chapter describes an example of a large construction project where NOA occurs and how the EMP database was utilized, with limited exposure information, to estimate missing dimensional data to assess the risk potential.

BACKGROUND

The presence of asbestiform amphiboles in rocks and soil in Clark County, Southern Nevada, was first reported by Buck et al. (2013). Baumann et al. (2015) mapped asbestos occurrences in the surface rocks in the region and, based on the higher frequency of occurrences of asbestos there, suggested that the higher-than-expected occurrences of mesothelioma among women and young adults in southern Nevada could be attributed to NOA. Pinheiro and Jin (2015) objected to this association on statistical grounds. Similarly, Pan et al. (2005) suggested a mesothelioma association between proximity to outcrops of asbestos in the surface rock in California. This association was thoroughly debunked, since the mesothelioma association was shown to be a statistically invalid conclusion in two papers by Berman et al. (2013) and Cox et al. (2013).

Despite the uncertainty that exists in the relationship between potential environmental exposures to NOA and mesothelioma, in an occupational setting where mineral dusts are generated from rock containing asbestos, the concentration of asbestos in an aerosol is important to know and understand. This is particularly true for road construction, where new exposures to the underlying rock and soil may occur daily. The recognition that mineral fiber could be found in many locations in Southern Nevada affected the construction progress of one of the largest projects in the area: the creation of the Boulder City Bypass for Interstate 11.

The project involved the construction of 14.75 miles of a four-lane highway with eighteen bridges. Phase I of the project involved the construction of 2.75 miles of highway and cuts in the soil and bedrock of 120 feet below the surface, and the placement of 45 feet of fill materials above ground. The second phase of the project involved six million cubic yards of blasted rock cutting 250 feet into a mountain ridge. A typical mile of a four-lane highway requires 85,000 tons of stone (Langer & Glanzman, 1993), so this project took over 1.25 million tons of stone and 350,000 tons of asphalt.

The construction work began in January 2013 with the removal and replanting of endangered cacti, installation of fences, and transmission lines. In late 2013, the presence of NOA in the soil and rock was reported (Buck et al., 2013). The project was delayed in November 2013 to reevaluate environmental and human health risks from possible exposure to NOA. In early 2014, the Nevada Department of Transportation (NDOT) (NDOT, 2014a) undertook site characterizations, including a preliminary risk assessment for workers. This site characterization was completed in November 2014, and construction began under a strict dust control protocol in April 2015. The Bypass was completed in the summer of 2018. The project cost was 318 million dollars, including 12.7 million dollars to deal with the NOA issue.

For quantitative carcinogenic risk assessment, NDOT utilized the inhalation unit risk (IUR) for asbestos at the level of 0.23 fibers per cubic centimeter of air (f/cc) (U.S. EPA, 1988). The IUR is a risk metric typically used by the U.S. Environmental Protection Agency (EPA). It is equal to the excess risk of cancer per unit of concentration, assuming lifetime exposure 24 hours per day, 7 days per week. The IUR by the EPA for asbestos is assumed to be applicable to any type of asbestos fibers, and therefore it does not take into consideration relevant toxicological characteristics of fibers. For example, the value of 0.23 f/cc is very high for chrysotile but may be low for some varieties of asbestiform amphiboles. The IUR value used in the NDOT risk assessment was developed based on initial dose-response studies in the 1980s from occupational cohort exposures to commercial asbestos. NDOT concluded that, based on the background exposure levels, the cancer risk for the workers ranges from 0.03 to 0.7 cases per 1,000,000 for the four separate air sampling locations, with an average of 0.2 cases per 1,000,000. It was determined that the risk level was lower than the EPA acceptable level of 1 in 100,000 for carcinogens. The obvious limitation of the risk assessment was that only airborne concentrations from 2014 (in the pre-construction phase of the project) were utilized. Also, only "ambient" air samples at the four established monitoring locations were considered for determining risk. The NDOT study did not utilize a probabilistic approach to risk determination, with only point estimations of parameters used instead of ranges. A comparatively short exposure duration (1 year) was considered for the workers. The project started in 2013 and ended in 2018, a period of five years.

It is important to understand what the risks are for people who may be exposed to a harmful agent so that proper precautions can be taken to minimize the risk. An active industrial hygiene monitoring program and, in the case of NOA, TEM analysis of air samples will provide the data necessary to assess the risk. Based on these determinations, adjustments to exposure controls can be implemented. This process is demonstrated in this and other chapters of this book.

In this chapter, we will demonstrate how mineral type and dimensional characteristics of the elongated actinolite particles from Southern Nevada can be used to estimate the carcinogenic potency of the particles. We have quantified and characterized risks for hypothetical exposures to the narrow particles in the aerosol to demonstrate the approach. The dimensional characteristics of elongate particles of a single mineral in an aerosol of rock dust can be used to predict potency, and in combination with exposure concentration scenarios, the risk. This demonstration of determining cancer risk is based on the assumptions in Table 10.5 for where data were missing from the original study.

DATA SOURCES

A) Airborne sampling and concentrations of amphibole asbestos

All data were provided by the Nevada Department of Transportation from reports to them by private contractors as part of their analysis to understand how to build a road in areas that contain unevenly distributed trace amounts of asbestos when they need to blast and move the rock. We recognize and appreciate their cooperation in this study.

Initial (background) measurements of ambient levels of asbestos in the area of the Boulder City bypass project were derived from samples collected at four air sample stations selected across the project area. The four stations were situated, respectively, on the north and south ends of Phase I of the project, near the center, and on the far eastern end, closest to Boulder City. Ambient air monitoring was performed in May-August 2014, on a regular 10-day schedule (5 days on and 5 days off), prior to the beginning of construction.

According to the available results, concentrations of amphibole (actinolite) determined throughout the sampling campaign were designated as asbestos fibers by TEM based only on NIOSH 7402 PCME criteria: particles longer than 5 μm, with an aspect ratio of at least 3, and wider than 0.25 μm, and had an average level of 0.00039 f/cc (95% CI 0.000176, 0.000603). The particle dimensions (length, width) and mineral type information are available for each particle.

The reason the NIOSH PCME method was used is the mistaken belief that particles thinner than 0.25 μm were not counted by optical phase contrast microscopy (PCM) because they were at or below the resolution limit and therefore, were not included in occupational exposure assessments made by electron microscopy. Today, NIOSH's PCM method 7400 states that amphibole particles as narrow as 0.05 and chrysotile fibers as narrow as 0.15 μm can be visible by PCM methods used for occupational monitoring (NIOSH 7400-Version 3, 2019). This basically means that some of the observable <0.25-micron width PCM count is being incorrectly removed from the PCME count.

The second stage of air monitoring for the full project area started in 2015 and lasted until 2017, during construction of the bypass.

The perimeter samples for the second stage were analyzed by TEM and are available for the period of observations from 2015 to 2017. The samples were collected from 10 sample locations. Ambient air samples were collected on an approximate 10-day schedule (5 days on and 5 days off). During sampling, each sampling station was checked twice to verify that the filters were not overloaded and to verify the proper pump flow rates. After each 5-day sampling, the stations were idle for approximately 5 days. The average PCME amphibole concentration was 0.000254 f/cc (95% CI 0.00099, 0.00108). The particle information (dimensions and mineral classification) is also available. This information shows that 94% of PCME particles were actinolite.

Personal air samples were also collected and analyzed by PCM in the period from 2015 to 2017. The sampling covered a wide range of construction operations including crushing, trenching, excavating, drilling, and different types of work assignments/operators. Both short-term and time-weighted average (TWA) samples were collected. The average PCM TWA concentration was 0.009 f/cc (95% CI 0.007, 0.010). While no mineral identification is available for PCM measurements, for purposes of our analysis, we assumed that the perimeter samples' mineralogy reflected the exposure mineralogy, with about 94% of the concentrations being actinolite.

B) Soil and Rock Sampling

The NDOT project to evaluate NOA in the Boulder City bypass project included two protocols for bulk soil and rock sampling and analysis.

Protocol 1

In the proposed construction area, soil and rock were sampled for the purpose of determining the presence (if any) and concentration of NOA. Samples were collected throughout the length and width of the construction site. Sample types included subsurface samples collected from the proposed excavation areas in soils either by backhoe trenching (20 samples) or hollow-stem auger drilling (6 samples). Samples of bedrock materials were collected by using either rock coring (5 samples) or rock outcrops (10 samples). Surface soil was collected from across the project area (65 samples). Also, "biased" or "targeted" rock sampling was performed at 15 locations.

Analytical results by PLM (EPA Method 600, 1993) include the presence of actinolite asbestos in some surface and subsurface soils, alluvium, and bedrock. The concentrations in the bulk materials were characterized as "low." All PLM results were below 0.25%, which is the lowest reporting level above non-detection for EPA method 600 and CARB method 435. Twelve of the 66 surface soil samples were selected from across the project area and submitted for additional TEM analysis. All TEM analyses were either non-detectable or below the analytical sensitivity of the analysis, except for one bedrock sample having 0.025% actinolite and one subsurface sample with a large chrysotile fiber (6.83%). Unfortunately, no particle dimensions were recorded for any of the minerals identified.

Overall, following Protocol 1, while asbestos was detected in some samples, it was in amounts too low to be quantified, and no dimensions of individual actinolite particles were provided. For this reason, the TEM measurements of individual actinolite particles made following Protocol 2 were used in our risk assessment process.

Protocol 2

A second sampling protocol for bulk rock and soil was undertaken by NDOT, with the principal objective being to obtain geologic and mineralogic data to assess the presence (if any) and concentration of NOA in surface and subsurface materials along the project alignment (NDOT, 2014b). In this protocol, seven distinct soil and overburden/rock units were identified within the project boundaries. Five additional rock units were mapped in limited areas along the alignment or within 300 feet of the boundaries. Geotechnical borings and NOA samples were spaced at intervals of 500 to 800 feet along the alignment. The NOA samples were obtained at regular intervals so that the number of tests for each unit would be approximately proportional to the relative prominence of each mapped geologic unit.

A total of 311 samples were analyzed by TEM, with 80 analyzed by PLM for "quality control." A total of 113 TEM tests were performed on samples obtained from a shovel, trowel, auger cuttings, or backhoe bucket, and 198 TEM tests were performed on rock core or hand samples of rock obtained from outcrops.

Soil materials were dried and sieved by the analytical lab to obtain a minus No. 200 sieve so that particles with a long dimension of less than 74 μm would dominate the sample. In this set of analyses, any actinolite longer than 5 μm with an aspect ratio of at least 3 would be labeled an actinolite asbestos fiber. EMP width measurements included all widths below 3 microns, abandoning the minimum 0.25 μm width as had been done in the aerosol study.

Rock materials were dried, crushed, and ground at the analytical lab using a disk pulverizer calibrated to achieve a nominal 200 mesh particle size. This method was selected because mechanical pulverization liberates fibrils from asbestos fiber bundles in ways that might be similar to processes during construction, including blasting. The target analytical sensitivity for total weight percent was 0.0002%.

Following the second protocol, actinolite particles meeting their fiber definition ($L > 5$ μm, $L/W \geq 3$, and $W < 3$) were detected in 45% of the samples, with the maximum level detected for each of the geologic units ranging from 0.014 to 6.38% w/w.

DIMENSIONAL CHARACTERISTICS OF THE AIRBORNE PCME EMPS

The 2014 ambient air sampling detected 384 PCME elongate actinolite particles from the background samples, with dimensions measured by TEM. We performed statistical analysis of the dimensional data. Frequency distributions of length and width of the actinolite PCME particles in the 2014 airborne samples are shown in Figure 10.1.

The dimensional characteristics of the PCME actinolite particles are listed in Table 10.1.

Aerodynamic diameter was calculated from the empirical formula of Timbrell (1965). The specific surface area was calculated by assuming a rectangular cross-section with measured width and thickness calculated from the models of Wylie et al. (1982). The fibrosity index is a measure of the uniformity of width across many ranges of length, such that the smaller the index, the less variability in particle width there is, and the more asbestiform nature of the particle population (Chapter 8). A fibrosity index of 0.64 suggests a population with high levels of non-asbestiform fragments. EMPA is the proportion of EMPs longer than 5 μm that are also less than or equal to 0.15 μm in width, and EMPB is the proportion with width less than 0.25 μm. EMPA and EMPB are not included in PCME tabulations. The fraction of asbestiform fibers was calculated from the discriminant function derived by Wylie et al. (2022) (see Chapter 9).

The background sample results show no particles in the EMPA category (Chapter 3) because no particles with width < 0.15 μm were counted by the TEM PCME

(a)

(b)

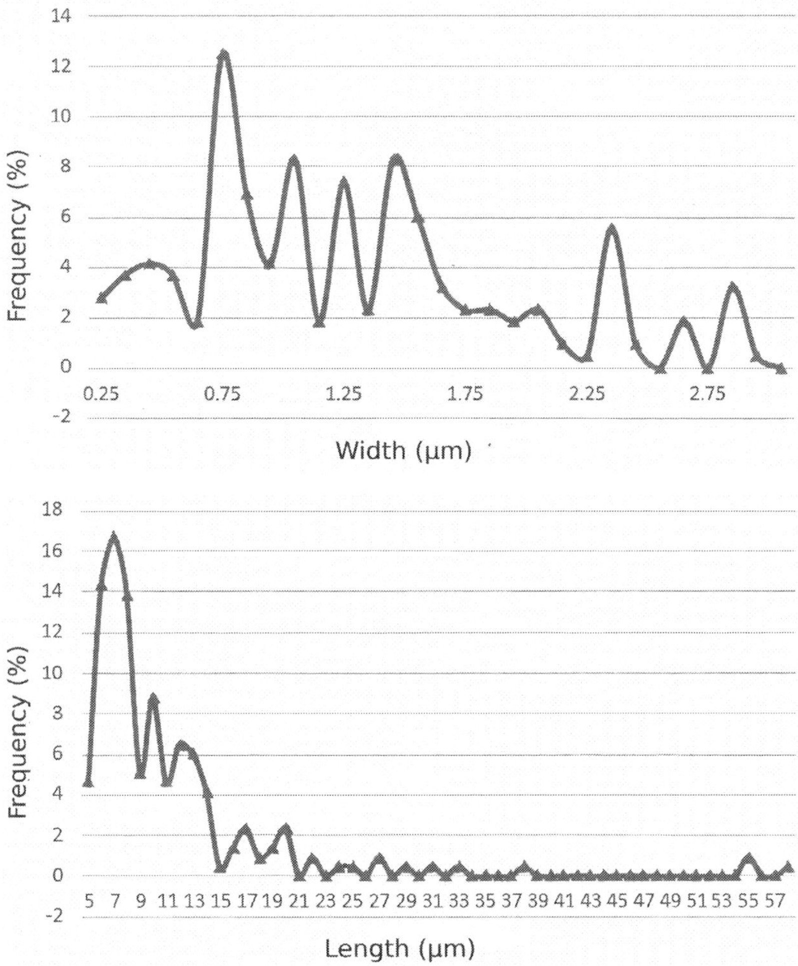

FIGURE 10.1 Dimensional frequency distribution of the 2014 airborne PCME particles for the pre-construction project phase by width (a) and length (b).

method. The fraction of EMPB particles was very low (1.9%), most probably signifying some laboratory reporting of the fibers with width close to 0.25 µm. (According to the method, no fibers with width <0.25 µm were supposed to be counted.) The fraction of the "borderline" EMPB fibers is higher, if we select only fibers that would adhere to the criteria of true asbestiform fibers by the model of Wylie et al. (2022) – in this case, the proportion of asbestiform fibers thinner than 0.25 µm increases to 8.3%.

The dimensional characteristics of the perimeter samples collected during the construction phase are given in Table 10.2. The frequency distribution of the particles is illustrated in Figure 10.2.

TABLE 10.1
Dimensional characteristics of airborne PCME actinolite particles (2014)

Parameter*	Value
Length, µm, GM (GSD)	9.71 (1.60)
Width, µm, GM (GSD)	1.08 (1.79)
Aspect ratio, µm, GM (GSD)	8.99 (1.86)
Aerodynamic diameter, µm, GM (GSD)	5.13 (1.86)
Specific surface area, µm (-1), GM (GSD)	8.01 (1.55)
Fibrosity index	0.64
Fraction of asbestiform EMPs (calculated from Wylie et al., 2022), %	22.7
EMPA, %	0
EMPB, %	1.9
EMPA, % for asbestiform fraction	0
EMPB, % for asbestiform fraction	8.3

* All dimensional characteristics assume L > 5 µm, L/W ≥ 3:1, W ≥ 0.25 µm, W < 3 µm, except for fibrosity index that is calculated for L >2 µm, L/W ≥ 3:1, W ≥ 0.25 µm.

TABLE 10.2
Dimensional characteristics of airborne PCME actinolite particles (2015–2017)

Parameter*	Value
Length, µm, GM (GSD)	9.03 (1.73)
Width, µm, GM (GSD)	0.76 (1.78)
Aspect ratio, µm, GM (GSD)	11.96 (1.83)
Aerodynamic diameter, µm, GM (GSD)	3.71 (1.71)
Specific surface area, µm (-1), GM (GSD)	10.47 (1.54)
Fibrosity index	0.51
Fraction of asbestiform EMPs (calculated from Wylie et al., 2022), %	40.7
EMPA, %	0
EMPB, %	6.0
EMPA, % for asbestiform fraction	0
EMPB, % for asbestiform fraction	14.7

* All dimensional characteristics assume L > 5 µm, L/W ≥ 3:1, W ≥ 0.25 µm, W < 3 µm, except for fibrosity index that is calculated for L > 2 µm, L/W ≥ 3:1, W ≥ 0.25 µm.

The fibrosity index for the construction stage airborne particles characterizes a higher proportion of the asbestiform habit for the samples. This fraction, based on Wylie et al. (2022), is 40.7% vs. 22.7% in the background (2014) samples. The perimeter sample results also show no particles in the so-called EMPA category, because no particles with width < 0.15 µm were counted by the TEM PCME method. The

(a)

(b)

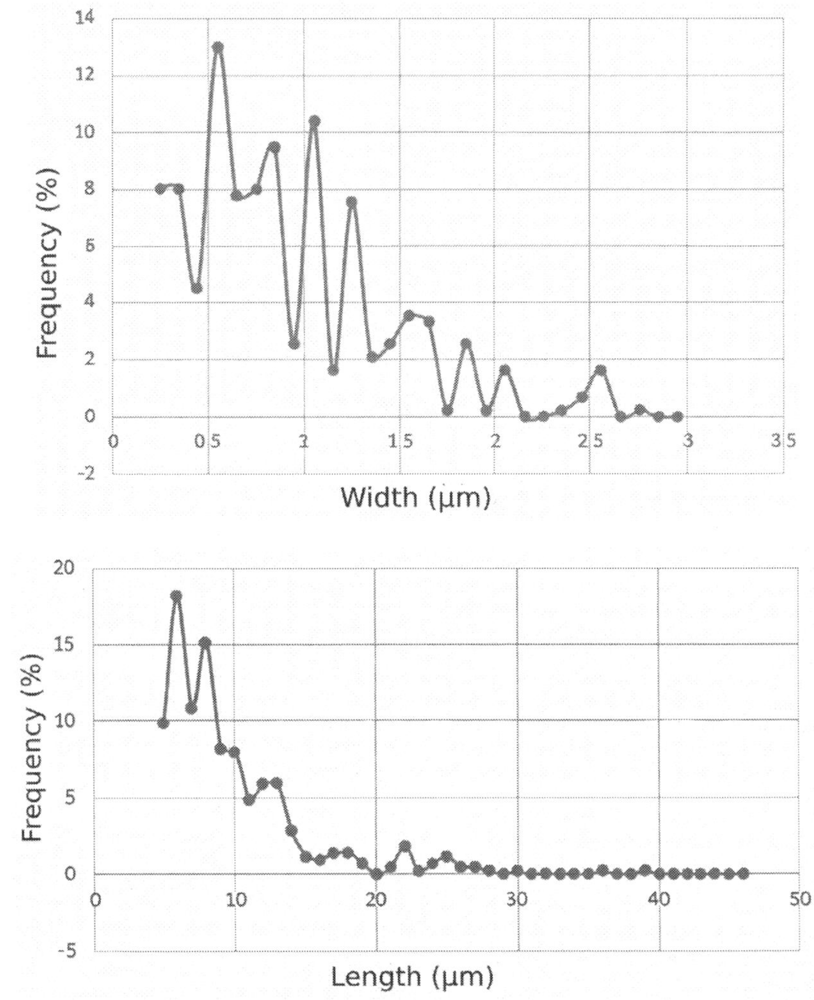

FIGURE 10.2 Dimensional frequency distribution of airborne PCME particles for the project construction perimeter samples (2015–2017) by width (a) and length (b).

fraction of EMPB particles was 6%. The EMPB fraction was higher for the particles defined as asbestiform by Wylie et al. (2022) (14.7%).

DIMENSIONAL CHARACTERISTICS OF THE FIBERS IN ROCK AND SOIL

Following Protocol 2, soil and rock sampling detected and measured 456 elongate actinolite particles. The distributions of their lengths and widths are shown in Figure 10.3, and the dimensional characteristics of the particles are listed in

(a)

(b)

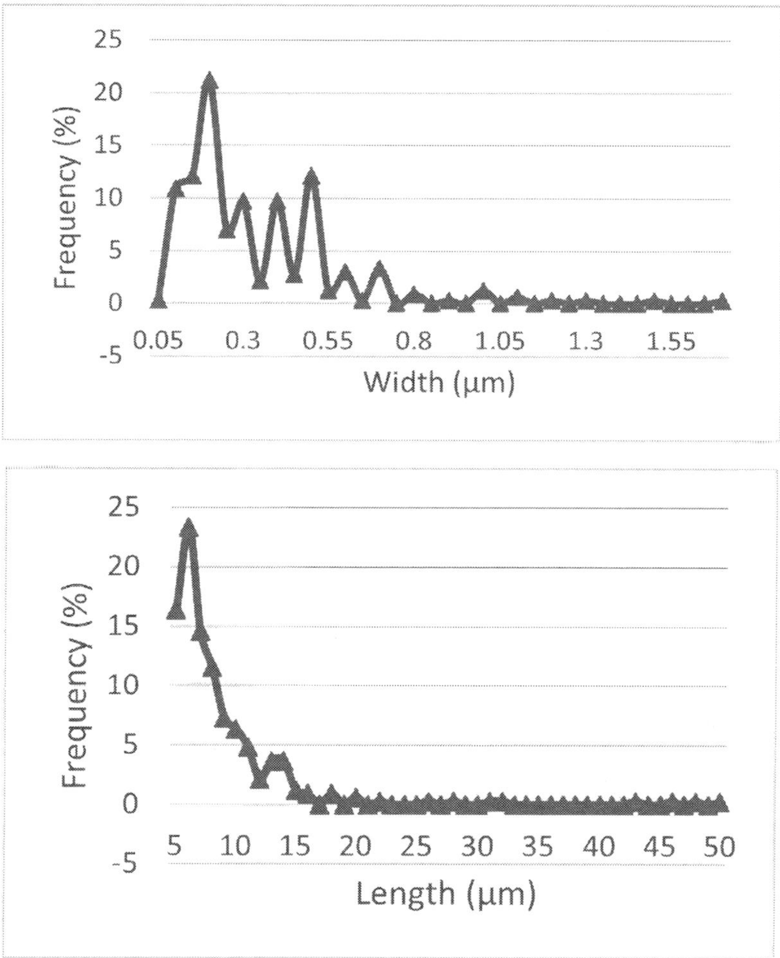

FIGURE 10.3 Dimensional distribution of actinolite EMP in rock/soil by width (a) and length (b).

Table 10.3. Here, the fibrosity index is consistent with a population dominated by asbestiform particles.

METHODS TO DETERMINE THE POTENCY OF THE AIRBORNE ACTINOLITE EMPS FROM THE BOULDER CITY BYPASS PROJECT

The standard PCME method, used in the analysis of the airborne samples at the Nevada bypass site, does not allow determination of the parameters defining the level of cancer potency for EMPs because it lacks information about the narrowest fibers.

The abundance of asbestos in the soil and rock samples collected under Protocol 2 is not fully comparable to the aerosol of Protocol 1 because they were specifically

TABLE 10.3
Dimensional characteristics of actinolite in soil and rock under Protocol 2

Parameter*	Value
Length, μm, GM (GSD)	8.17 (1.49)
Width, μm, GM (GSD)	0.36 (2.15)
Aspect ratio, μm, GM (GSD)	22.80 (2.20)
Aerodynamic diameter, μm, GM (GSD)	1.84 (2.06)
Specific surface area, μm (-1), GM (GSD)	18.65 (1.81)
Fibrosity index	0.44
Fraction of asbestiform EMPs (by Wylie et al., 2022), %	77.9
EMPA, %	14.8
EMPB, %	39.8
EMPA, % for asbestiform fraction	19.0
EMPB, % for asbestiform fraction	51.1

* All dimensional characteristics assume L > 5 μm, L/W ≥ 3:1, W < 3 μm, except for fibrosity index that is calculated for L > 2 μm, L/W ≥ 3:1, W < 3 μm.

selected in the area where asbestos would most likely be present from a mineralogical standpoint. In this case, asbestiform particles would be collected with a higher probability than non-asbestiform particles. To the contrary, the air samples represent a "random" dispersion of particles, including both asbestiform and non-asbestiform varieties of elongate mineral particles. However, non-asbestiform EMPs are generally thicker than their asbestiform counterparts and would not be expected to stay airborne in a similar fashion to the thinner asbestiform EMPs. Air samples are therefore more likely to contain a higher portion of asbestiform EMPs in an equally mixed dust aerosol.

This fact can be confirmed quantitatively. More than 75% of the actinolite EMPs from the Protocol 2 samples could be characterized as asbestiform by discriminant analysis vs. about 22% of the airborne actinolite PCME EMPs. One of the reasons for this striking difference is the rejection of thin EMPs during PCME counting. However, even if only EMPs from the soil and rock samples wider than 0.25 μm were counted, the fraction of actinolite EMPs in the soil sample would still be 63%.

Given these limitations, the following methodology has been used in this study to estimate the carcinogenic potency of airborne actinolite EMPs from Boulder City bypass:

1. Asbestiform particles (with dimensional characteristics typically found in asbestiform amphibole populations) are identified by a discriminant function that separates EMPs into asbestiform and non-asbestiform populations (Wylie et al., 2022). While the misclassification rate for discriminant analysis was about 15%, this methodology was demonstrated to be sufficient for toxicological assessment, with the fraction of correctly identified asbestiform actinolite fibers being as high as 96.7% (Van Orden, 2023). In this

chapter, particles are identified as one or the other by the discriminant equation. As can be seen from Table 10.1, the proportion of EMPs classified as asbestiform in the aerosol is 22.4%.

2. EMPA and EMPB from the soils, as determined specifically for those particles classified as asbestiform (77.9% of the actinolite soil EMPs), will be 19% and 51.1%, respectively.
3. To apply the distribution of asbestiform fibers in the bulk samples to the PCM air samples, a model that relates the proportion of asbestiform fibers as a function of the minimum width was developed. From this model, we can extrapolate to estimate abundances of particles with widths between 0.05 and 0.25 μm, those making up the missing EMPA and EMPB.
4. Potency factors R_M for mesothelioma and R_L for lung cancer are calculated based on the Hodgson and Darnton (2000) method. For specific actinolite fibers in soil/rock from the Boulder bypass project area, the potency factors are estimated from the EMPA and EMPB components of the asbestiform fraction of the aerosol.

The potency factors are then applied to the asbestiform particles in the airborne EMPs. In this case, the potencies of all particles that do not meet the EMP criteria or are not identified as asbestiform are assumed to be negligible. These steps are discussed in more detail below.

POTENCY DETERMINATION FOR ASBESTIFORM EMPS

Models for potency factors based on the EMPA and EMPB parameters are derived as follows. The fractions of EMPA and EMPB were determined for the following mineral types: crocidolite, amosite, Libby amphiboles, and glaucophane (all airborne datasets), and anthophyllite and balangeroite (bulk datasets). The potency factors for mesothelioma and lung cancer were used as described in Chapter 3 and in Wylie and Korchevskiy (2023).

Carcinogenic potency for mesothelioma is expressed as R_M, the percentage of the expected mortality from all causes due to mesothelioma, adjusted to the age of first exposure of 30, per unit of cumulative exposure in fibers per year, and R_L as a percent excess mortality of lung cancer from baseline lung cancer mortality (Hodgson & Darnton, 2000).

Only fibers longer than 5 μm, with an aspect ratio of at least 3 meeting asbestiform EMP criteria (discriminant function Wylie et al., 2022), were included in the calculations.

The following linear and non-linear regression equations (Equations 10.1 through 10.8) have been determined for this mineral set as follows:

A. Linear regression equations

Linear regression I

$$R_M = -0.03 + 0.011\ \text{EMPA} \tag{10.1}$$

$$\left(R = 0.96,\ R^2 = 0.92,\ p < 0.00070\right).$$

Linear regression II

$$R_M = -0.098 + 0.0073 \text{ EMPB} \tag{10.2}$$

$$\left(R = 0.94,\ R^2 = 0.89,\ p < 0.0013\right).$$

Linear regression III

$$R_L = 0.85 + 0.080 \text{ EMPA} \tag{10.3}$$

$$\left(R = 0.85,\ R^2 = 0.72,\ p < 0.03\right).$$

Linear regression IV

$$R_L = 0.58 + 0.059 \text{ EMPB} \tag{10.4}$$

$$\left(R = 0.92,\ R^2 = 0.84,\ p < 0.01\right).$$

B. Non-linear regression equations

Non-linear regression I

$$R_M = 0.0065 \text{ EMPA}^{1.05} \tag{10.5}$$

$$\left(R = 0.83,\ R^2 = 0.69,\ p < 0.02\right).$$

Non-linear regression II

$$R_M = 0.00049 \text{ EMPB}^{1.52} \tag{10.6}$$

$$\left(R = 0.84,\ R^2 = 0.699,\ p < 0.019\right).$$

Non-linear regression III

$$R_L = 0.488 \text{ EMPA}^{0.61} \tag{10.7}$$

$$\left(R = 0.83,\ R^2 = 0.69,\ p < 0.04\right).$$

Non-linear regression IV

$$R_L = 0.11 \text{ EMPB}^{0.90} \tag{10.8}$$

$$(R = 0.89,\ R^2 = 0.80,\ p < 0.016).$$

Figure 10.4 illustrates the linear regression equations for both lung cancer and mesothelioma, using EMPA and EMPB as independent predictors. The relationships on the non-linear scale are similar.

The potency of the mixed particle cloud, however, depends on the fraction of asbestiform fibers. This fraction is unknown for the airborne material because the thinnest fibers were excluded from the count. However, we can reconstruct the fraction of asbestiform fibers in the air samples based on the following method.

Figure 10.5 demonstrates the relationship between the fraction of asbestiform fibers and the minimum width defining the set, the width cutpoint. As can be seen, the fraction of asbestiform EMPs linearly depends on the width cutpoint, as shown in Equation 10.9:

$$AF = 30.33 - 31.76 \text{ WC}, \qquad (10.9),$$

where AF is the fraction of asbestiform EMPs (%), and

WC is the lowest width cutpoint (μm) ($R = 0.995$, $R2 = 0.991$, $p < 0.000001$).

A similar relationship can be found for airborne samples from 2015 to 2017.

$$AF = 58.36 - 69.46 \text{ WC}, \qquad (10.10),$$

where AF is the fraction of asbestiform EMPs (%), and

WC is the lowest width cutpoint (μm) ($R = 0.989$, $R2 = 0.978$, $p < 0.00002$).

The statistical significance of the model demonstrates that the fraction of asbestiform EMPs greater than the width cutpoint follows a linear relationship across different samples and allows confidence in estimates of the fraction outside the analytical range, for example, 0.05 < widths < 0.25 μm.

We can examine the robustness of this relationship on a wider scale by applying it to our EMP database (the database is described in Chapter 2).

Based on these data, a similar regression equation was calculated with 0.25 μm as the lowest cutpoint (as for Boulder City Bypass actinolite), as shown in Equation 10.11:

$$AF = 62.08 - 76.13 \text{ WC} \left(R = 0.984, R2 = 0.967, p < 0.0004\right) \qquad (10.11).$$

The coefficients in the equations obviously depend on the specific sample characteristics. However, based on the equation, we can predict the fraction of asbestiform EMPs for the entire database by using 0.05 μm as a cutpoint. The predicted value is 57.5%, while the actual fraction is 58.9%, showing good agreement.

Utilizing Equation 10.9, we can conclude that the asbestiform fraction of actinolite in the air samples for Boulder City Bypass actinolite will be 28.4% for 2014 (prior to the major project activities) and 54% for 2015–2017 (during the construction project).

From this information, we can approximate the potency factor for the airborne samples, as shown in Equation 10.12:

$$\text{Potency of pure asbestiform mineral (\%)} \times \text{Fraction of asbestiform fibers} \qquad (10.12).$$

(a)

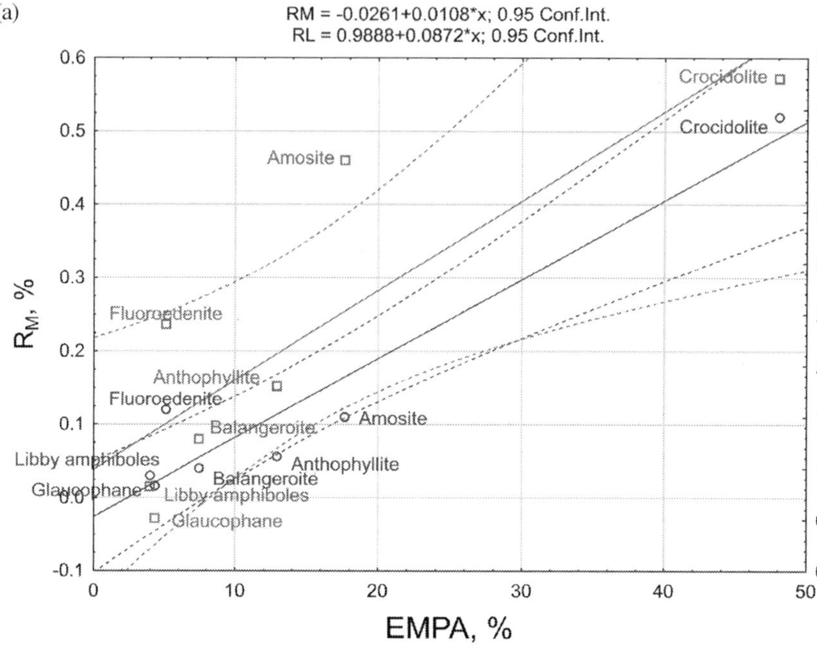

(b)

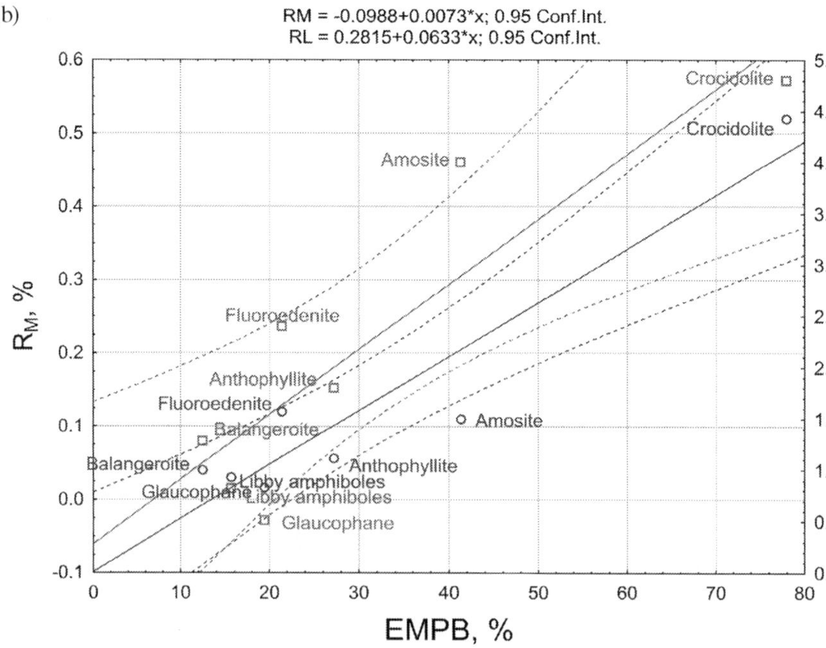

FIGURE 10.4 The linear relationships between mesothelioma (R_M) and lung cancer (RL) potency with (a) EMPA and (b) EMPB parameters. Red squares – represent lung cancer potency levels and blue circles represent mesothelioma potency levels.

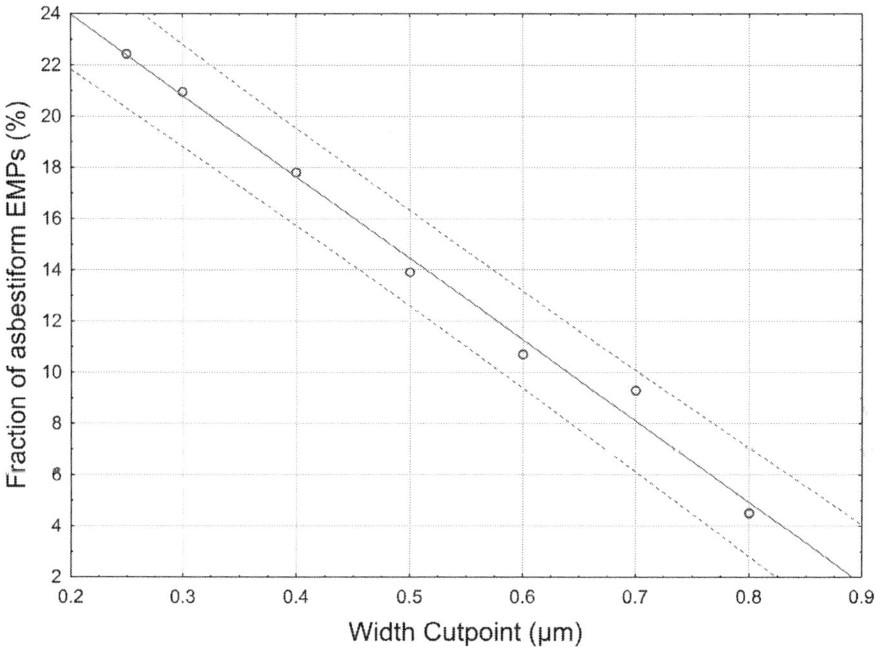

FIGURE 10.5 The relationship between the fraction of asbestiform EMPs in the 2014 PCME actinolite data set and the lowest width cutpoint.

Table 10.4 contains the estimations of potency values R_M and R_L for the asbestiform fraction of the elongate mineral particles, calculated from regression Equations 10.1 through 10.8.

Averaging the values of linear and non-linear models for mesothelioma and lung cancer potency factors, we can conclude that according to Equation 10.12, R_M=0.11% and R_L=2.01%, for airborne Boulder City Bypass actinolite during the active project period (2015–2017).

DETERMINATION OF THE INHALATION UNIT RISK VALUE

Korchevskiy et al. (2020) proposed a simple method to determine asbestos IUR based on mesothelioma and lung cancer potency factors, as shown in Equation 10.13:

$$IUR = 2.265R_M + 0.073R_L \quad (10.13).$$

According to this equation, IUR for the Boulder City Bypass actinolite is calculated as

$$IUR = 2.265 \times 0.11 + 0.073 \times 2.01 = 0.39 \text{ (per f/cc)}.$$

It is higher than the average value used by NDOT.

TABLE 10.4
The estimations of potency factors

Regression equations	R_M, %	R_L, %
Eq. 10.1	0.179	N/A
Eq. 10.2	0.275	N/A
Eq. 10.3	0.143	N/A
Eq. 10.4	0.193	N/A
Eq. 10.5	N/A	2.37
Eq. 10.6	N/A	3.59
Eq. 10.7	N/A	5.37
Eq. 10.8	N/A	3.79

TABLE 10.5
The general methodological assumptions for risk characterization

#	Assumption
1.	The fraction of asbestiform fibers in air samples can be reconstructed for all ranges of widths based on the distribution of widths > 0.25 μm.
2.	The fraction of actinolite asbestos EMPs in PCM personal air samples is identical to the fraction of actinolite asbestos EMPs in TEM perimeter air samples.
3.	The mesothelioma and lung cancer potency factors for asbestiform airborne actinolite fibers are identical to potency factors for asbestiform actinolite fibers found in soil and rock samples in the area.
4.	The mesothelioma and lung cancer potency factors for asbestiform actinolite fibers found in soil and rock samples in the area can be reconstructed by using regression analysis based on EMPA and EMPB fractions (as in Wylie et al., 2020).
5.	Asbestiform actinolite fibers can be distinguished from non-asbestiform (cleavage fragments) particles by the discriminant function methodology (as in Wylie et al., 2022).

RISK CHARACTERIZATION FOR THE BOULDER CITY BYPASS WORKERS

The general methodological assumptions for the risk characterization are listed in Table 10.5.

We utilized Monte Carlo simulation to evaluate the risk for hypothetical workers who might be exposed to the Boulder City Bypass aerosol. As a first approximation, the following assumptions were made: 1) the exposure duration was assumed to fluctuate uniformly between 1 and 5 years, with a daily exposure period from 4 to 8 hours; 2) inhalation unit risk was assumed to follow a lognormal distribution, with a geometric mean of 0.39 (per f/cc) and geometric standard deviation of 1.6 (typical for various applications of a lognormal distribution); 3) the airborne concentration of asbestiform actinolite particles was assumed to correspond to the personal sample

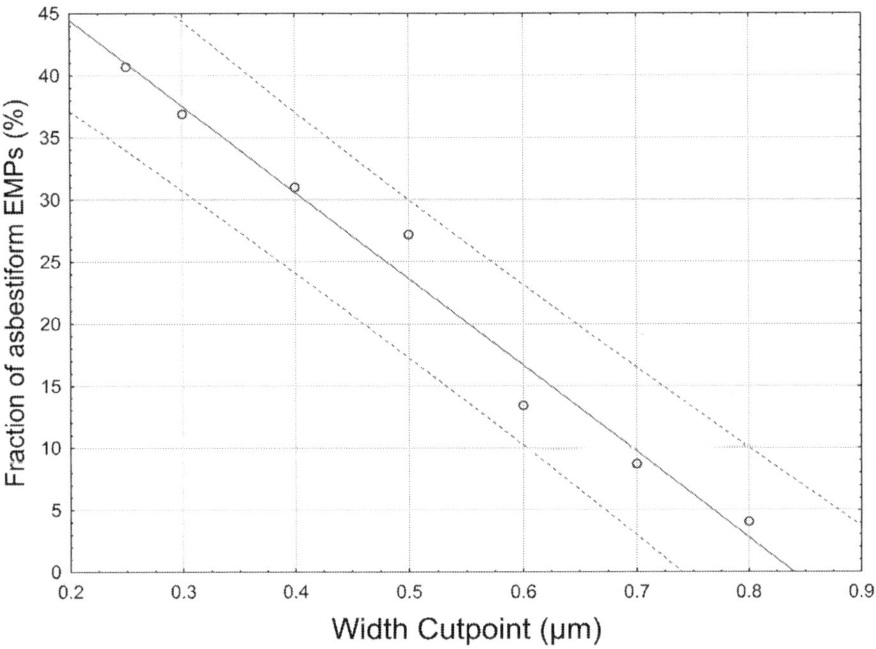

FIGURE 10.6 demonstrates the relationship between the fraction of asbestiform fibers and the minimum width defining the set, the width cutpoint. As can be seen, the fraction of asbestiform EMPs linearly depends on the width cutpoint, as shown in Equation 10.10:

results, and to follow a normal distribution with 10th percentile of 0.000569 f/cc and 95th percentile of 0.031 f/cc. (Usually, industrial hygiene data follow a log-normal distribution. In this case, specifically for asbestos, the assumption of normal distribution was made to account for possible undetected fibers in the samples. Using zero values instead of other statistical estimations for non-detects is consistent with the U.S. EPA risk assessment approach.); and 4) the average exposure onset age for workers was estimated as 18 to 30 years.

The results of 100,000 simulations are demonstrated in Figure 10.7.

As we can see, the total excess cancer risk for workers is not expected to exceed 1.95 cases per 10,000 workers per lifetime. It is higher than U.S. EPA and NIOSH target criteria for acceptable risk of cancer. However, the central tendency level of risk is 0.62 cases per 10,000 workers, which is within the acceptable level.

The risk of cancer will be higher if the exposure extends beyond 5 years of assumed project construction duration. However, in the NDOT risk assessment, the duration of exposure was assumed to be 1 year, potentially assuming a short duration of employment for the project workforce. The shorter duration would imply a lower risk of cancer.

Also, we considered the combination of mesothelioma and lung cancer excess mortality in our risk characterization. It can be derived from Equation 10.12 that the mesothelioma risk for Nevada actinolite comprises about 64% of the total respiratory

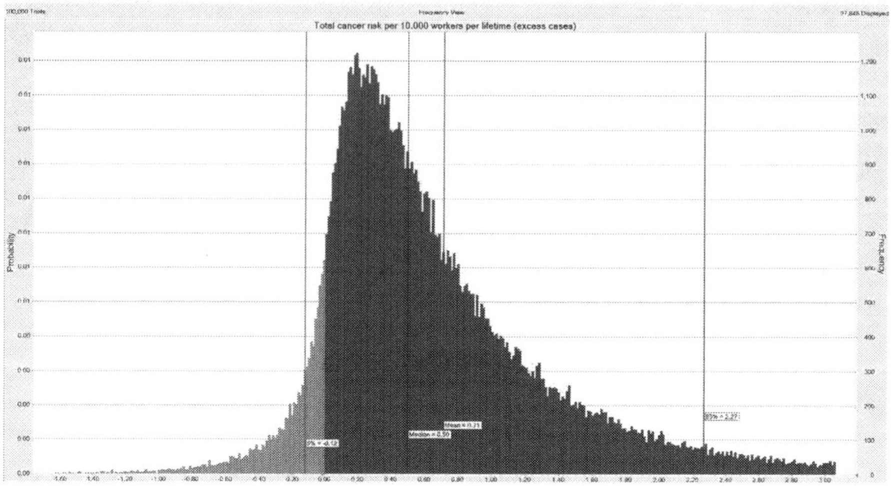

FIGURE 10.7 Total cancer excess risk per 10,000 workers per lifetime. The "negative" part of the risk distribution is highlighted in red. The "negative" values are obviously a statistical artifact.

cancer risk, while lung cancer would be responsible for 36% of cases. In this case, the excess mesothelioma risk for workers per lifetime would be about 1.24 cases per 10,000 workers per lifetime, or 124 cases per lifetime per 1,000,000. This level would be less than the possible maximum baseline rate of mesothelioma in the population, which is usually assumed to fluctuate between 75 and 210 cases per 1,000,000 per lifetime (Price & Ware, 2009).

DISCUSSION

From animal studies and human epidemiology, it seems clear that elongate particles of durable minerals that are both longer than 5 µm and have widths that range from 0.05 to <0.2 µm possess the greatest potency for mesothelioma and lung cancer. To assess risk from an aerosol containing respirable elongate mineral particles (f/cc) quantitatively, the component that is very narrow must be known or estimated. We have demonstrated a method to estimate a missing component if the dimensions of the rest are known so that the best risk model can be developed.

Our study has significant uncertainties and limitations. We used a classification discriminant analysis model for asbestiform and non-asbestiform particles to determine the asbestiform fraction of Nevada actinolite, which appears to be a mixed variety of fibers with true asbestiform fibers and non-asbestiform fragments included (Wylie et al., 2022). We assigned a definite asbestiform habit to the particles with a discriminant function value higher than 0; however, this approach has an error rate. In any case, our approach is consistent because we developed potency determination models specifically for particles with positive discriminant function values (and not for other methods to distinguish asbestiform particles from cleavage fragments).

We determined the potency of the asbestiform fraction for the Boulder City Bypass actinolite as R_M=0.11% (for mesothelioma) and R_L=2.01% (for lung cancer). In comparison, mesothelioma potency for crocidolite fibers (assumed to be prevailingly asbestiform) is 0.52%, and lung cancer potency for crocidolite is 4.8%.

Ideally, the data sets to be used in this type of risk analysis would include TEM exposure data with no minimum width restriction and sufficient results over the course of the work project so that an ongoing assessment of the risk could be determined.

REFERENCE LIST

Baumann, F., Buck, B. J., Metcalf, R. V., McLaurin, B. T., Merkler, D. J., & Carbone, M. (2015). The presence of asbestos in the natural environment is likely related to mesothelioma in young individuals and women from Southern Nevada. *Journal of Thoracic Oncology*, *10*(5), 731–737. https://doi.org/10.1097/JTO.0000000000000506

Berman, D. W., Cox, L. A., Jr., & Popken, D. A. (2013). A cautionary tale: The characteristics of two-dimensional distributions and their effects on epidemiological studies employing an ecological design. *Critical Reviews in Toxicology*, *43*(Suppl 1), 1–25. https://doi.org/10.3109/10408444.2013.777688

Buck, B. J., Goossens, D., Metcalf, R. V., McLaurin, B., Ren, M., & Freudenberger, F. (2013). Naturally occurring asbestos: Potential for human exposure, Southern Nevada, U.S.A. *Soil Science Society of America Journal*, *77*(6), 2192–2204. http://dx.doi.org/10.2136/sssaj2013.05.0183

CDC/NIOSH (NIOSH). (2019). *Asbestos and other fibers by PCM, method 7400, issue 3: NIOSH manual of analytical methods (NMAM)* (5th ed.). https://www.cdc.gov/niosh/nmam/pdf/7400.pdf

Cox, L. A., Jr., Popken, D. A., & Berman, D. W. (2013). Causal vs. spurious spatial exposure-response associations in health risk analysis. *Critical Reviews in Toxicology*, *43*(Suppl 1), 26–38. https://doi.org/10.3109/10408444.2013.777689

Hodgson, J. T., & Darton, A. (2000). The quantitative risks of mesothelioma and lung cancer in relation to asbestos exposure. *Annals Of Occupational Hygiene*, *44*(8), 565–601.

Korchevskiy, A., Rasmuson, J. O., Rasmuson, E. J., & Strode, R. D. (2020). Inhalation unit risk (IUR) of asbestos based on available science. *Inhalation Toxicology*, *32*(9–10), 372–374. https://doi.org/10.1080/08958378.2020.1829210

Kuryvial, R. J., Wood, R. A., & Barrett, R. E. (1974). *Identification and assessment of asbestos emissions from incidental sources of asbestos* (Report EPA-650/2-74-087). Environmental Protection Agency.

Langer, W. H., & Glanzman, V. M. (1993). *Natural aggregate, building America's future* (U.S. Geological Survey Circular 1110). U.S. Government Printing Office.

Nevada Department of Transportation (NDOT). (2014a). *Final phase I site characterization report for Boulder city bypass naturally occurring asbestos (NOA) project phase I (railroad pass to Silverline road), prepared by Tetra Tech, Helena, MT.* https://m.moam.info/ndot-naturally-occurring-asbestos-final-report-regional-_647a2b97097c476d028c87ed.html

Nevada Department of Transportation (NDOT). (2014b). *Interstate 11 – Boulder city bypass phase 2 design build project geologic evaluation, sampling and testing for naturally-occurring asbestos, Boulder City, Clark County, Nevada* (Kleinfelder Project 137120). NDOT.

Occupational Safety and Health Administration (OSHA). (1995). *Safety and health regulations for construction: Subpart Z – toxic and hazardous substances: Asbestos* (29 CFR 1926.1101). https://www.osha.gov/laws-regs/regulations/standardnumber/1926/1926.1101

Occupational Safety and Health Administration (OSHA). (2016). *Respirable crystalline silica for construction, part 1926 subpart Z 1926.1153*. https://www.osha.gov/laws-regs/regulations/standardnumber/1926/1926.1153

Pan, X., Day, H. W., Wang, W., Beckett, L. A., & Schenker, M. B. (2005). Residential proximity to naturally occurring asbestos and mesothelioma risk in California. *American Journal of Respiratory Critical Care Medicine*, *172*(8), 1019–1025. https://doi.org/10.1164/rccm.200412-1731oc

Pinheiro, P. S., & Jin, H. (2015). No increased risk for mesothelioma in relation to natural-occurring asbestos in Southern Nevada. *Journal of Thoracic Oncology*, *10*(7), e62–e63. https://doi.org/10.1097%2FJTO.0000000000000564

Price, B., & Ware, A. (2009). Time trend of mesothelioma incidence in the United States and projection of future cases: An update based on SEER data for 1973 through 2005. *Critical Reviews in Toxicology*, *39*(7), 576–588. https://doi.org/10.1080/10408440903044928

Timbrell, V. (1965). Human exposure to asbestos: Dust controls and standards. The inhalation of fibrous dusts. *Annals of the New York Academy of Sciences*, *132*(1), 255–273. http://dx.doi.org/10.1111/j.1749-6632.1965.tb41107.x

U.S. EPA. (1988). *Integrated risk information system (IRIS)* (Online Database). Office of Research and Development, National Center for Environmental Assessment. Retrieved October 19, 2023, from http://www.epa.gov/iris

U.S. EPA. (1993, July). *Test method: Method for the determination of asbestos in bulk building materials* (R. L. Perkins & B. W. Harvey, Eds., EPA/600/R-93/116). United States Environmental Protection Agency. https://www.nist.gov/system/files/documents/nvlap/EPA-600-R-93-116.pdf

Van Gosen, B. S. (2005). *Reported historic asbestos mines, historic asbestos prospects, and natural asbestos occurrences in the Eastern United States* (U.S. Geological Survey Open-File Report 2005-1189). http://pubs.usgs.gov/of/2005/1189/

Van Gosen, B. S. (2006). *Reported historic asbestos prospects and natural asbestos occurrences in the Central United States* (U.S. Geological Survey Open-File Report 2006-1211). http://pubs.usgs.gov/of/2006/1211/

Van Gosen, B. S. (2007). *Reported historic asbestos mines, historic asbestos prospects, and natural asbestos occurrences in the Rocky Mountain States of the United States (Colorado, Idaho, Montana, New Mexico, and Wyoming)* (U.S. Geological Survey Open-File Report 2007-1182). http://pubs.usgs.gov/of/2007/1182/

Van Gosen, B. S. (2008). *Reported historic asbestos mines, historic asbestos prospects, and natural asbestos occurrences in the Southwestern United States (Arizona, Nevada, and Utah)* (U.S. Geological Survey Open-File Report 2008-1095). http://pubs.usgs.gov/of/2008/1095/

Van Gosen, B. S. (2010). *Reported historic asbestos mines, historic asbestos prospects, and other natural occurrences of asbestos in Oregon and Washington* (U.S. Geological Survey Open-File Report 2010-1041). http://pubs.usgs.gov/of/2010/1041/

Van Gosen, B.S., & Clinkenbeard, J.P. (2011). *Reported historic asbestos mines, historic asbestos prospects, and other natural occurrences of asbestos in California* (U.S. Geological Survey Open-File Report 2011-1188). http://pubs.usgs.gov/of/2011/1188/

Van Orden, D. R. (2023). Discriminant analysis of amphiboles: Additional considerations. *Environmental Research*, *230*, 114579. http://dx.doi.org/10.1016/j.envres.2022.114579

Wylie, A. G., & Korchevskiy, A. A. (2023). Dimensions of elongate mineral particles and cancer: A review. *Environmental Research*, *230*, 114688. https://doi.org/10.1016/j.envres.2022.114688

Wylie, A. G., Korchevskiy, A. A., Segrave, A. M., & Duane, A. (2020). Modeling mesothelioma risk factors from amphibole fiber dimensionality: Mineralogical and epidemiological perspective. *Journal of Applied Toxicology*, *40*(4), 515–524. https://doi.org/10.1002/jat.3923

Wylie, A. G., Korchevskiy, A. A., Van Orden, D. R., & Chatfield, E. J. (2022). Discriminant analysis of asbestiform and non-asbestiform amphibole particles and its implications for toxicological studies. *Computational Toxicology*, *23*, 100233. https://doi.org/10.1016/j.comtox.2022.100233

Wylie, A. G., Shedd, K. B., & Taylor, M. E. (1982, August 9–13). Measurement of the thickness of amphibole asbestos fibers with scanning electron microscope and transmission electron microscope. In K. F. J. Heinrich (Ed.), *Microbeam analysis: Proceedings of the annual 17th annual conference of the microbeam analysis society*. https://archive.org/details/1982-mas-proc-washington-dc/page/n1/mode/2up

11 The soil contamination by asbestos in Armley, Leeds (U.K.)

Dimensional characteristics as a "footprint" of exposure

Andrey Korchevskiy, Arseniy Korchevskiy, Jr. and Ann Wylie

"Legacy" asbestos contamination and related public health risks remain a significant concern requiring environmental and toxicological assessment. Based on Virta (2006), about 181 million metric tons of asbestos were produced worldwide from 1900 to 2003. A significant part of this asbestos has not degraded or been removed, and it remains in the built environment. It is important to develop approaches for evaluating this environmental legacy, including a potential retrospective reconstruction of the sources and comparative estimation of the toxic potential for different types and sources of asbestos.

The asbestos factory in the Armley district of Leeds, United Kingdom (U.K.), is one of the oldest in the world. The facility was opened around 1898 and produced asbestos textiles. Chrysotile asbestos was used for this purpose at least until the first decades of the twentieth century. The factory then manufactured asbestos insulation, including limpet spray formulation based on crocidolite asbestos, until the closure of the factory in 1958.

Arblaster et al. (1995) explored occupational and environmental links to mesothelioma deaths occurring in Leeds from 1971 to 1987. From 180 cases of mesothelioma deaths in Leeds, the authors found that 26% had potential occupational links to the Armley factory, and 48% had direct or indirect links to other jobs with likely occupational exposure to asbestos. About 21% of the cases had no recognized asbestos exposure. The authors were cautious in attributing them to potential environmental exposure from the factory but mentioned that such a relationship was suspected by the locals.

It should be noted that there are numerous publications in the media about the so-called Armley asbestos disasters, claiming that a significant number of homes in the area around the Armley factory are still contaminated with "blue" asbestos dust (apparently, crocidolite). In 2001, the Institute of Occupational Medicine (IOM, 2001) issued a report evaluating future cancer risks from asbestos contamination in

DOI: 10.1201/9781003424277-12

wider Armley and other areas of West Leeds. The report referred to the results of bulk dust sampling on the properties in the area; specifically in 15 properties within 40 meters of the former factory site, where detectable quantities of asbestos were found in seven (47%). The authors noted that crocidolite asbestos was not generally found in the samples. Also, IOM measured the activity-based airborne asbestos concentrations in several properties in Armley and concluded that the maximum possible exposure level was not expected to exceed 0.00001 f/cc. No mineralogical characteristic of the exposure was provided.

In June 2023, we collected three soil samples around one of the former factory buildings still preserved on Canal Road in Armley. Not intended to be a representative assessment, the sampling was performed as an attempt to see what information can be obtained about the types of mineral fibers that persist in the environment around the historical sources of asbestos emission. Two of the samples were obtained from pavement cracks close to the building, and one from the soil across Canal Road.

The samples were analyzed for asbestos content by transmission electron microscopy (TEM) by EMSL laboratory. For each of the samples, a sub-sample of the material was placed in an unused specimen container. In total, 100 mL of deionized fiber-free water was added to the container, which underwent vigorous agitation for 10 seconds to break up any clumps of bulk material. The sample was then placed in a sonicator for 10 minutes. A final vigorous agitation was applied to the sample for 10 seconds. The sample was allowed to settle for 2 minutes to allow agglomerations of consolidated material to fall to the bottom of the container. A 10-mL aliquot was then taken from the center of the sample and placed in a new unused sample container and brought up to 100 mL with deionized fiber-free water. After homogenization, dilutions were made until a proper loading was achieved for TEM analysis.

The filters prepared for each sample were dried and mounted onto glass microscope slides. Wedges of the filter were collapsed by hot acetone vapor and plasma etched in an oxygen plasma. A thin layer of carbon was then deposited on the surface of the filter, thus embedding the fibers of the sample in the carbon. The carbon-coated sample was then positioned onto a copper TEM grid and placed into an acetone Jaffe wick where the filter membrane was dissolved. The sample replica embedded in the carbon film and suspended on the grid was placed in the TEM for analysis.

A total of 200 fibers were recorded for each sample. The fiber counting rules and documentation requirements from the ISO 10312:2019 method (ambient air – determination of asbestos fibers – direct transfer transmission electron microscopy method) were used to size and identify the fibers. The samples were analyzed on a JEOL 1011 analytical TEM equipped with a digital camera and Oxford energy-dispersive X-ray analyzer (EDXA).

Chrysotile asbestos fibers were detected in two samples collected close to the Armley factory building. No fibers were detected in the soil sample from across the street.

The size distribution of chrysotile asbestos in the Armley samples is demonstrated in Figure 11.1.

The microphotograph of one of the detected chrysotile fibers for sample 2 is demonstrated in Figure 11.2.

To characterize the origin of the detected fibers, we compared the size distribution of asbestos with the length and width of fibers from several chrysotile samples.

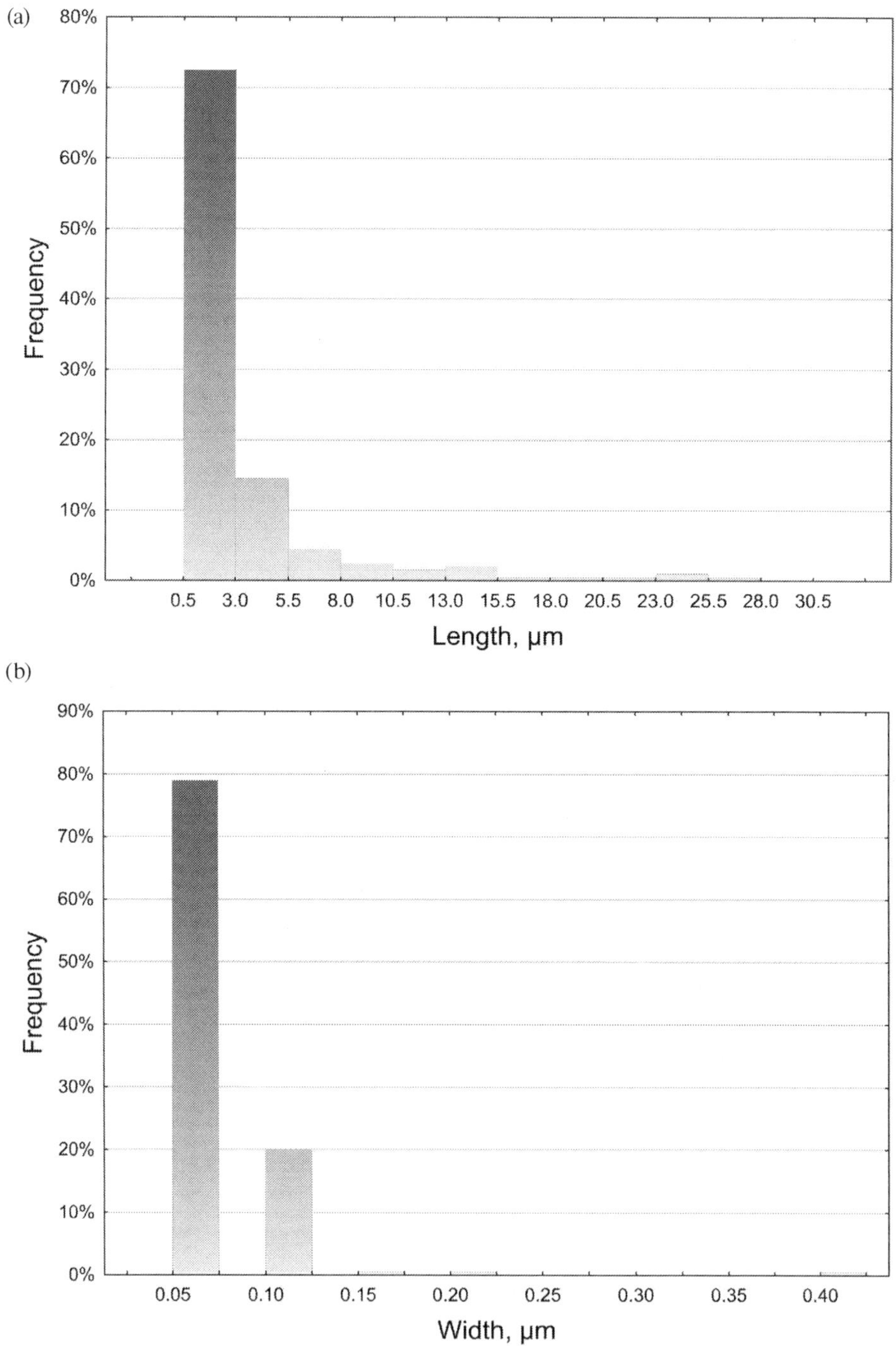

FIGURE 11.1 The distribution of length (a) and width (b) of chrysotile fibers in Armley samples (length/width ≥3:1).

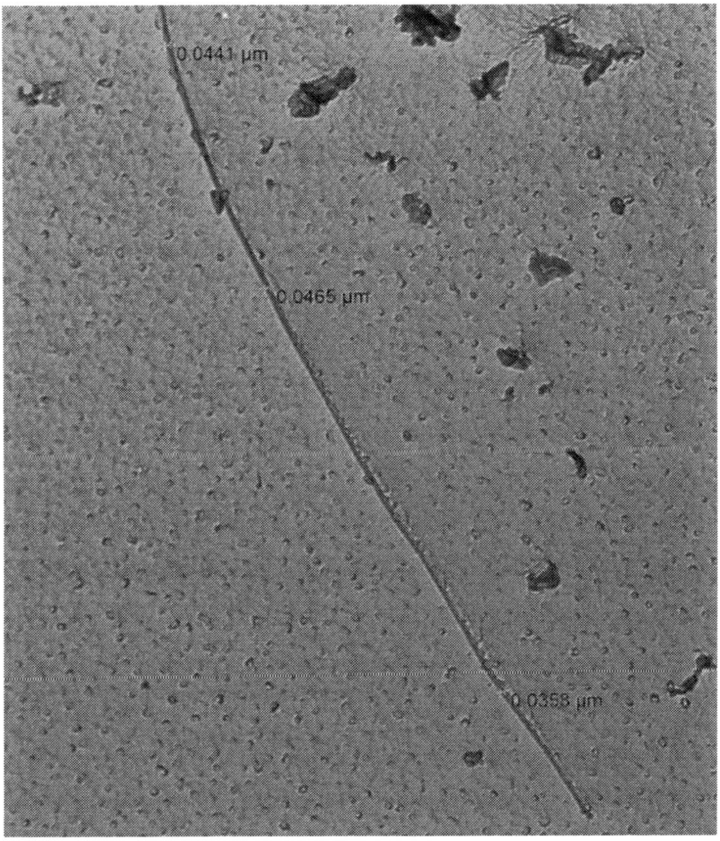

FIGURE 11.2 Microphotograph of one of the detected chrysotile structures

For bulk samples, we used our results of the dimensional characteristics of the fibers from the following sources:

1. Jeffrey mine, Quebec (Canada) (unspecified type of chrysotile)
2. Jeffrey mine, Quebec (long, thin chrysotile of "Plastibest" variety)
3. Thetford mine, Quebec (unspecified type of chrysotile)
4. Balangero, Italy (chrysotile found in the sample of balangeroite)
5. Quebec (chrysotile of textile variety, from Bell Group)
6. Quebec (chrysotile of textile variety, from J.M. Asbestos Inc., grade 3T-12)
7. Quebec (chrysotile of textile variety, from S.A.L. Group)
   Samples 5 through 7 were provided by Eric Chatfield. All bulk samples, except for samples 2 and 4, were analyzed by the EMSL laboratory, while samples 2 and 4 were analyzed by the BVNA laboratory (following the methodology described above for the Armley samples).
   For airborne chrysotile dimensional distribution, several simulations were performed to reconstruct the original fiber-by-fiber data from published

statistical characteristics. The following samples 8 through 10 were reconstructed with Monte Carlo simulation:

8. Quebec (data from Hwang, 1983)
9. South Carolina (U.S.A.) textile factory (data from Dement et al., 2008)
10. South Carolina textile factory (data from Dement & Harris, 1979)

Statistical results for the dimensional characteristics of samples are provided in Table 11.1.

This analysis of proximity can be performed on a quantitative basis. We used the Wasserstein distance as a metric of proximity between two-dimensional size distributions. The description of the methodology and the formula for the distance can be found, for example, in Panaretos and Zemel (2019).

TABLE 11.1
Statistical characteristics of dimensions for chrysotile samples (all length and width included length/width ≥ 3:1) (mean, standard deviation, geometric mean, geometric standard deviation)

Sample	Length (μm)	Width (μm)	Aspect ratio (μm)
Armley sample	3.52 (4.45) 2.19 (2.51)	0.07 (0.04) 0.06 (1.48)	57.9 (78.2) 33.9 (2.63)
Comparison samples			
Bulk			
1. Jeffrey mine, Quebec	2.1 (1.74) 1.66 (1.90)	0.09 (0.19) 0.08 (1.55)	28.8 (27.78) 21.9 (1.99)
2. Jeffrey mine, Quebec (long, thin chrysotile of "Plastibest" variety)	5.20 (8.66) 2.57 (2.95)	0.06 (0.09) 0.03 (2.63)	167.4 (283.9) 77.62 (3.31)
3. Thetford mine, Quebec (unspecified type of chrysotile)	2.55 (2.57) 1.90 (2.04)	0.08 (0.12) 0.07 (1.41)	32.3 (27.53) 25.7 (1.94)
4. Balangero, Italy (chrysotile found in the sample of balangeroite).	5.47 (6.66) 3.81 (2.21)	0.21 (0.64) 0.11 (2.12)	57.79 (86.02) 35.58 (2.53)
5. Quebec (chrysotile of textile variety, from Bell Group).	5.07 (5.73) 3.03 (2.70)	0.11 (0.09) 0.09 (1.81)	55.90 (67.95) 32.82 (2.73)
6. Quebec (chrysotile of textile variety, from J.M. Asbestos Inc., grade 3T-12)	3.06 (3.48) 4.09 (2.48)	0.09 (0.06) 0.10 (1.84)	37.95 (45.57) 39.94 (2.65)
7. Quebec (chrysotile of textile variety, from S.A.L. group)	6.13 (6.06) 4.09 (2.48)	0.13 (0.11) 0.10 (1.84)	65.07 (74.35) 39.94 (2.65)
Airborne			
8. Quebec (data from Hwang, 1983)	0.91 (1.24) 0.58 (2.42)	0.06 (0.03) 0.05 (1.72)	19.23 (33.29) 11.60 (2.41)
9. South Carolina textile factory (data from Dement et al., 2008)	11.93 (17.19) 5.01 (3.89)	0.47 (0.77) 0.23 (2.95)	65.12 (134.12) 21.87 (4.27)
10. South Carolina textile factory (data from Dement & Harris, 1979)	4.45 (6.38) 2.13 (3.27)	0.25 (0.43) 0.14 (2.52)	28.97 (50.06) 15.38 (2.82)

The unitless distances between various size distributions of chrysotile fibers are demonstrated in Table 11.2. The lowest distance corresponds to closer proximity of the size distributions.

Based on Table 11.2, the bulk sample of Armley chrysotile shows the closest similarity distribution with the 3T-12 textile grade of Quebec asbestos among all bulk samples. While bulk and airborne size distributions of fibers are not fully comparable, the closest airborne sample to Armley's chrysotile is South Carolina asbestos textile fibers as reported by Dement and Harris (1979).

We also used correlation coefficients as a measure of distribution similarities. The length and width of fibers were divided into 32 categories (as in Pooley & Clark, 1980). The correlations between vectors of categories were found for all pairs of chrysotile sources. Then, factor analysis was used to determine the proximity of various sources to each other and the source of interest (Armley chrysotile).

The results of the data projection in two-factor space are demonstrated in Figure 11.3.

Based on the factor analysis results, Armley chrysotile appears to be proximate to Plastibest asbestos from the Jeffrey mine and to the textile-grade 3T–12. From airborne samples, South Carolina data from 1979 seems to be the closest.

It can be concluded that the asbestos in the Armley samples is most probably related to textile production, similar to that used in the South Carolina asbestos textile plants. Therefore, the Armley chrysotile might be from the textile grade of Quebec origin. However, the "Plastibest" variety from the Jeffrey Mine can also be a source. It is also noteworthy that the asbestos factory in Armley was apparently owned by the same company as the Havelock asbestos mine in Swaziland, which reportedly also produced a textile grade of chrysotile, so the source mine remains uncertain.

Quantitative structure-activity relationship (QSAR) modeling can be used to estimate carcinogenic potency for airborne Armley chrysotile. Korchevskiy et al. (2019) related mesothelioma potency R_M (%) (see previous chapters of this book for an explanation of this metric) to the chemical composition of fibers and their aspect ratio. In particular, it can be demonstrated that for a specific chemical composition of fibers, mesothelioma potency is proportional to the power of the aspect ratio, following the equation

$$R_M \sim (AR\text{-}3)^K \quad (11.1),$$

where AR is the median aspect ratio of airborne fibers with length/width ≥ 3:1 (all lengths and widths included).

Table 11.3 demonstrates the geometric mean aspect ratio for airborne fibers included in our study, along with available published estimations of mesothelioma potency.

Assuming that the chemical composition of chrysotile from different locations is close enough (if not fully identical), we can estimate the mesothelioma potency using one of the chrysotile types as a baseline. We assumed that geometric mean aspect ratios can be used as a surrogate for median values. We utilized the potency of Quebec airborne chrysotile (R_M=0.0009%) as a baseline (as in Darnton, 2023).

TABLE 11.2
Wasserstein distances between size distributions of asbestos fibers (length/width ≥ 3:1).

	Armley, bulk	Jeffrey mine, bulk	Plastibest, bulk	Thetford mine, bulk	Balangero, bulk	Bell group, bulk	3T-12, bulk	S.A.L. bulk	Quebec, airborne	SC, 2008	SC, 1979
Armley, bulk	0	0.73	0.87	0.53	1.07	0.80	0.25	1.33	1.31	4.66	0.58
Jeffrey mine, bulk	0.73	0	1.60	0.23	1.76	1.51	0.53	2.04	0.60	5.37	1.31
Plastibest, bulk	0.87	1.60	0	1.38	0.83	0.65	1.09	1.05	2.16	3.83	0.55
Thetford mine, bulk	0.53	0.23	1.38	0	1.53	1.28	0.33	1.82	0.83	5.15	1.09
Balangero, bulk	1.07	1.76	0.83	1.53	0	0.85	1.27	0.76	2.36	3.82	1.03
Bell group, bulk	0.80	1.51	0.65	1.28	0.85	0	1.02	0.56	2.11	3.86	0.52
3T-12, bulk	0.25	0.53	1.09	0.33	1.27	1.02	0	1.55	1.09	4.88	0.79
S.A.L., bulk	1.33	2.04	1.05	1.82	0.76	0.56	1.55	0	2.64	3.44	0.96
Quebec, airborne	1.31	0.60	2.16	0.83	2.36	2.11	1.09	2.64	0	5.97	1.86
South Carolina, Dement et al., 2008 airborne	4.66	5.37	3.83	5.15	3.82	3.86	4.88	3.44	5.97	0	4.11
South Carolina, Dement & Harris, 1979, airborne	0.58	1.31	0.55	1.09	1.03	0.52	0.79	0.96	1.86	4.11	0

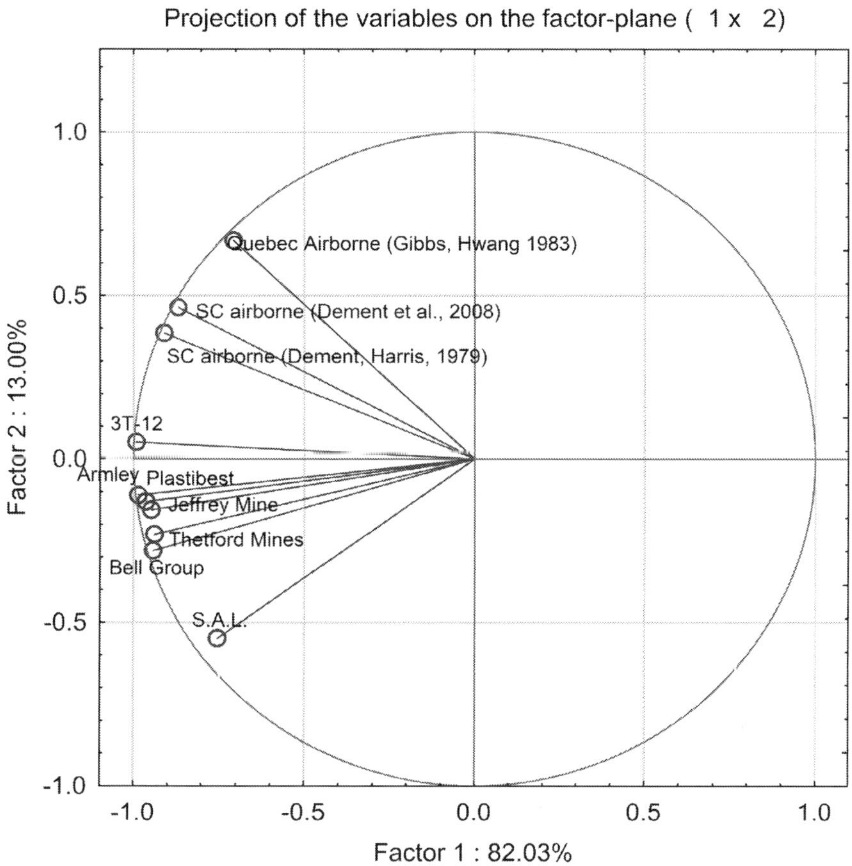

FIGURE 11.3 The results of factor analysis for the proximity of various types/sources of chrysotile

TABLE 11.3
Geometric mean aspect ratio for airborne chrysotile fibers (length/width ≥ 3:1)

Sample	Aspect ratio
Quebec (Gibbs & Hwang, 1980)	11.6
South Carolina, textile (Dement et al., 2008)	21.87
South Carolina, textile (Dement & Harris, 1979)	14.49
Armley, soil sample	33.9
Balangero, soil sample	35.58

*Darnton (2023)**Korchevskiy and Wylie (2023)

TABLE 11.4
Comparison of modeled and published potency factors for varieties of chrysotile

Chrysotile variety	Modeled R_M (%)	Published R_M (%)
Quebec (Gibbs & Hwang, 1980)	0.0009 (baseline)	0.0009*
South Carolina, textile (Dement et al., 2008)	0.003	0.008 (average between male and female data) *
South Carolina, textile (Dement & Harris, 1979)	0.0014	0.008 (average between male and female data)*
Armley, soil sample	0.006	–
Balangero, soil sample	0.006	0.0043**

* Darnton, 2023 ** Korchevskiy and Wylie (2023)

Table 11.4 contains estimations of potency factors calculated based on Equation (11.1) for several types of chrysotile in comparison to published values.

It can be seen that our reconstruction is very close for the Quebec and Balangero estimations. Apparently, the model underestimates the reported mesothelioma potency for South Carolina textile cohorts. This may be a result of crocidolite contamination of textile chrysotile in this locality.

Also, a risk assessment methodology can be used to estimate possible airborne concentrations and human health risk from potential exposure to Armley chrysotile. Table 11.5 contains the soil concentrations of chrysotile in samples collected in Armley, based on the HSE report. It should be noted that the weight % of chrysotile in the sample is not a representative metric because it does not fully account for the change in the weight of the matrix during bulk sample preparation. However, we used the weight percent of asbestos structures in the Armley samples as an illustration of a wider risk assessment methodology and concept, assuming that the "true" weight fraction of the soil contamination in Armley would be uniform and available for our evaluation.

Empirically, the airborne concentrations of asbestos based on concentrations in soil can be estimated as follows:

$$C_{\text{air, asbestos, PCME}}\ (\text{f/cc}) = F_S/100 \times C_{\text{air, respirable dust}}\ (\mu\text{g/m}^3)/1000 \times \lambda \times C_{\text{soil, asbestos, PCME}}\ (\%)\ /100,$$

where

F_S (%) is the fraction of soil emission in the airborne respirable dust concentrations,

$C_{\text{air, asbestos, PCME}}$ (f/cc) is the airborne asbestos concentration produced by soil emission,

$C_{\text{air, respirable dust}}$ (μg/m^3) is the respirable dust concentration produced by soil emission,

$C_{\text{soil, asbestos, PCME}}$ (%) is the weight fraction of asbestos in soil,

λ (f/cc per mg/m^3 per asbestos % in soil) is the soil-to-air coefficient of asbestos release from soil (Korchevskiy & Strode, 2024).

TABLE 11.5
Results of the TEM analysis for the soil samples from Armley, Leeds, with detected asbestos (data from IOM, 2001)

Sample #	Asbestos type	Total number of detected structures	Analytical sensitivity (structures/g)	Concentration (structures/g)	Weight %, all structures	Weight %, PCME structures (length >5 μm, width ≥0.15 μm, length/width ≥≥3)*
1	Chrysotile	201	7,654,004	1,538,454,715	0.007	0.0031
2	Chrysotile	203	61,601,267	12,505,057,162	0.073	0.029

* PCME is a concentration of airborne fibers detected by TEM but supposed to be visible by optical microscope. We use the definition of PCME according to the NIOSH 7400 standard, Issue 3.

The soil-to-air coefficients for asbestos were estimated by different authors; in particular, Addison et al. (1988) published the data allowing us to estimate an average λ for chrysotile asbestos and "intermediate" soil type as 316 f/cc per mg/m^3 per asbestos % in soil.

Conditionally assuming the soil fraction in airborne respirable dust (F_S) as 10%, respirable dust concentration in Leeds at the level of about 15 μg/m^3, and taking the average PCME asbestos % between sample 1 and sample 2, we get the asbestos concentration:

$$C_{\text{air, asbestos}}\ (\text{f/cc}) \approx 10/100 \times 15\ \mu\text{g/m}^3 /1000 \times 316 \times 0.016 /100 = 0.000075\ \text{f/cc}.$$

This is about one order of magnitude higher than the upper bound estimation of the activity-based exposure level estimated by IOM (2001).

Based on the Hodgson and Darnton (2000) methodology, and assuming the potency factor R_M=0.006%, with exposure from birth for 75 years, 24 hours/7 days per week, we would estimate mesothelioma risk from hypothetical soil contamination in Armley, Leeds at the level of 1 case per 1,000,000 (see Korchevskiy & Rasmuson, 2024 for the methodology and examples of risk calculations). This risk value is usually evaluated as negligible.

Our study has obvious uncertainties and limitations. In particular, only a few soil samples were collected in Armley, and the representativeness of the obtained data is unknown. However, even a limited number of samples can provide important insights regarding the dimensional distribution and potential health-related risk for detected fibers. Our approach demonstrates consistency and illustrates the utilization of QSAR modeling for the purposes of human health risk assessment.

In any case, the contamination around the Armley asbestos factory is an interesting example of "legacy" asbestos impact. Additional monitoring in the area might be beneficial to reassure public confidence in adequate preventive measures, but also for further investigation of the historical origin of asbestos fibers in current environments.

REFERENCE LIST

Addison, J., Davies, L. S. T., Robertson, A., & Willey, R. J. (1988). *Release of dispersed asbestos fibres from soils* (Technical Report # PB-89-170716/XAB; TM-88/14, United Kingdom. PB-89-170716/XAB; TM-88/14). https://www.osti.gov/etdeweb/biblio/6084614

Arblaster, L., Hatton, P., Howel, D., Renvoize, E., Schweiger, M., & Swinburne, L. M. (1995). Occupational and environmental links to mesothelioma deaths occurring in Leeds during 1971–1987. *Journal of Public Health Medicine*, *17*(3), 297–304. https://doi.org/10.1093/oxfordjournals.pubmed.a043122

Darnton, L. (2023). Quantitative assessment of mesothelioma and lung cancer risk based on phase contrast microscopy (PCM) estimates of fibre exposure: An update of 2000 asbestos cohort data. *Environmental Research*, *230*, 114753. https://doi.org/10.1016/j.envres.2022.114753

Dement, J. M., & Harris, R. (1979). *Estimates of pulmonary and gastrointestinal deposition for occupational fiber exposures* (Issue 79–135 of DHEW). NIOSH Publication.

Dement, J. M., Kuempel, E. D., Zumwalde, R. D., Smith, R. J., Stayner, L. T., & Loomis, D. (2008). Development of a fibre size-specific job-exposure matrix for airborne asbestos fibres. *Occupational & Environmental Medicine*, *65*(9), 605–612. https://doi.org/10.1136/oem.2007.033712

Gibbs, G. W., & Hwang, C. Y. (1980). Dimensions of airborne asbestos fibres. *IARC Scientific Publications*, *1980*(30), 69–78. PMID: 7239672.

Hodgson, J. T., & Darnton, A. (2000). The quantitative risks of mesothelioma and lung cancer in relation to asbestos exposure. *Annals of Occupational Hygiene*, *44*(8), 565–601. PMID: 11108782.

Hwang, C. Y. (1983). Size and shape of airborne asbestos fibres in mines and mills. *British Journal of Industrial Medicine*, *40*(3), 273–279. https://doi.org/10.1136/oem.40.3.273

Institute of Occupational Medicine (IOM). (2001). *An evaluation of the likely future cancer risks from asbestos contamination in Wider Armley and other areas of West Leeds* (Research Report TM/01/06). http://www.iom-world.org/pubs/IOM_TM0106.pdf

Korchevskiy, A., & Rasmuson, J. (2024). Theoretical and practical aspects of asbestos dose-response assessment. In A. Korchevskiy, J. Rasmuson, & E. Rasmuson (Eds.), *Health risk assessment for asbestos and other fibrous minerals*. John Wiley & Sons. ISBN: 978-1-119-43843-4. https://doi.org//10.1002/9781119438397

Korchevskiy, A., & Strode, R. (2024). Asbestos in soil: Risk characterization for Occupational and Environmental Exposures. In A. Korchevskiy, J. Rasmuson, & E. Rasmuson (Eds.), *Health risk assessment for asbestos and other fibrous minerals*. John Wiley & Sons. ISBN: 978-1-119-43843-4. https://doi.org//10.1002/9781119438397

Korchevskiy, A., & Wylie, A. (2023). Toxicological and epidemiological approaches to carcinogenic potency modeling for mixed mineral fiber exposure: The case of fibrous balangeroite and chrysotile. *Inhalation Toxicology*, *35*(7–8), 185–200. https://doi//10.1080/08958378.2023.2213720

Korchevskiy, A., Rasmuson, J. O., & Rasmuson, E. J. (2019). Empirical model of mesothelioma potency factors for different mineral fibers based on their chemical composition and dimensionality. *Inhalation Toxicology*, *31*(5), 180–191. https://doi.org/10.1080/08958378.2019.1640320

National Institute of Occupational Safety and Health (NIOSH). (2019). *Asbestos and other fibers by PCM, method 7400, issue 3*. NIOSH.

Panaretos, V. M., & Zemel, Y. (2019). Statistical aspects of Wasserstein distance. *Annual Review of Statistics and Its Applications*, *6*, 405–431. https://doi.org/10.1146/annurev-statistics-030718-104938

Pooley, F. D., & Clark, N. J. (1980). A comparison of fibre dimensions in chrysotile, crocidolite and amosite particles from samples of airborne dust and from post-mortem lung tissue specimens. *IARC Scientific Publications*, *1980*(30), 79–86. PMID: 7239673.

Virta, R. L. (2006). *Worldwide asbestos supply and consumption trends from 1900 through 2003* (U.S. Geological Survey Circular 1298, p. 80). https://pubs.usgs.gov/circ/2006/1298/c1298.pdf

12 Peritoneal mesothelioma hazard rate as a function of mineralogical parameters

Revisiting the results of the experimental study

A. Korchevskiy & A. Wylie

INTRODUCTION

Mesothelioma remains an important subject for epidemiological and toxicological studies. This malignancy is distinctly different from other tumors in humans, a fact that is particularly manifested in the difficulties in controlling and treating this condition (Testa, 2017). Though asbestos and other asbestiform mineral fibers are widely implicated in a majority of human mesotheliomas, there is growing evidence for spontaneous mesothelioma cases (Carbone et al., 2019), as well as mesotheliomas caused by other factors, like ionizing radiation (Pelnar, 1988; Attanoos et al., 2018). Peritoneal mesothelioma is a comparatively rare type of malignant mesothelioma, comprising not more than 15–20% of new cases. Among the hallmarks of peritoneal mesothelioma are equal distribution among men and women (vs. pleural mesothelioma predominance in men), the variability of tumor aggressiveness and disease progression, the tendency of the disease to stay within the peritoneal cavity, and other factors (Greenbaum & Alexander, 2020).

The attempts to explore the biological mechanisms of the development of peritoneal mesothelioma by creating an experimental model in laboratory animals have a substantial history. Okada et al. (1989) demonstrated mesothelioma cases in male Wistar rats by colloidal iron deposition in the peritoneum. Miller et al. (1999) induced peritoneal mesothelioma in male SPF Wistar rats by instillation of different kinds of man-made vitreous fibers, glass microfibers, silicon carbide whiskers, and amosite asbestos, concluding that mesothelioma potency depends on dimensions and the biosolubility of the fibers. Adachi et al. (2001) observed peritoneal mesothelioma induction in rats with intraperitoneal administration of suspended solutions of silicon carbide whiskers, chrysotile asbestos, potassium titanate whiskers, and refractory fibers.

One of the most famous experiments on intraperitoneal instillation of asbestos fibers was performed by Davis et al. (1991). The importance of Davis' study was the

DOI: 10.1201/9781003424277-13

attempt to use not just bulk samples of the materials, but specifically the elutriated dust, to analyze the carcinogenic potency of the most relevant, respirable fraction of the agent. Davis also used samples of the same mineral (tremolite) derived from various locations around the world, all with pronounced differences in dimensional characteristics. The following samples of tremolite were used by Davis:

(1) Asbestiform tremolite from Jamestown, California
(2) Asbestiform tremolite from Korea
(3) Asbestiform tremolite from an unknown source, labeled Swansea, Scotland
(4) Non-asbestiform tremolite from Ala di Stura, Italy
(5) Non-asbestiform tremolite from Carr Brae, Dornie, Scotland
(6) Non-asbestiform tremolite from Shinness, Scotland

Based on the information from Davis' study, three asbestiform tremolites (Jamestown, Korea, and Swansea) were prepared in the following way. The materials were packed into the dust dispensers, and airborne dusts were generated. Respirable fractions of these dusts were collected with a vertical elutriator. No further purification was required.

The tremolite from Ala di Stura had to be broken by hand to separate the thicker, longer fibers before packing into the dust dispenser, but the material was then treated in the same manner as the asbestiform varieties. It is fibrous, but the large bundles of fiber were very easy to split and separate because of their brittle nature. This type of mineral fiber is referred to as byssolite.

The Dornie tremolite also required different treatment. The crumbled crystal powder was washed free of organic material by repeated sedimentation in distilled water. The tremolite was collected by decanting off the water and drying the powder at 110°C overnight. This loose material consisted mainly of small needle-like crystals which were used for dust preparation as above.

The prismatic crystals of the Shinness tremolite were reported to be hand-picked for purity from a roughly crushed preparation and ground in distilled water for 5 minutes in a corundum micronizing mill. The resulting powder was collected by filtration, dried at 110°C overnight, and then used for dust generation. Shinness, Dornie, and Italian tremolite samples were distinctly different from the first three varieties and are usually referred to as "non-asbestiform" types.

For the animal studies, weighed amounts of tremolite dust were suspended in phosphate-buffered saline (PBS) so that the planned dose of 10 mg was contained in a saline volume of 2.0 ml. This dose was administered to groups of either 33 or 36, 3-month-old rats of the AF/Han strain as a single intraperitoneal injection.

Davis reported the results of the analysis of the injected materials performed by X-ray diffraction on a Philips X-ray powder diffractometer, by infrared spectrophotometry with a Perkin Elmer spectrophotometer (PE 580), and by polarized light microscopy. Small samples of minerals were also evaluated by scanning electron microscopy (SEM) (Cambridge Instruments S250 Mark 2) and transmission electron microscopy (TEM) (Hitachi H7000), with individual particles analyzed semi-quantitatively by energy-dispersive X-ray spectroscopy (Link Analytical 860.200, AN10).

Davis et al. (1991) reported that from 216 animals in the study, 133 developed peritoneal mesothelioma. The authors calculated the relative hazard of the tremolite samples and attempted to relate the hazard estimation with dimensional characteristics of the material. The conclusion was that carcinogenicity is related to the number of long, thin fibers, though "the relationship was by no means exact." Actually, although Davis suggested that the abundance of fibers with length greater than 8 μm and width smaller than 0.25 μm would predict mesothelioma potency better than other size categories, no statistically significant relationship with a specific size of fibers was established in the study.

In 2018, Eric Chatfield published the results of the re-sampling of the materials used by Davis to create improved estimations of dimensional characteristics of the tremolite samples in the experiment (Chatfield, 2018, 2021). Chatfield noted that "the resolution and image contrast that could be achieved by scanning electron microscopes in 1991 were limited . . . and in the light of more recent work, improved measurement accuracy for the thinnest EMPs would be desirable."

Also, recently, various advanced statistical methods have been used to explore the impact of dimensional and chemical composition characteristics of elongate mineral particles on their carcinogenic potency (Korchevskiy et al., 2019; Wylie et al., 2020). In particular, it was demonstrated that mesothelioma potency of various types of elongate mineral particles can be modeled by using such parameters as specific surface area, fiber width, Wylie's fibrosity index, and others (Korchevskiy & Wylie, 2022). High correlation was found between mesothelioma and lung cancer potency factors and fractional parameters, such as the fraction of fibers ≤0.15 μm among all fibers longer than 5 μm (Wylie et al., 2020; Korchevskiy & Wylie, 2021). The database of elongate mineral particle dimensionality contains information on more than 570,000 particles, enabling determination of the relationships between various dimensional metrics. It was shown that asbestiform and non-asbestiform elongate mineral particles have distinct dimensional characteristics, clearly discriminating the particle with different morphology by the level of carcinogenicity (Wylie et al., 2022; Korchevskiy & Wylie, 2025a, 2025b). Newly available methodology and data open additional opportunities to characterize tremolite particles from Davis' study.

It should be noted that various hypotheses have been formulated to explain the differences between types of elongated mineral particles (EMPs) in the development of peritoneal mesothelioma compared to pleural tumors. In particular, Okada et al. (1989) described the induction of peritoneal mesothelioma in male Wistar rats by injection of ferric saccharate. The iron-induced peritoneal mesothelioma was further explored by Hu et al. (2010). Korchevskiy et al. (2019) demonstrated that iron content in asbestos fibers (along with other characteristics) can serve as a predictor for mesothelioma risk.

It seems important to utilize mathematical modeling for the determination of predictive parameters that can be used to explain the differences in mesothelial carcinogenicity of various types of tremolite by combining original particle-by-particle data from the Chatfield study with the mesothelioma hazard estimations reported by Davis. It is possible to determine analogies and differences in hazard rates determined in animal experiments with observations from human epidemiological studies.

The objectives of this study are (1) to evaluate the role of long, thin fibers in the development of peritoneal mesothelioma in rats; (2) to estimate the relationship between the relative hazard for different varieties of tremolite EMPs and the fraction of long, thin fibers (the EMPA category); (3) to verify the hypothesis that iron in the fibers is a predictor of peritoneal mesothelioma potency factors; (4) to develop regression models relating peritoneal mesothelioma hazard values with chemical composition and dimensional characteristics of particles; and (5) to compare the patterns for peritoneal mesothelioma risk modeling in animals and humans.

The hypothesis is that the relative hazard in the Davis study can be modeled from chemical composition and dimensional characteristics, with parameters similar to those derived from human studies. We also hypothesize that the asbestiform and non-asbestiform habit of tremolite particles used for the experimental study of Davis can be determined from dimensional data, and that there is a significant difference in the propensity of particles in various habits to produce mesothelioma risk. We anticipate that, along with similarities, the differences in the peritoneal mesothelioma response between rats and humans should be observed.

MATERIALS AND METHODS

Estimation of mesothelioma potency

The particle-by-particle information for six tremolite samples utilized by Davis, as reanalyzed by Chatfield, was included in the database on fibrous minerals that was earlier characterized in several publications (Korchevskiy & Wylie, 2021, 2022) and described in Chapter 2. The methodological details of the re-testing of the tremolite materials are described in Chatfield (2021).

We evaluated four parameters: EMPA, iron content, biopersistence, and the dimensional coefficient of carcinogenicity for the tremolite samples in comparison with other known carcinogens to predict their mesothelioma potency.

1. The EMPA characteristic was quantified for each tremolite sample, as the fraction of EMPs with width ≤0.15 μm among fibers longer than 5 μm.
2. The dimensional coefficient of carcinogenicity (DCC) was calculated for each of the tremolite samples, according to the formula (see Chapter 4 of this book):

$$DCC = 1\text{-}\exp\left(-0.1 * \text{Surface Area} / (1000\ \text{Width}^3+1)\right).$$

3. The weight percent of iron oxides in the fibers was based on Verkouteren and Wylie (2000)
4. A biopersistence measure was used as in Gualtieri et al. (2018).

The peritoneal mesothelioma hazard data along with dimensional characteristics and iron oxide content of fibers are provided in Table 12.1.

We also used a similar approach for modeling peritoneal mesothelioma potency in human cohorts.

TABLE 12.1
Relative hazard, along with EMPA, DCC, and iron content

Source of tremolite	Relative hazard, logged	DCC parameter	EMPA (%)	Iron oxides content (wt %)
Shinness	–4.71	0.003	0	1.4
Dornie	–3.9	0.0016	0	1.5
Ala di Stura	–1.61	0.0049	0	3.6
Swansea	0.56	0.0059	0	4.25
Jamestown	0.83	0.025	6.4	3.1
Korea	0	0.057	14.7	0.6

We used the peritoneal mesothelioma potency factor R_M-Per, defined as a percent of peritoneal mesothelioma cases to expected mortality from all causes (adjusted to the age of first exposure of 30) per unit of cumulative exposure, as shown in Equation 12.2:

$$R_{M\text{-}Per}r = 100\frac{PerO_M}{\left(E_{Adj} \times X\right)}, \qquad (12.2),$$

where $PerO_M$ is the number of peritoneal mesothelioma deaths, E_{Adj} the total expected deaths from all causes adjusted to the age of first exposure of 30, and X is the mean cumulative exposure in PCM fibers/cubic centimeter-years (f/cc-years).

For chrysotile, amosite, crocidolite, and Libby amphiboles, data from Darnton (2023) were used to estimate peritoneal mesothelioma potency. Fluoro-edenite potency in peritoneal mesothelioma was utilized based on total mesothelioma mortality calculations from Korchevskiy et al. (2019), and the fraction of peritoneal mesotheliomas in the population exposed to fluoro-edenite (7.69%) was based on data from Bruno et al. (2014). It should be noted that the risk assessment method by Darnton utilizes cumulative exposure concentrations based on PCM methodology. We assume that concentration X is compatible with PCM values. In particular, for amphiboles, PCM fibers would include fibers longer than 5 μm and not thinner than 0.05 μm. For chrysotile, fibers thinner than 0.15 μm may not be visible by PCM. See Chapter 2 for more explanation. We will use fibers longer than 5 μm, with width ≥0.05 μm and width ≤3 μm for our analysis in this chapter.

The data for modeling are provided in Table 12.2. The table also contains an estimate of fiber biopersistence (in terms of the year lifetime of fibers in acellular dissolution process) (based on Gualtieri et al., 2018).

The biosolubility of tremolite in Davis' studies was assumed to be 49 years. Biopersistence of fluoro-edenite was assumed to be the average of all biopersistence values for amphiboles as reported in Gualtieri et al. (2018) (108 years).

The peritoneal mesothelioma potency for erionite is not published, and there is disagreement on the possible fraction of peritoneal mesothelioma in exposed

TABLE 12.2

Peritoneal mesothelioma potency, EMPA, DCC, iron content, and biopersistence

Mineral type, source	Peritoneal mesothelioma potency factor (%)	DCC parameter (average for length >5 μm, length/width ≥3, width ≥0.05 μm, width ≤3 μm)	EMPA fraction (%)	Iron oxides content (%)	Biopersistence (years)
Chrysotile, Quebec, Canada	0.000051	0.08	37.0	1.5	0.3
Amosite, South Africa	0.0425	0.064	16.0	37.31	74
Crocidolite, Australia and South Africa	0.08	0.093	33.0	33.9	66
Libby amphiboles, Libby, Montana, U.S.A.	0.002	0.0195	3.0	6.74	49
Fluoro-edenite, Italy	0.00923	0.034	1.9	2.63	108
Anthophyllite, Russia	N/A	0.02	4.0	10.1	245
Glaucophane, California, U.S.A.	N/A	0.013	2.0	9.01	N/A
Erionite, Turkey	N/A	.097	41.1	1.25	181
Balangeroite, Italy	N/A	0.03	5.0	25.84	55.6

populations. For example, Boffetta (2007) quoted several sources where the fraction of peritoneal mesothelioma among all mesothelioma cases fluctuated from 6.6 to 12%. In the study of Baris in the village of Karain with the highest level of erionite exposure, 4.4% of mesothelioma cases were peritoneal. We will attempt to estimate the potency of erionite for peritoneal mesothelioma based on quantitative structure-activity relationship (QSAR) modeling and then compare the estimated potency with the reported values.

Also, balangeroite potency for peritoneal mesothelioma is not known. Ferrante et al. (2020) listed 6 cases of death from pleural cancer and 2 cases of death from malignant neoplasms of the peritoneum in a cohort of Balangero chrysotile mine and mill workers, but it is unclear if these cases can be interpreted as mesothelioma. Also, balangeroite was just a contaminant in the possible exposure of workers at the Balangero mine. Korchevskiy and Wylie (2023) demonstrated that in the cohort of Balangero chrysotile mine and mill workers, among 7 cases of mesothelioma, about 3 cases can be attributed to balangeroite contamination.[1] We will explore what fraction of this estimated number of cases should be expected to have a peritoneal origin.

Predicting habit of particles

Criteria particles were defined according to the formula from Wylie et al. (2022):

$C=2.99\log_{10}(\text{length})-5.82\log_{10}(\text{width})-3.80$ (positive for criteria particles, negative for non-criteria particles, assuming EMPs longer than 5 μm, with an aspect ratio greater than 3:1, and width less than 3 μm). The fraction of criteria particles was determined for each of the samples of tremolite in the Davis study.

The Pearson index, a linear correlation coefficient in the regression between $\log_{10}$-transformed width and length of EMPs, was also calculated for EMPs longer than 2 μm, with an aspect ratio greater than 3:1, and width less than 3 μm (see Chapters 8 and 9.)

The combined habit of each tremolite sample was predicted based on the following discriminant function specifically developed for tremolite:

$$\text{CritFraction} \geq 0.67 \times \text{PearsonIndex} + 0.133,$$

where CritFraction is the fraction of criteria particles for each mineral sample, and

PearsonIndex is the Pearson index, as described above (Korchevskiy & Wylie, 2025a, 2025b).

Regression analysis was used to determine the relationships between potency factors and various characteristics of mineral EMPs. Statistica 14.0 by Tibco was utilized for the calculations.

RESULTS

We determined that the relative hazard of EMP-5 in Davis' experiment can be reconstructed based on the EMPA parameter and iron content of the fibers.

The regression Equation 12.1 is as follows:

$$\text{Hazard} = -8.4305 + 1.608\text{Fe} + 0.392\text{EMPA} + 0.9987\log_{10}(\text{Bioper}), \quad (12.1),$$

where Hazard is the relative hazard of peritoneal mesothelioma in Davis' experiment,

EMPA is the fraction of fibers ≤0.15 μm among fibers longer than 5 μm (%),

Bioper – Biosolubility, assumed to be equal to 49 (years) for tremolite (see Chapter 5), and

Fe is the iron content in fibers (wt %).

$$\left(R = 0.984, R^2 = 0.968, p < 0.00565\right)^{\cdot}$$

The relationship between the modeled and observed hazard rate of peritoneal mesothelioma in Davis' experiment is demonstrated in Figure 12.1.

It can be demonstrated that the dimensional criteria for EMPA (0.15 μm) maximizes the correlation for Equation 12.1. Figure 12.2 demonstrates the linear correlation and P values for analogies to Equation 12.1, if other width cutpoints were

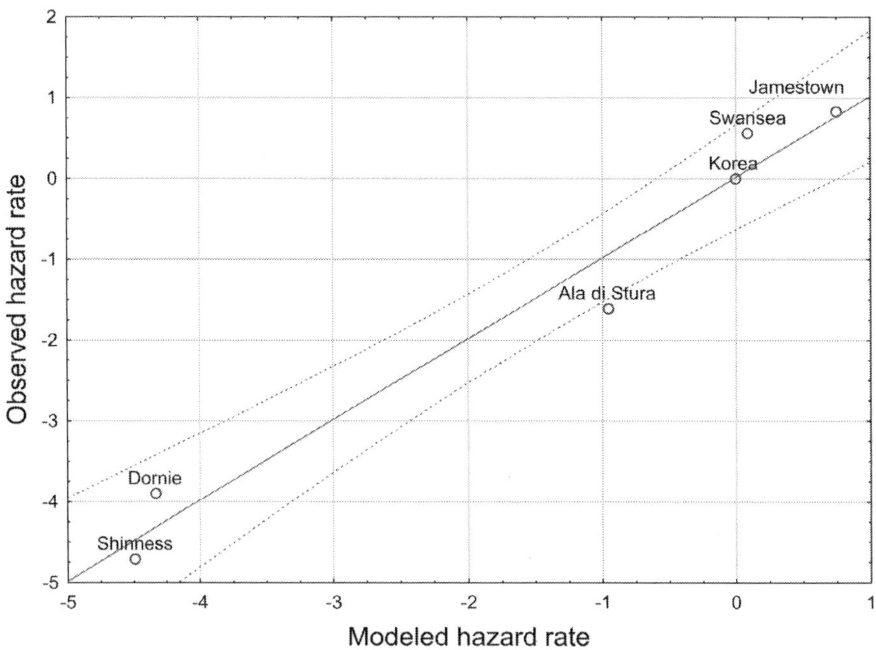

FIGURE 12.1 The relationship between modeled and observed peritoneal mesothelioma hazard rate in rats.

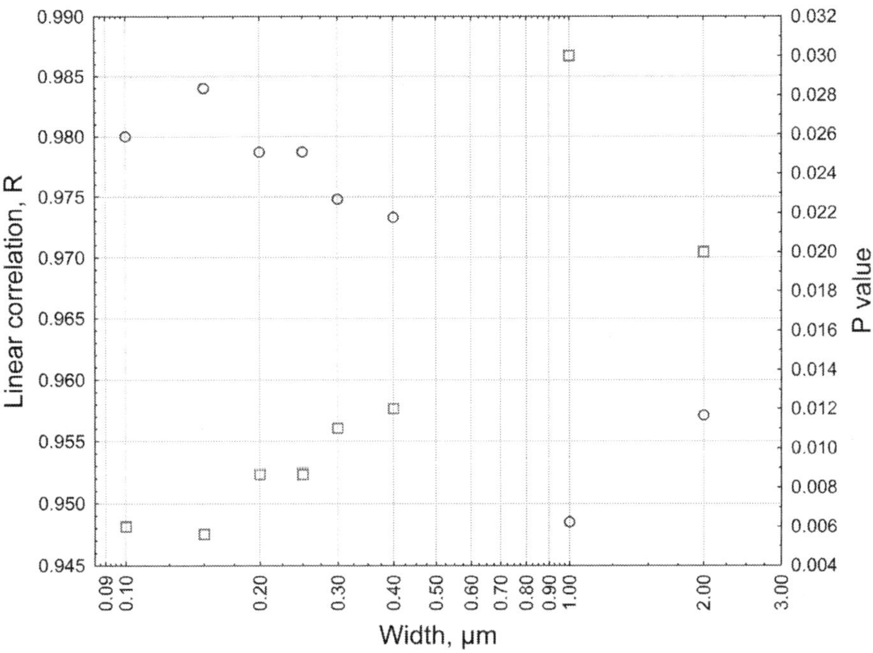

FIGURE 12.2 Relationship between linear correlation and P value with the width cutpoint when the hazard rate in Davis data is regressed by iron content, dimensional fraction (fibers thinner than a certain width among fibers longer than 5 μm), and biosolubility (assumed to be constant for tremolite varieties). Blue circles denote the correlation values and red dots indicate P values.

used for the dimensional fraction. The lowest value of P and highest correlation are achieved for the EMPA fraction.

A similar, though slightly less precise, relationship exists between the hazard rate of peritoneal mesothelioma in Davis' experiment and the dimensional coefficient of carcinogenicity (DCC), described in Chapter 5.

We determined the following regression equation:

$$\text{Hazard} = -8.55 + 1.52\text{Fe} + 106.45\text{DCC} + 1.00\log_{10}(\text{Bioper}),$$

where Hazard is the relative hazard of peritoneal mesothelioma in Davis' experiment,

DCC is the dimensional coefficient of carcinogenicity,

Bioper is biosolubility, assumed to be equal to 49 (years) for tremolite (see Chapter 5), and

Fe is the iron content in fibers (%).

($R = 0.979$, $R^2 = 0.959$, $p < 0.00841$).

It is possible to evaluate the habit (asbestiform vs. non-asbestiform) of the minerals in Davis experiment based on dimensional characteristics.

TABLE 12.3
The Pearson index and criteria particle content

Type of tremolite	Pearson index	Fraction of criteria particles
Shinness	0.552	0.10
Dornie	0.813	0.04
Ala di Stura	0.529	0.19
Swansea	0.601	0.23
Jamestown	0.228	0.57
Korea	0.132	0.91

Table 12.3 contains the Pearson index and criteria particle fraction for six mineral subtypes in the study.

Based on the proposed criteria, for combined datasets (see Materials and Methods section), the following classification was performed:

Non-asbestiform	*Asbestiform*
Shinness	Korea
Dornie	Jamestown
Ala di Stura	
Swansea	

Using the same set of independent variables, we can model the potency factor for peritoneal mesothelioma in human cohorts.

The regression equation we determined is as follows:

$$R_{M\text{-}Per} = -0.07 + 0.00018Fe + 0.0023EMPA + 0.035\log_{10}(Bioper)$$

where $R_{M\text{-}Per}$ is the peritoneal mesothelioma potency factor (%),

EMPA is the fraction of fibers with width ≤ 0.15 μm among fibers longer than 5 μm (%),

Bioper is the Biopersistence (Years), and

Fe is the iron content in fibers (%).

($R = 0.9998$, $R^2 = 0.9996$, $p < 0.02$).

The relationship is illustrated in Figure 12.3.

It should be noted that the hazard rate in animals and the potency factor in humans are not expected to belong to a similar scale or be comparable. It is remarkable, though, that these characteristics can be modeled by using the same predictors.

The observed and modeled potency factors for peritoneal mesothelioma in humans are demonstrated in Table 12.4.

Generally, the model provides an acceptable level of predictive accuracy. The model estimated the potency of Libby amphiboles for peritoneal mesothelioma in

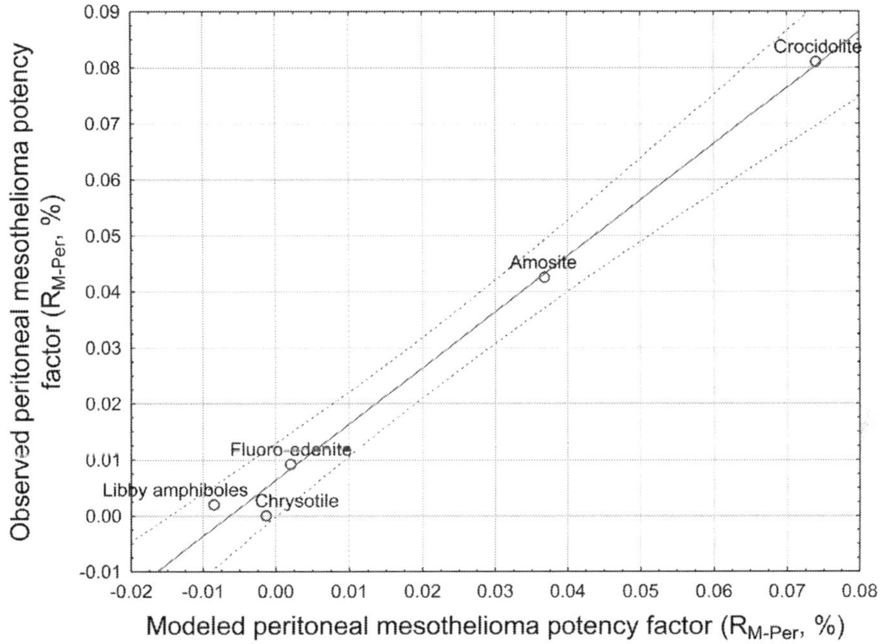

FIGURE 12.3 The relationship between the modeled and observed peritoneal mesothelioma potency factor in humans.

TABLE 12.4
Observed and modeled peritoneal mesothelioma potency in humans

Mineral type	Peritoneal mesothelioma potency factor (%), observed	Peritoneal mesothelioma potency factor (%), modeled
Chrysotile	0.000051	<0
Amosite	0.0425	0.039
Crocidolite	0.08	0.076
Libby amphiboles	0.002	<0
Fluoro-edenite	0.00923	0.006
Anthophyllite	-	0.024
Erionite	-	0.10
Balangeroite	-	0.007

humans as negligible. That may require additional confirmation. Only one case from 15 mesothelioma cases in Darnton's cohort for Libby amphiboles was of peritoneal origin. Potentially, it could be a case of spontaneous mesothelioma.

Anthophyllite mesothelioma potency (0.056% for all types of mesotheliomas) was initially estimated by Korchevskiy et al. (2013) for Russian anthophyllite workers and the population; no data specifically for peritoneal mesotheliomas were available.

Meurman et al. (1994) reported that among four cases of mesothelioma among Finnish anthophyllite workers, one was of peritoneal origin. In this case, we can estimate the peritoneal mesothelioma potency for anthophyllite as 0.014%, slightly lower but of the same order as our predicted value (0.024%).

The potency of fibrous balangeroite is estimated as 0.007% by our model. As previously noted, our published analysis found about three balangeroite-related cases of mesothelioma in the cohort of asbestos workers in Balangero, from a total of seven cases. The total mesothelioma potency of balangeroite is 0.045% (Korchevskiy & Wylie, 2023). In this case, the number of peritoneal mesothelioma cases in the same cohort can be estimated as 0.46 (<1), explaining why no actual peritoneal mesothelioma cases were recorded.

The peritoneal mesothelioma potency of erionite is estimated as 0.10%. Assuming that the total mesothelioma potency factor for erionite is 2.58% as predicted by the "blind" model in the Korchevskiy et al. (2019) study, about 3.87% of mesothelioma cases related to erionite in Karain, Turkey, should be peritoneal. As we mentioned earlier, the lowest fraction of peritoneal mesotheliomas in the total mesothelioma count of erionite-related cohorts was 4.4%, very close to our estimation.

The biopersistence of glaucophane is unknown, so it is impossible to estimate peritoneal mesothelioma potency based on our model.

It is also possible to evaluate peritoneal mesothelioma potency of non-asbestiform varieties of fibrous minerals. For example, if amosite peritoneal mesothelioma potency is 0.04%, the potency of its non-asbestiform grunerite variety is predicted to be less than 0 (negligible).

We can also use DCC as one of the independent variables. In this case, the regression equation will be as follows:

$$R_{M\text{-}Per} = -0.06 + 0.0003Fe + 0.92DCC + 0.02\log_{10}(Bioper),$$

where $R_{M\text{-}Per}$ is the peritoneal mesothelioma potency factor (%),

DCC is the dimensional coefficient of carcinogenicity,
Bioper is the biosolubility, and
Fe is the iron content in fibers (weight %).
($R = 0.983$, $R^2 = 0.997$, $p < 0.23$).

This shows that DCC appears to be a less efficient predictor of peritoneal mesothelioma potency than EMPA.

Based on the developed regression equations, peritoneal mesothelioma potency in humans can be estimated for six samples of tremolite in Davis' study. The results are shown in Table 12.5.

According to the modeling results, all four types of tremolite, characterized as non-asbestiform according to dimensional characteristics, demonstrate negligible peritoneal mesothelioma potency in humans.

DISCUSSION

For decades, animal experiments were one of the limited sources of knowledge about the toxicity of elongate mineral particles. However, many questions remain regarding

TABLE 12.5
Modeled peritoneal mesothelioma potency in the fibers tested by Davis' experiment (based on the EMPA regression).

Type of tremolite	Modeled peritoneal mesothelioma potency (%), EMPA-based
Shinness	<0
Dornie	<0
Ala di Stura	<0
Swansea	<0
Jamestown	0.001
Korea	0.019

the interpretation of both *in vivo* and *in vitro* laboratory results for human toxicology and risk assessment. For example, Saffiotti (2005) listed numerous agents causing mesotheliomas in laboratory animals, while in humans, mesothelioma is seen as prevailingly related to asbestos exposure. Berman and Crump (2003) addressed the differences in observations on asbestos carcinogenicity between animals and humans, suggesting that "different mechanisms drive the effects observed in the animal studies than those that dominate for asbestos-induced cancers in humans and that such mechanisms depend more strongly on mineralogy."

The peritoneal injection study in rats by Davis is an example of a landmark experiment that has been a matter of scientific discussion for years. In our paper, we revisited the results of Davis' study based on the retesting of the tremolite samples that he utilized for the induction of peritoneal mesothelioma. We considered the methodology for analyzing and modeling the impact of the dimensional parameters of these tremolite samples on the toxicity level, as outlined in several recent publications (Wylie & Korchevskiy, 2023; Korchevskiy & Wylie, 2021, 2022).

We modeled the hazard rate of peritoneal mesothelioma in the Davis study utilizing three variables: wt % iron oxide content of the fibers, EMPA parameter (reflecting the fraction of very thin fibers among the particles longer than 5 μm), biopersistence (based on Gualtieri et al., 2018), and estimation of the acellular dissolution rate of various fiber-forming minerals, with several assumptions made about fibers not included in the Gualtieri study, as described in Chapter 4. We also utilized a new variable, the dimensional coefficient of carcinogenicity (DCC), introduced in Chapter 4 and in Korchevskiy and Wylie (2025a, 2025b). The dimensional coefficient of carcinogenicity is a metric estimating the relative probability of fibers to induce mesothelioma, based on the sequence of events proposed for pleural mesothelioma, as described in Chapter 5. We explored whether the DCC would also be a good predictor of peritoneal mesothelioma potency factors.

It should be noted that EMPA and iron content are not statistically related in Davis' tremolite sample ($R = -0.23$, $p > 0.05$). For various types of mineral fibers, EMPA is also unrelated to iron content ($R = 0.0015$, $p > 0.05$).

We determined that the hazard rate of malignant peritoneal mesothelioma in rats can be efficiently approximated by a regression on EMPA, total wt % iron content, and biopersistence, with a correlation coefficient of $R = 0.984$, $R^2 = 0.968$, $p < 0.00565$. If EMPA is replaced by the DCC parameter, a regression equation can also be developed with $R = 0.979$, $R^2 = 0.959$, $p < 0.00841$.

We also utilized a method for estimating the habit of mineral samples from the Davis study. We demonstrated that four samples in the study were non-asbestiform: Shinness, Dornie, Swansea, and Ala di Stura; while two were asbestiform: Jamestown and Korea. With the exception of Swansea tremolite, which the original team characterized as asbestiform, this classification is identical to that provided by Davis in the qualitative analysis of habit.

The hazard rate of peritoneal mesothelioma in rats from Davis' experiments cannot be considered a direct predictor of potency in human exposure. The direct instillation of fibers into the peritoneal cavity does not replicate the process of fiber transfer to this area that begins with inhalation, requiring additional steps, each with its own probability. However, we hypothesized that EMPA, iron content, and biopersistence can be predictors of peritoneal mesothelioma in humans.

We estimated the peritoneal mesothelioma potency in humans of different mineral sources based on the updated information for the Hodgson and Darnton method (Darnton, 2023). The mentioned dimensional database was used to calculate selected dimensional parameters to analyze along with the mesothelioma potency information.

It should be noted that peritoneal mesothelioma potency has not been directly calculated and published until this study, although the data for calculations were available from Hodgson and Darnton (2000). First, we showed that the difference in peritoneal mesothelioma potency between various samples of the same mineral can be explained by the same variables that best explained the difference in peritoneal mesothelioma relative hazard in rats. We explored the prediction of observed peritoneal potency factors for crocidolite, amosite, chrysotile, fluoro-edenite, and Libby amphiboles, and confirmed the accuracy of the predictions. We also calculated peritoneal mesothelioma potency factors for anthophyllite and balangeroite and demonstrated that the available information is consistent with the results of our modeling. For example, the data from the Finland study (as reported by Meurman et al., 1994) suggest an approximate peritoneal mesothelioma potency of anthophyllite at the level of about 0.014%, with our model estimating it as 0.024%, a close approximation. Our model showed the potency factor of balangeroite, reasonably approximating the data for balangeroite potency as reconstructed in Korchevskiy and Wylie (2023). We confirmed very low (negligible) peritoneal mesothelioma potency for chrysotile asbestos.

Our estimation of the peritoneal mesothelioma potency factor for erionite is slightly lower than expected, with the fraction of peritoneal mesothelioma in the erionite-exposed cohort quantified as about 3.7%, while the lowest estimation of this fraction derived from various sources is about 4.4%. Further studies are warranted to clarify the role of various factors impacting the mesothelioma potency of zeolites.

Based on the developed model, we were also able to reconstruct the peritoneal mesothelioma potency for the six samples of tremolite. All four tremolite samples determined to be non-asbestiform are determined to have negligible peritoneal mesothelioma potency, while two asbestiform samples have statistically significant potency to produce peritoneal mesothelioma.

We see differences in the level of factors and characteristics that cause pleural and peritoneal mesothelioma in humans vs. the effects observed in animals. Several of the tremolite populations characterized as non-asbestiform still produced some rates of peritoneal mesothelioma in Davis' experiment on rats. However, all non-asbestiform fibers had negligible (<0) peritoneal mesothelioma potency, as determined by our modeling.

Also, Carbone et al. (2019) emphasized the substantial differences in mechanisms and clinical manifestations of pleural and peritoneal mesothelioma, suggesting that peritoneal mesothelioma is much less often associated with asbestos exposure. However, non-asbestos-related peritoneal mesotheliomas in humans are, for the most part, a result of spontaneous processes (like the case study described in Yoo et al., 2019, where idiopathic or spontaneous peritoneal mesothelioma is characterized).

Our study has significant uncertainties and limitations. In fact, it would be beneficial to replicate the full study of Davis with higher numbers of animals and samples of fibrous minerals. Comparing tremolite potency with other types of asbestiform and non-asbestiform materials in the same experiment would be very interesting. It would also be extremely useful to compare intraperitoneal and inhalation studies in animals. However, the organization of large studies on animals is even less realistic now than previously, as the toxicological community considers further limitations on animal testing. While modeling cannot substitute for actual real-life observations, it is obvious that in the future, toxicology will rely on *in silico* tools to a large scale. In our paper, we demonstrated that the spectrum of information derived from historical animal studies (like Davis' experiment in rats) can be significantly expanded even without replicating the original test. The insights from the peritoneal mesothelioma induction in rats can, with due limitations, be utilized in human toxicology, epidemiology, and risk assessment.

NOTE

1 Chatfield (personal communication) has found very thin pyroxene fibers in the chrysotile samples from Balangero which may be a factor in potency.

REFERENCE LIST

Adachi, S., Kawamura, K., & Takemoto, K. (2001). A trial on the quantitative risk assessment of man-made mineral fibers by the rat intraperitoneal administration assay using the JFM standard fibrous samples. *Industrial Health*, *39*(2), 168–174. https://doi.org/10.2486/indhealth.39.168

Attanoos, R. L., Churg, A., Galateau-Salle, F., Gibbs, A. R., & Roggli, V. L. (2018). Malignant mesothelioma and its non-asbestos causes. *Archives of Pathology & Laboratory Medicine*, *142*(6), 753–760. https://doi.org/10.5858/arpa.2017-0365-RA

Berman, D. W., & Crump, K. S. (2003). *Final draft: Technical support document for a protocol to assess asbestos-related risk* (EPA #9345.4-06). Document Display, NEPIS, US EPA.

Boffetta, P. (2007). Epidemiology of peritoneal mesothelioma: A review. *Annals of Oncology*, *18*(6), 985–990. https://doi.org/10.1093/annonc/mdl345

Bruno, C., Tumino, R., Fazzo, L., Cascone, G., Cernigliaro, A., De Santis, M., Giurdanella, M. C., Nicita, C., Rollo, P. C., Scondotto, S., Spata, E., Zona, A., & Comba, P. (2014). Incidence of pleural mesothelioma in a community exposed to fibres with fluoro-edenitic composition in Biancavilla (Sicily, Italy). *Annali dell'Istituto Superiore di Sanita*, *50*(2), 111–118. https://doi.org/10.4415/ANN_14_02_02

Carbone, M., Adusumilli, P. S., Alexander, H. R., Jr., Baas, P., Bardelli, F., Bononi, A., Bueno, R., Felley-Bosco, E., Galateau-Salle, F., Jablons, D., Mansfield, A. S., Minaai, M., de Perrot, M., Pesavento, P., Rusch, V., Severson, D. T., Taioli, E., Tsao, A., Woodard, G., . . . Pass, H. I. (2019). Mesothelioma: Scientific clues for prevention, diagnosis, and therapy. *CA: A Cancer Journal for Clinicians*, *69*(5), 402–429. https://doi.org/10.3322/caac.21572

Chatfield, E. J. (2018). Measurement of elongate mineral particles: What we should measure and how do we do it? *Toxicology and Applied Pharmacology*, *361*, 36–46. https://doi.org/10.1016/j.taap.2018.08.010

Chatfield, E. J. (2021). Size distributions of amphibole EMPs used in two independent intraperitoneal injection studies on rats. In J. R. Millette & J. S. Webber (Eds.), *Asbestos and other elongate mineral particles – new and continuing challenges in the 21st century*. ASTM International.

Darnton, L. (2023). Quantitative assessment of mesothelioma and lung cancer risk based on phase contrast microscopy (PCM) estimates of fibre exposure: An update of 2000 asbestos cohort data. *Environmental Research*, *230*, 114753. https://doi.org/10.1016/j.envres.2022.114753

Davis, J. M., Addison, J., McIntosh, C., Miller, B. G., & Niven, K. (1991). Variations in the carcinogenicity of tremolite dust samples of differing morphology. *Annals of the New York Academy of Sciences*, *643*, 473–490. https://doi.org/10.1111/j.1749-6632.1991.tb24497.x

Ferrante, D., Mirabelli, D., Silvestri, S., Azzolina, D., Giovannini, A., Tribaudino, P., & Magnani, C. (2020). Mortality and mesothelioma incidence among chrysotile asbestos miners in Balangero, Italy: A cohort study. *American Journal of Industrial Medicine*, *63*(2), 135–145. https://doi.org/10.1002/ajim.23071

Greenbaum, A., & Alexander, H. R. (2020). Peritoneal mesothelioma. *Translational Lung Cancer Research*, *9*(Suppl 1), S120–S132. https://doi.org/10.21037/tlcr.2019.12.15

Gualtieri, A. F., Pollastri, S., Gandolfi, N. B., & Gualtieri, M. L. (2018). In vitro acellular dissolution of mineral fibres: A comparative study. *Scientific Reports*, *8*, 7071. https://doi.org/10.1038/s41598-018-25531-4

Hodgson, J., & Darnton, A. (2000). The quantitative risks of mesothelioma and lung cancer in relation to asbestos exposure. *Annals of Occupational Hygiene*, *44*(8), 565–601. https://pubmed.ncbi.nlm.nih.gov/11108782/

Hu, Q., Akatsuka, S., & Yamashita, Y. (2010). Homozygous deletion of *CDKN2A/2B* is a hallmark of iron-induced high-grade rat mesothelioma. *Laboratory Investigation*, *90*(3), 360–373. https://doi.org/10.1038/labinvest.2009.140

Korchevskiy, A. A., Rasmuson, E. J., Rasmuson, J. O., & Strode, R. D. (2013, February 24–27). *Asbestos mining in Russia: Approaches to public health risk assessment* (Preprint 13–117). Mining: It's All About People. Pre-Prints of the Society for Mining, Metallurgy & Exploration Annual Meeting, Denver, CO.

Korchevskiy, A. A., Rasmuson, J. O., & Rasmuson, E. J. (2019). Empirical model of mesothelioma potency factors for different mineral fibers based on their chemical composition and dimensionality. *Inhalation Toxicology*, *31*(5), 189–191. https://doi.org/10.1080/08958378.2019.1640320

Korchevskiy, A. A., & Wylie, A. G. (2021). Dimensional determinants for the carcinogenic potency of elongate amphibole particles. *Inhalation Toxicology*, *33*(6–8), 244–259. https://doi.org/10.1080/08958378.2021.1971340

Korchevskiy, A. A., & Wylie, A. G. (2023). Toxicological and epidemiological approaches to carcinogenic potency modeling for mixed mineral fiber exposure: The case of fibrous balangeroite and chrysotile. *Inhalation Toxicology*, *35*(7–8), 185–200. https://doi.org/10.1080/08958378.2023.2213720

Korchevskiy, A. A., & Wylie, A. G. (2025a). Habit of elongate amphibole particles as a predictor of mesothelial carcinogenicity. *Toxicology Reports*, *14*, 101908. https://doi.org/10.1016/j.toxrep.2025.101908

Korchevskiy, A. A., & Wylie, A. G. (2025b, April 24). The empirical metric of mesothelial carcinogenicity for carbon nanotubes and elongate mineral particles. *Inhalation Toxicology* (online). https://doi.org/10.1080/08958378.2025.2486087

Korchevskiy, A. A., & Wylie, A. G. (2022). Dimensional characteristics of the major types of amphibole mineral particles and the implications for carcinogenic risk assessment. *Inhalation Toxicology*, *34*(1–2), 24–38. https://doi.org/10.1080/08958378.2021.2024304

Meurman, L. O., Pukkala, E., & Hakama, M. (1994). Incidence of cancer among anthophyllite asbestos miners in Finland. *Occupational and Environmental Medicine*, *51*(6), 421–425. https://doi.org/10.1136/oem.51.6.421

Miller, B. G., Searl, A., Davis, J. M., Donaldson, K., Cullen, R. T., Bolton, R. E., Buchanan, D., & Soutar, C. A. (1999). Influence of fibre length, dissolution and biopersistence on the production of mesothelioma in the rat peritoneal cavity. *Annals of Occupational Hygiene*, *43*(3), 155–166. PMID: 10366897.

Okada, S., Hamazaki, S., Toyokuni, S., & Midorikawa, O. (1989). Induction of mesothelioma by intraperitoneal injections of ferric saccharate in male Wistar rats. *British Journal of Cancer*, *60*, 708–711. https://doi.org/10.1038/bjc.1989.344

Pelnar, P. V. (1988). Further evidence of nonasbestos-related mesothelioma. A review of the literature. *Scandinavian Journal of Work and Environmental Health*, *14*(3), 141–144. https://doi.org/10.5271/sjweh.1939

Saffiotti, U. (2005). Mesothelioma carcinogenesis: In vivo models. In H. I. Pass, N. J. Vogelzang, & M. Carbone (Eds.), *Malignant mesothelioma*. Springer. https://doi.org/10.1007/0-387-28274-2_4

Testa, J. R. (2017). Malignant mesothelioma: An asbestos legacy. In J. R. Testa (Ed.), *Asbestos and mesothelioma*. Current Cancer Research Book Series. https://doi.org/10.1007/978-3-319-53560-9_1

Verkouteren, J. R., & Wylie, A. G. (2000). The tremolite-actinolite-ferro-actinolite series: Systematic relationships among cell parameters, composition, optical properties, and habit, and evidence of discontinuities. *American Mineralogist*, *85*(9), 1239–1254. https://doi.org/10.2138/am-2000-8-917

Wylie, A. G., & Korchevskiy, A. A. (2023). Dimensions of elongate mineral particles and cancer: A review. *Environmental Research*, *230*, 114688. https://doi.org/10.1016/j.envres.2022.114688

Wylie, A. G., Korchevskiy, A. A., Segrave, A., & Duane, A. (2020). Modeling mesothelioma risk factors from amphibole fiber dimensionality: Mineralogical and epidemiological perspective. *Journal of Applied Toxicology*, *40*(4), 515–524. https://doi.org/10.1002/jat.3923

Wylie, A. G., Korchevskiy, A. A., Van Orden, D. R., & Chatfield, E. J. (2022). Discriminant analysis of asbestiform and non-asbestiform amphibole particles and its implications for toxicological studies. *Computational Toxicology*, *23*, 100233. https://doi.org/10.1016/j.comtox.2022.100233

Yoo, S. H., Kim, H. M., Park, J. K., Kim, M. S., & Yi, S. Y. (2019). A case of peritoneal sarcomatoid mesothelioma with absence of occupational exposure to asbestos. *Kosin Medical Journal*, *34*(2), 146–151. https://doi.org/10.7180/kmj.2019.34.2.146

13 Asbestos terminology

How to combine mineralogical, toxicological, and analytical information for the purpose of standardization

A. Korchevskiy & A. Wylie

INTRODUCTION

Asbestos terminology has developed organically in several scientific areas over the past decades, with terms that have different meanings in the mineralogical literature, causing significant discrepancies and controversies that continue today. The term "asbestos" is a historical commercial term related to a specific type of mined mineral dating back to Roman times. The overwhelming evidence of the toxicity of mineral fibers among asbestos industry workers means that every toxic mineral fiber has been referred to as "asbestos." The regulatory definition of asbestos in the United States usually includes a list of minerals covered by the term, namely chrysotile, crocidolite, amosite, anthophyllite asbestos, tremolite asbestos, and actinolite asbestos. However, the U.S. EPA, in its toxicological review of 2014, used the term "Libby amphibole asbestos" for the solid solution series of several minerals, including winchite and richterite, that occur together in the vermiculite mine in Libby, Montana (U.S. EPA, 2014). In 2011, NIOSH developed a research roadmap for "asbestos fibers and other elongate mineral particles," raising the idea that there is a wider class of minerals that might be "asbestos or at least asbestos-like in carcinogenicity," and suggesting that structures resulting from the crushing or fracturing of non-fibrous minerals (e.g., cleavage fragments) might be significantly different in toxicity from commercial asbestos fibers, recommending additional research (NIOSH, 2011). NIOSH also introduced a new term: "elongate mineral particle (EMP)," defined by a ratio of length to width, the aspect ratio, of 3:1 or greater, to cover both fiber and fragment. In 2002, Lowers and Meeker attempted to tabulate asbestos-related terminology from various bibliographic sources, listing dozens of definitions for the terms acicular, asbestiform, asbestos, cleavage, cleavage fragments, fiber, fibril, fibrous, and parting (Lowers & Meeker, 2002). Organizations that produce standard protocols for laboratory analysis, such as ASTM International and the International Organization for

DOI: 10.1201/9781003424277-14

Standardization (ISO), have standards with definitions of key terms that vary among their own methods.

The inconsistency in terminology affects science, regulations, and public perceptions of the problem. The majority of toxicological information for mineral fibers is available only for elongate mineral particles longer than 5 μm, which we denote as EMP-5 (Hodgson & Darnton, 2000; Berman & Crump, 2008a, 2008b; Darnton, 2023). The toxicological difference between cleavage fragments and asbestiform fibers is well established in scientific literature (Mossman, 2008; Wylie & Korchevskiy, 2023). Some sources, however, argue that biological systems may not distinguish between asbestos and cleavage fragments because they are only affected by "shape, size dimensions and surface charge" (Gordon, 2018). Such arguments overlook the fact that cleavage fragments, belonging to the category of elongate mineral particles, have statistically confirmed significant differences in size and shape compared to asbestiform fibers (Korchevskiy & Wylie, 2021), and the net surface charge of cleavage fragments is also different from asbestos (Schiller et al., 1980). Also, the ASTM and ISO approaches to define asbestos fibers as structures longer than 0.5 μm with an aspect ratio equal to or greater than 5:1 make it incompatible with toxicological literature and risk assessment. To avoid misunderstandings in the characterizations of exposure for workers and communities, and to help advance research efforts, better definitions of asbestos-related terms are needed to ensure that the real mineralogical and toxicological meanings for the terminology are clear and interrelated.

We suggest the following basis for sound asbestos terminology:

a) ***Elongate mineral particles (EMP)*** is an umbrella term for a class of particulates that have a length at least three times greater than width. Some EMPs are associated with potential adverse toxicological outcomes following inhalation.
b) Such interrelated characteristics as dimensions, shape, mechanical properties, and mineral composition of EMPs define the level of carcinogenic potency for EMPs.
c) Cleavage fragments are non-asbestiform particles making up a class of EMPs produced by mechanical forces and not by mineral growth. Cleavage fragments have distinct dimensional characteristics compared to asbestiform fibers, affecting the difference in their carcinogenicity, even when the mineral composition is the same.
d) Only a specific sub-class of EMPs can be defined as "carcinogenic" EMPs, signifying differences between fibers that are carcinogenic and nuisance dust.

Basic definitions of asbestos-related terms were proposed in Chapter 1 of this book. This chapter will revisit the content of the book and demonstrate how the toxicology of elongate mineral particles affects the establishment of a set of definitions that would be scientifically based and efficient in application to various fields of theory and practice.

OBJECTIVES

To establish a version of asbestos terminology that is consistent with mineralogical and toxicological observations and principles.

To explore the relationship between the habit of EMP datasets (asbestiform vs. non-asbestiform) and their dimensional characteristics.

To relate the toxic potential and carcinogenicity of EMPs with parameters reflecting their dimensions and habit.

MATERIALS AND METHODS

1. As described elsewhere in this book (Chapter 2), the database with dimensional characteristics of elongate mineral particles, now containing 569,090 records for 240 asbestiform, non-asbestiform, and mixed datasets for various mineral types, deposits, sources, and analytical methods, was utilized. The information was reorganized into 78 datasets for specific minerals and locations, assuming known asbestiform or non-asbestiform habit.
2. Criteria particles were defined according to the formula from Wylie et al. (2022):

$$C = 2.99\log_{10}(\text{length}) - 5.82\log_{10}(\text{width}) - 3.80$$

   which is positive for criteria particles and negative for non-criteria particles, assuming EMP–5. To define mesotheliomagenic EMP-5s, various width fractions of EMP-5 were correlated with potency factor R_M (Darnton, 2023). The cutpoint of 0.15 μm was demonstrated as a possible cutpoint for mesotheliomagenic particles (so-called EMPA particles) (as in Wylie et al., 2020). Because of possible measurement error in the size of particles, however, the upper cutpoint can fluctuate from about 0.10 to 0.20 μm. Nevertheless, we hypothesize that a fraction of such thin particles longer than 5 μm is a necessary condition and predictor of mesotheliomagenicity.
3. The relationship between criteria particle classification, mesotheliomagenic particles, and specific surface area was demonstrated.
4. The fraction of criteria particles and Pearson index (a linear correlation coefficient in the regression between $\log_{10}$-transformed width and length of EMP-2) were tested for classification of datasets as asbestiform vs./non-asbestiform.
5. The fraction of criteria particles was correlated with mesothelioma potency factors/hazard rates based on human occupational data by Darnton (2023), pleural mesothelioma in rats by Cook et al. (2016), and peritoneal mesothelioma in rats by Davis et al. (1991).
6. The mesothelioma potency factor R_M (%) was correlated with the fraction of EMPA particles and biopersistence measured as acellular dissolution lifetime of fibers with a width of 0.25 μm (Gualtieri et al., 2018) for chrysotile, crocidolite, amosite, erionite, and Libby amphiboles.
7. The combined classification of datasets as asbestiform/non-asbestiform and definitely mesotheliomagenic/other particles was performed.

RESULTS

1. Figure 13.1 demonstrates the correlation between mesothelioma and lung cancer potency factors and the size fraction of EMP-5 particles. To take into

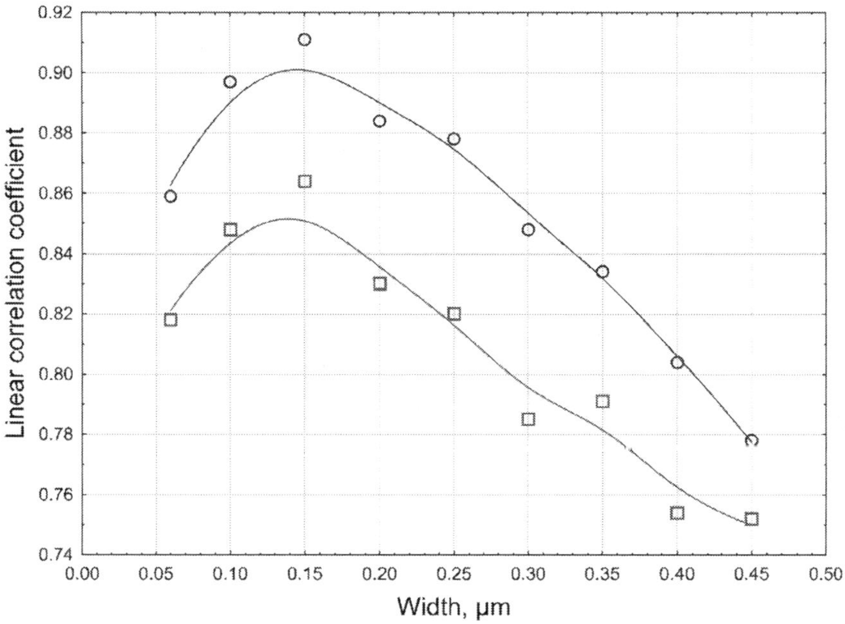

FIGURE 13.1 The relationship between the linear correlations between mesothelioma (blue circles) and lung cancer (red squares) potency factors and the fraction of elongate mineral particles fitting the width criteria (less than a certain cutpoint).

account possible measurement error (see Chapter 2), the correlations were averaged for intervals of cutpoints with a size of 0.05. It was determined that the width level of 0.15 to 0.20 μm maximizes the linear correlation between the fraction of EMP-5 fitting the width criteria and both the mesothelioma and lung cancer potency factors. We determined that the objective meaning of this relationship is that EMPs are carcinogenic when their width is less than the cutpoint, maximizing the correlation (value in the interval 0.15 to 0.20 μm). Earlier, we demonstrated that 0.15 or 0.17 μm can serve as a value of width maximizing the correlation with potency. We assume that the interval 0.15 to 0.20 μm serves as a conservative estimation of the upper cutpoint for maximizing the correlation, considering possible measurement error. The decrease of the correlation after this interval can be explained by the hypothesis that fibers are mesotheliomagenic up to the upper width of 0.2 μm and not for the higher values of the width (see Chapter 4 for additional explanations.) Earlier (Korchevskiy & Wylie, 2021), we suggested that the width cutpoint for lung cancer is slightly higher than for mesothelioma, but combining correlations by width intervals shows that the difference may be absent, and approximately the same interval contains maxima for both lung cancer and mesothelioma potency factors.

There are several reasons why particles longer than 5 μm and thinner than 0.15 to 0.20 μm are mesothelial carcinogens and other particles have much lower or non-existent potential to produce mesothelial cancer. Apparently, EMPA particles have an aerodynamic diameter in the range that would allow them to reach the pleura with higher probability. They also seem to have sufficient specific surface area to produce inflammation and, at the same time, to be able to pierce cell membranes or activate size and shape-related reactions for the survival of damaged cells.

As we demonstrated in Chapter 4, several biological events are needed for pleural cancer to develop: the particles should reach the pleura; they should be able to cause expanded chronic inflammation in pleural tissue; and the particles should have qualities of length, width, chemical composition, and rigidity that cause cell damage and, at the same time, counteract autoimmunity and repair mechanisms. This chain of events, causing malignant pleural mesothelioma, as we suggested, should have a probability proportional to particle biopersistence, surface area, and reciprocal width with a certain power. When the probability of particles to cause cancer decreases below statistical significance, no risk elevated above a baseline would be observed in epidemiological studies. For this reason, mineralogically asbestiform particles can produce cancer with various levels of potency, while non-asbestiform cannot.

Table 13.1 shows the difference between particles longer than 5 μm with width ≤0.2 μm vs. width >0.2 μm for key parameters characterizing their toxicity potential. As we can see, particles with width ≤0.2 μm have significantly higher specific surface area, length and dimensional coefficient of carcinogenicity (DCC), and significantly lower surface area, width, and aerodynamic diameter. All differences are statistically significant at $p<0.001$.

2. All elongate mineral particles can be subdivided into four groups based on two dichotomies: definitely mesotheliomagenic – all other particles; and criteria – non-criteria particles, as demonstrated in Figure 13.2. Both

TABLE 13.1
Characteristics of particles with width ≤0.2 μm vs. particles with width >0.2 μm (average/standard deviation).

	Surface area (μm^2)	Specific surface area per volume (μm^{-1})	Length (μm)	Width (μm)	Aerodynamic diameter (μm)	Dimensional Coefficient of Carcinogenicity (DCC)
Length >5 μm, width ≤0.20 μm	6.23 (9.27)	41.55 (12.39)	14.23 (19.81)	0.14 (0.04)	0.76 (0.22)	0.15 (0.14)
Length >5 μm, width >0.20 μm	29.66 (57.36)	11.43 (6.68)	10.94 (18.28)	0.90 (0.68)	4.2 (2.68)	0.01 (0.03)

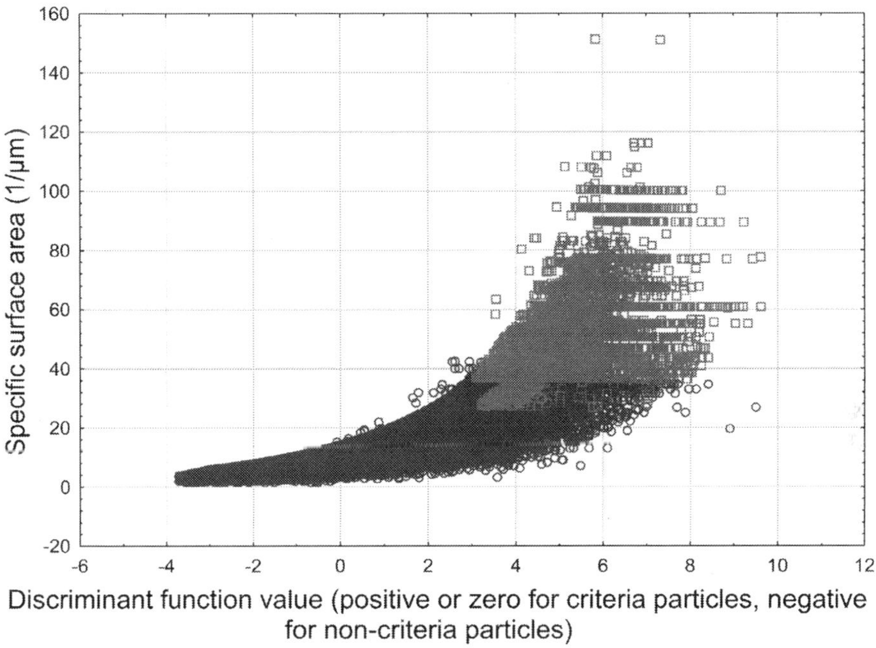

FIGURE 13.2 Relationship between specific surface area of particles and the value of the discriminant function for the determination of criteria particles. Red squares denote definitely mesotheliomagenic EMPA particles and blue circles denote other types of particles. (All mineral types except chrysotile included.)

classifications are discussed in Chapters 3, 4 and 9. Amphibole particles with a width ≤0.15 µm and length >5 µm are "definitely carcinogenic," though their carcinogenic potential depends on the exposure level and chemical composition, rigidity, and/or biopersistence. All other amphibole particles are considered not classifiable for carcinogenicity based on our models (though their classification for carcinogenicity should also be analyzed in the context of all involved characteristics). Figure 13.2 illustrates that non-criteria particles do not belong to the "definitely carcinogenic category." Specific surface area (surface area divided by volume) is one of the predictors of mesotheliomagenicity (Korchevskiy & Wylie, 2022). As can be seen in Figure 13.2, the specific surface area of definitely mesotheliomagenic particles longer than 5 µm (interpreted as a ratio of surface area to volume) is always higher than 26 (μm^{-1}) and, in most cases, higher than 36 μm^{-1}. The specific surface area of particles correlates with the dimensional coefficient of carcinogenicity (DCC) as described in Chapter 4 ($R=0.649$, $R^2=0.42$, $p<0.0003$), although the correlation is not very high (showing that specific surface area is just one of the parameters that affects carcinogenicity).

3. The habit is a mineralogical parameter characterizing the origin and nature of individual particles in asbestiform and non-asbestiform datasets, each of which has a distinctive distribution of dimensional parameters; however, there is some overlap in dimensional characteristics. In Chapter 9, we showed that different combined dimensional characteristics can be utilized to determine the habit of particles. Such characteristics can include, for example, the fraction of criteria particles in the dataset and the fibrosity index (see Chapters 8 and 9), or the Pearson index calculated as a linear correlation coefficient between log-transformed length and width of EMP–2.

   Incorporating this information, another classification of asbestiform vs. non-asbestiform can be performed by the following method:

   If $F \geq 0.34R+0.35$, asbestiform;
   otherwise, if $0.1 \leq R \leq 0.4$ and $0.2 \leq F \leq 0.4$, unclassified,
   otherwise, non-asbestiform,
   where F is the criteria particle fraction.
   R is the Pearson index.

   The classification method was tested on a selection of 143 datasets (79 asbestiform, 51 non-asbestiform, and 13 with uncertain classification). From the asbestiform and non-asbestiform datasets, 2 datasets were misclassified, comprising a 1.5% error rate. From asbestiform datasets, 1 was misclassified as non-asbestiform, and 1 non-asbestiform dataset was misclassified as asbestiform. The precision of the method was found to be 98.7%, accuracy 98.4%. From mixed samples, 31% were determined to be unclassified by the method. No asbestiform or non-asbestiform sets were assessed as unclassified. No tremolite datasets were misclassified. Figure 13 illustrates the classification of the datasets. Figure 13.3(a) demonstrates it for all types of amphiboles, and 13.3(b) only for tremolite.
4. The fraction of criteria particles is also one of the predictors of carcinogenicity for elongate mineral particles, which can be demonstrated based on several different sources of data. For example, the fraction of criteria particles for various types of amphiboles and single-chain silicates (crocidolite, amosite, anthophyllite, fluoro-edenite, Libby amphiboles, glaucophane, balangeroite) correlates with Darnton's (2023) mesothelioma potency factors R_M with $R=0.908$, $R^2=0.82$, $p<0.0046$ (Figure 13.4a). The fraction of criteria particles of crocidolite, amosite, anthophyllite, ferro-actinolite asbestos, tremolite asbestos, aluminum silicate, dawsonite, fybex, silicon carbide, and non-fibrous grunerite correlates with the relative mesothelioma potency of fibers from intrapleural instillation experiments in rats based on the data from Cook et al. (2016) ($R=0.858$, $R^2=0.74$, $p<0.003$) (Figure 13.4b). The peritoneal mesothelioma hazard rate in rats for six varieties of tremolite correlates with the fraction of criteria particles ($R=0.864$, $R^2=0.75$, $p<0.026$) (Figure 13.4c).
   a) Correlation with Darnton (2023) mesothelioma potency in various occupational cohorts.

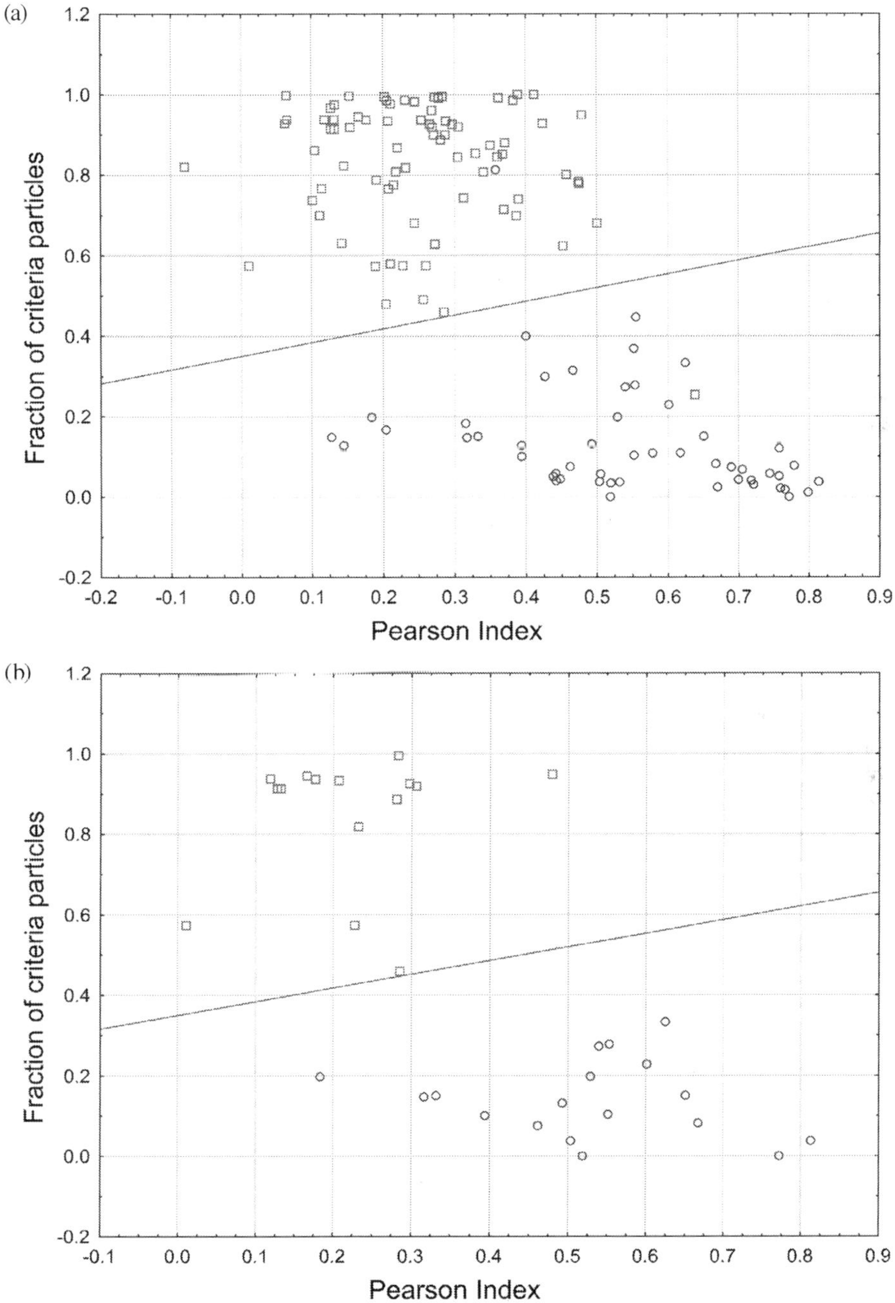

FIGURE 13.3 The classification of EMP datasets by habit, based on the dimensional parameters. Red squares denote asbestiform datasets and blue circles denote non-asbestiform datasets. a) All mineral types. b) Tremolite.

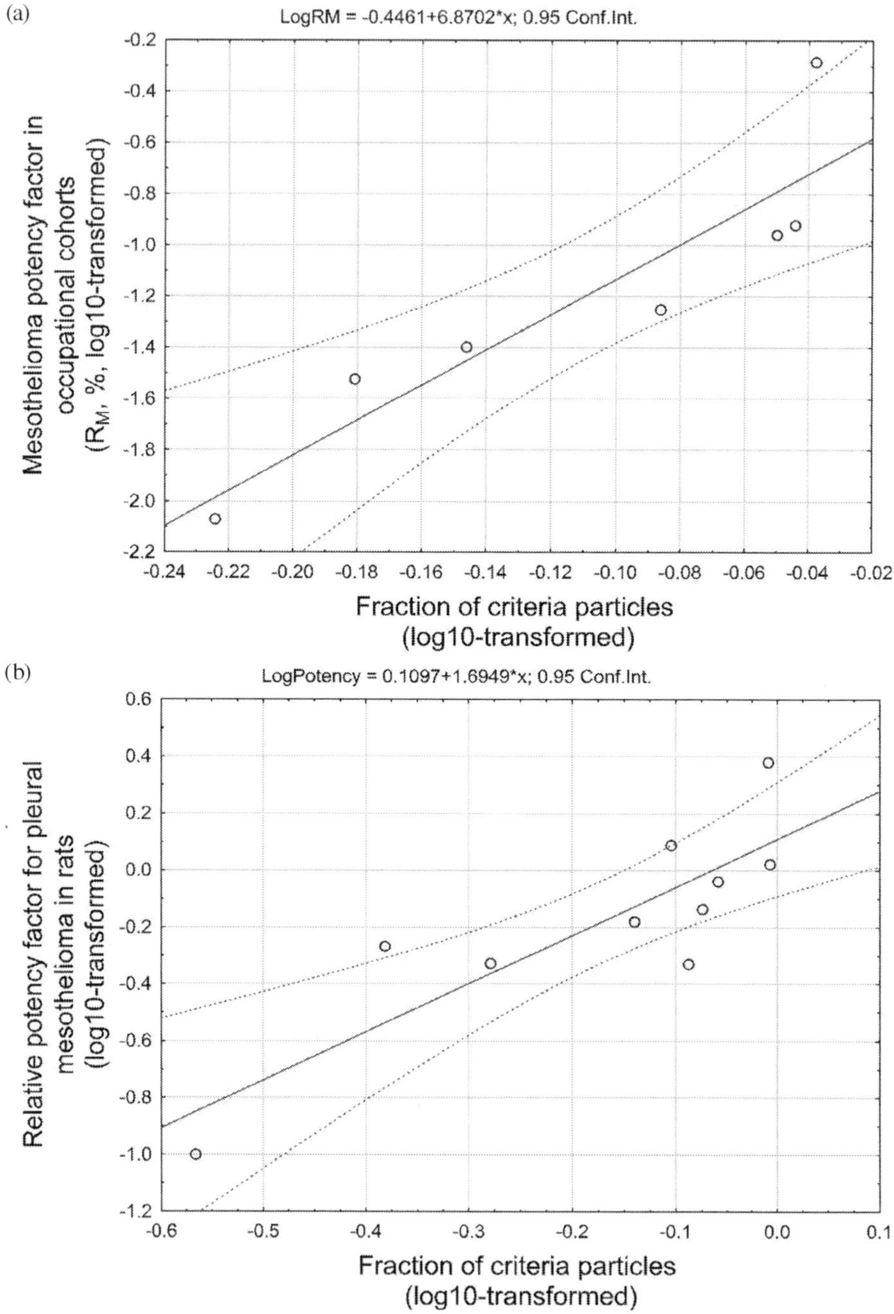

FIGURE 13.4 The relationship between mesothelioma potency and the fraction of criteria particles in exposure to EMPs. Red line denotes regression relationship and dotted lines denote 95% confidence intervals. a) Human occupational cohorts. b) Experiments with pleural instillation in laboratory animals. c) Experiments with peritoneal instillation in laboratory animals.

(c)

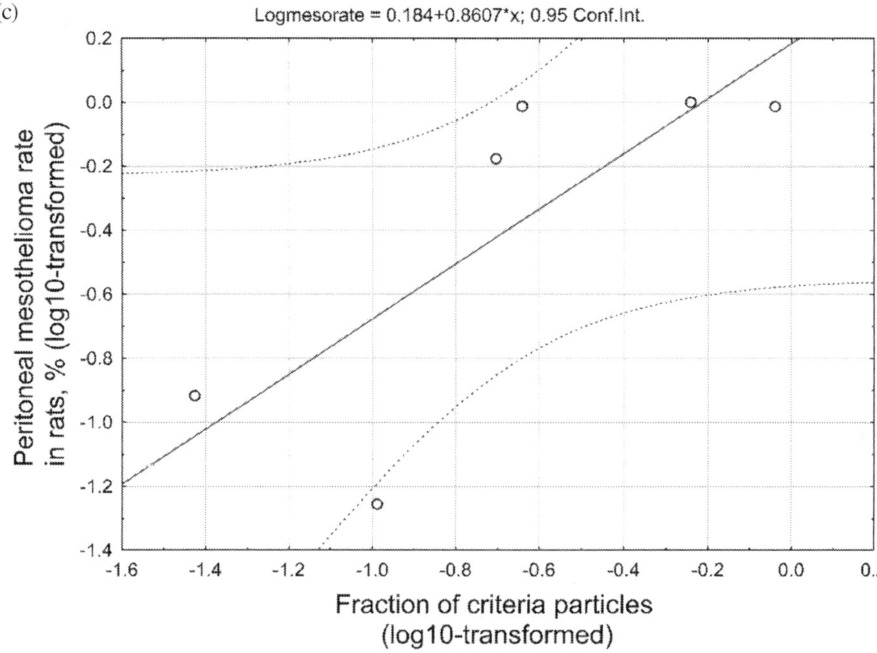

FIGURE 13.4 (Continued)

b) Correlation with potency factors for pleural instillation in rats.
c) Correlation with mesothelioma hazard rate in peritoneal instillation experiments in rats.

It should be noted that carbon nanotubes (CNTs) are an example of a "third habit" of elongate particles, with "engineered" origin instead of natural geological growth (as in asbestiform particles) or creation by mechanical force from the bulk minerals (as in cleavage fragments). CNTs cannot be classified as "asbestiform" or "nonasbestiform."

However, as we demonstrated in Chapter 4, a dimensional coefficient of carcinogenicity (DCC) can be used to distinguish between definite carcinogenic categories and other types of particles for both CNTs and EMPs. This metric is defined as:

$$DCC=1-\exp(-0.1*\text{Surface Area}/(1000\ \text{Width}^3+1)).$$

We can demonstrate a relationship between various parameters estimating particle carcinogenicity and their habit. Figure 13.5 demonstrates several average characteristics for sets in our database, grouped by location and mineral type of particles into 78 subgroups.

As we conclude, the absolute majority (94%) of datasets determined to be definite mesotheliomagenic by EMPA criteria have a fraction of particles with DCC ≥0.05 higher than 8%. There are only two sets with a DCC

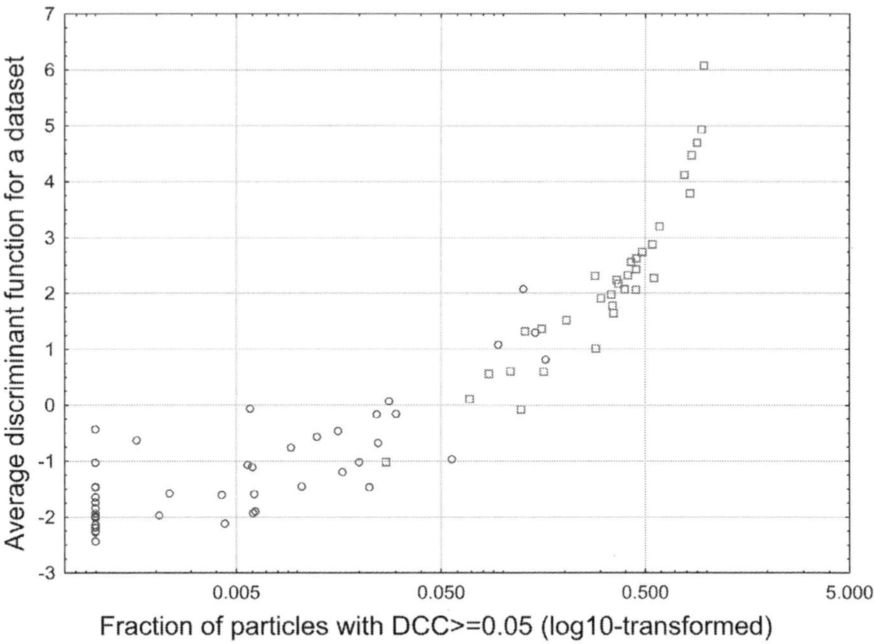

FIGURE 13.5 Relationship between the fraction of particles with DCC ≥0.05 and the average discriminant function for criteria/non-criteria EMP-5 particles (as in Chapter 9). Red squares represent datasets with EMPA statistically significantly higher than 0, while blue circles represent other datasets.

≥0.05 fraction below 8% anthophyllite from India (fraction of 2.7%) and California glaucophane (fraction of 6.7%). Anthophyllite from India could be a mixed population or outlier, requiring additional studies. Glaucophane from California has a very low mesothelioma potency compared with other amphiboles, if any (about 0.0085% as projected by Korchevskiy et al., 2019). See Korchevskiy and Wylie (2025b) for more observations about DCC and its distribution in various populations of fibers.

5. As demonstrated in Chapter 3, two factors affect the relative potency of elongate mineral particles for mesothelioma: the fraction of fibers longer than 5 μm with a width less than or equal to 0.15 μm, and biopersistence. We use the term "biopersistence" in a broad sense, combining several characteristics such as durability in a biological environment, stiffness, half-life in the lungs, and other similar parameters. In Chapter 3, we showed that the potency factor R_M (%) correlates with the EMPA parameter and biopersistence measured in terms of Gualtieri's acellular lifetime of dissolving fibers, for two types of crocidolite (from Australia and South Africa), amosite, Libby amphiboles, chrysotile, and erionite (Gualtieri et al., 2018). The relationship is demonstrated in Figure 13.6. The log-log regression is

$$Log_{10}(RM) = -4.06 + 1.01Log_{10}(EMPA) + 1.21Log_{10}(Bioper),$$

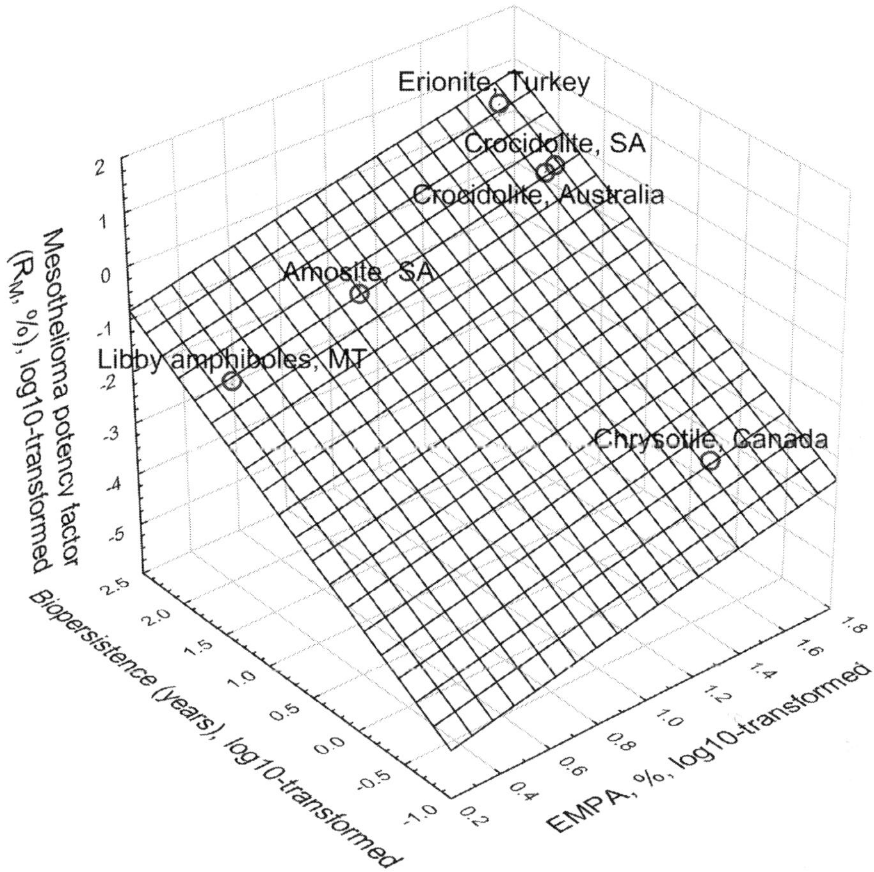

FIGURE 13.6 The regression of the mesothelioma potency factor by EMPA and biopersistence.

where R_M is the mesothelioma potency factor from Darnton's meta-analysis (Darnton, 2023),

EMPA is the fraction of fibers longer than 5 μm and not thicker than 0.15 μm, and

Bioper is the lifetime of fibers dissolved by Gualtieri's method (years) ($R = 0.983$, $R^2 = 0.966$, $p < 0.006$).

6. The Rigidity Index is another parameter characterizing the stiffness of elongate mineral particles and CNTs (see Chapter 7). Particles should be rigid, biopersistent, long, and thin to produce a significant effect on pleural cells. In Chapter 7, we used a combined parameter (average rigidity index for particles with DCC ≥0.05) as one of the predictors of mesothelioma potency.

We can also propose a model where this parameter (average rigidity index for particles with DCC ≥0.05) would be used along with biopersistence and EMPA to predict mesotheliomagenicity.

It can be demonstrated that

$Log_{10}(R_M) = -4.95+1.15Log_{10}(EMPA) + 1.29Log_{10}(Bioper) + 1.29Log_{10}$ (RigidityIndex),

where R_M is the mesothelioma potency factor from Darnton's meta-analysis (Darnton, 2023),

EMPA is the fraction of fibers longer than 5 μm and not thicker than 0.15 μm,

Bioper is the lifetime of fibers dissolved by Gualtieri's method (years), and

RigidityIndex is the average rigidity index for particles with DCC ≥0.05 (μm^2GPa x 10^4).

($R = 0.99$, $R^2 = 0.97$, $p < 0.008$).

The model predicts chrysotile potency of $R_M = 0.0013\%$ (vs. published average value of 0.0014% for all types of chrysotile), 0.29% for crocidolite (0.52% published), 0.09% for amosite (0.1% published), 0.1% for asbestiform anthophyllite (0.056% published), 0.02% for Libby amphiboles (0.03% published), 0.035% for balangeroite (0.045% published), and 6.4% for erionite (4.5% published). If we assume that the biopersistence of non-asbestiform minerals is the same as for the asbestiform variety (which might be an overestimation), we would get a mesothelioma potency of non-asbestiform riebeckite as 0.0002% and non-asbestiform grunerite as 0.00014%. Assuming the biopersistence of fibrous talc is 4.1 years (as follows from experimental data in Jurinski & Rimstidt, 2001), we would estimate its mesothelioma potency as 0.00003% (lower than for any other known type of elongate particles, and statistically negligible).

7. The length of elongate mineral particles is another relevant factor impacting carcinogenicity. It is widely accepted by many epidemiologists and toxicologists that particles with length<=5 μm should not be considered mesotheliomagenic.

   For example, the approach proposed under the EU CLH (Harmonized Classification and Labeling) regulations for the determination of the carcinogenicity of carbon nanotubes included the following criteria:

   1. Length >5 μm,
   2. Length/width ≥3:1,
   3. Width ≥30 nm and < 3 μm (BAuA 2021).

   Various authors have demonstrated that 5 μm can be a good parameter distinguishing mesotheliomagenic and non-mesotheliomagenic EMPs. For example, Wylie and Korchevskiy (2023) showed that for the length categories L < 5 μm, no statistically significant correlations with the potency of dimensional fractions were found (contrary to dimensional fractions for fibers with length > 5 μm). Roggli (2015) stated that studies in both experimental animal models and human tissue samples do not support a pathogenic role for fibers 5 μm or less in length. Claims concerning the numerical majority of such fibers in tissues carry no weight with respect to the causation of disease, and in vitro studies of possible pathogenic mechanisms do not override the findings in inhalational animal models or human epidemiological studies. Bernstein (2022) concluded that while short asbestos fibers are present in most occupational or environmental exposures, the large body of studies strongly supports that they do not contribute to the health effects of asbestos exposure.

While initially the lower bound of length for potency estimation seems based on available analytical techniques, rather than underlying toxicological studies, it seems that the guess was not wrong. However, the lower bound of length may be even higher. Berman and Crump (2008b) argued that only fibers longer than 10 μm have the potency to produce cancer. Further studies are needed to see what the true lower bound of length can be as a threshold of potency.

Also, the lower bound of width for mesotheliomagenic fibers apparently exists, as well as upper bound of length. In particular, data for carbon nanotubes show no potency at widths below 37 nm (the diameter typical for carbon nanotubes, but too low a value for EMPs to be significant with the exception of single fibrils of chrysotile). Based on the theory described in Chapter 7, particles with length > 100 μm and width=0.15 μm would not have substantial rigidity for significant biological effects. For narrower fibers, the maximum length for biological rigidity would be much smaller.

8. Table 13.2 contains a characterization of the selected terms and definitions (previously listed in Chapter 1) from the position of toxicological science. The comments on the current regulatory practice and possible changes are also listed.

CONCLUSIONS

1. The asbestiform fibers and cleavage fragments may have similar chemical compositions, but they differ in dimensions, and the corresponding datasets (or individual particles) can be efficiently separated by length and width data.
2. Other dimensional characteristics (like specific surface area) for cleavage fragments and asbestiform fibers are also significantly distinct, which makes their behavior in the environment and in human lungs different.
3. The samples of elongate mineral particles can be classified by their habit (asbestiform vs. non-asbestiform) based on two major characteristics: the fraction of criteria particles, determined by a quantitative method (discriminant function), and the correlation between width and length. This method allows for the determination of the habit of tremolite datasets with 100% certainty; the error for all mineral types is less than 3 %.
4. The fraction of criteria particles by the Wylie et al. (2022) method appears to be a good predictor of various characteristics of EMPs. In particular, the mesothelioma potency of amphiboles in human cohorts, as well as in intrapleural and intraperitoneal injection studies in animals, seems to correlate with this parameter.
5. The fraction of particles longer than 5 μm that have a width of ≤0.15 μm (EMPA) serves as a strong predictor of mesothelioma potency for a sample of fibers. The limitations of measurement methods would most provably make particles with a width of ≤0.20 μm to also be counted as EMPA. The EMPA fraction should be significantly different from 0 to assure

TABLE 13.2
Scientific basis for major asbestos-related definitions.

Term	Suggested definition	Relevant quantitative characteristics and toxicological meaning	Current regulatory understanding
Elongate mineral particle (EMP)	Any mineral particle with a length-to-width ratio (aspect ratio) of 3:1 or greater.	From all types of elongate mineral particles, about 73% have an aspect ratio of 5:1 or greater, and about 47% have an aspect ratio of 10:1 or greater. Only elongate mineral particles are demonstrated to cause pleural mesothelioma (vs. other shapes and sizes of particulates).	NIOSH defined elongate particles as "any particle with a minimum aspect ratio of 3:1," emphasizing that they focus on inhalable, thoracic, or respirable size particles. The term EMP is more reasonable than the definition of "structures." While the cut point of 3:1 in the aspect ratio is just conventional, most toxicological and risk assessment data are available only for a minimum aspect ratio of 3:1.
Mineral fiber	An elongate mineral particle that attained its shape during formation in nature with an aspect ratio sufficiently large to impart flexibility in hand samples.	From the particles in mineralogically asbestiform datasets (see "Asbestiform"), about 30% of counted particles are longer than 5 μm with an aspect ratio of at least 3:1. Mineral fiber should be further interpreted from a toxicological perspective based on its size and morphology, as well as methods applied for its microscopy determination.	OSHA defines fiber as a "particular form of asbestos 5 μm or longer, with a length-to-diameter ratio of at least 3 to 1," though the term "fiber" mineralogically has obvious qualitative, rather than quantitative meaning. The ASTM and ISO definition of fiber as a structure with a minimum length of 0.5 μm and an aspect ratio of 5:1 and greater lacks a toxicological basis.
Asbestos fibril	A naturally formed single crystal fiber of asbestos that cannot be further separated longitudinally into smaller components.	The fibril width is about 10–40 nm for chrysotile, 20–200 nm for amosite, and 10–100 nm for crocidolite.	Current definitions are adequate.
Acicular	Straight and rigid with cross-sectional dimensions that are small relative to its length; like a needle.		

Term	Suggested definition	Relevant quantitative characteristics and toxicological meaning	Current regulatory understanding
Cleavage fragment	An elongate mineral particle created by fragmentation that is bound in whole or in part by inherent planes of weakness.	From the cleavage fragments population with an aspect ratio of ≥3:1, the particles with an aspect ratio greater than 10:1 comprise 10–17% vs. about 70% for asbestos fibers, and greater than 20:1 comprise 1–3% vs. 45% for fibers. Cleavage fragments are significantly different from asbestiform fibers by size and various parameters impacting biological activity. No studies have ever demonstrated that cleavage fragments are mesotheliomagenic for humans in the absence of asbestiform fibers.	OSHA does not require counting of cleavage fragments (non-asbestiform minerals) in the framework of the asbestos standard, whatever their size and aspect ratio. The non-asbestiform particles are regulated as dust. OSHA defines cleavage fragments as "mineral particles formed by comminution of minerals, especially those characterized by parallel sides and a moderate aspect ratio (usually less than 20:1)."
Fibrous	The mineral habit that describes particles having the appearance of fiber ***or*** being composed of fiber.		
Asbestiform	A naturally occurring, polyfilamentous mineral growth habit in which fibers are formed of parallel fibrils in bundles that can be separated into smaller fibers and fibrils with hand pressure; asbestiform minerals are flexible in hand samples and fibers have higher tensile strength than other habits of the same mineral.	Populations of asbestiform fibrils typically have widths in the range of 0.01 to 0.5 micrometers. On average, the width of asbestiform EMP-5s increases by 0.008 μm per 1 μm of length, vs. 0.14 μm per 1 μm of length for cleavage fragments. Not all asbestiform fibers are able to produce mesothelioma in humans, but fibers with proved mesotheliomagenicity are always asbestiform.	The term needs further adjustment to account for the difference between "asbestiform minerals" and "asbestiform particles." For example, asbestiform minerals can produce airborne asbestiform fibers and potentially cleavage fragments. Other types of minerals (non-asbestiform) cannot produce airborne asbestos fibers.
Criteria particles	The particles fitting the dimensional criteria for the asbestiform variety.	The dimensional rule for criteria particles corresponds to the discriminant function equation (Wylie et al., 2022) and can be expressed as $Length^{2.99}/Width^{5.82} > 6{,}300$. Some criteria particles can be definitely mesotheliomagenic.	

(Continued)

Table 13.2 (*Continued*)
Scientific basis for major asbestos-related definitions.

Term	Suggested definition	Relevant quantitative characteristics and toxicological meaning	Current regulatory understanding
Asbestos	A generic term applied to the asbestiform variety of serpentine (chrysotile) and the asbestiform variety of amphibole group minerals (including anthophyllite, grunerite, tremolite, actinolite, and riebeckite) that have been exploited, prospected, described in the literature, traded, and sold commercially for their unique physical properties of high tensile strength, flexibility, and durability in the built environment.	Commercial asbestos has been demonstrated to be carcinogenic, though potency factors depend on various characteristics (like size, chemical composition, and rigidity of fibers).	The term asbestos should be used only in relationship to commercial asbestos; otherwise, the term "asbestiform mineral" is suitable.
PCM equivalent fibers	Particles with an aspect ratio of 3:1 or greater and a length longer than 5 micrometers, visible by PCM that are also visible by TEM, including chrysotile fibers of 0.15 micrometer and amphibole fibers of 0.05 micrometer in diameter or more.	The previous criteria for PCM fibers (width>0.25 micrometers) would discount about 25% of typical amphibole fibers and 30% of chrysotile fibers, with a significant fraction of them being of potential toxicological relevance.	The current PCM 7400 method by NIOSH assumes that chrysotile fibers of 0.15 micrometer and amphibole fibers of 0.05 micrometer in diameter or more are countable by optical microscopy.

Term	Suggested definition	Relevant quantitative characteristics and toxicological meaning	Current regulatory understanding
Carcinogenic EMPs	Elongate mineral particles that can produce asbestos-related cancers in humans when exposed in substantial quantities.	The EMP exposure is suspected to be carcinogenic for mesothelioma if EMFA (fraction with width of ≤0.15 μm among particles with length of >5 μm) is statistically significantly different from zero. Also, the fraction of fibers with DCC ≥0.05 in the mesotheliomagenic population is typically more than 8%. The level of potency increases when biopersistence and the fraction of thin fibers increases. The length of mineral particles with mesotheliomagenic potential appears to range from more than 5 μm to less than 60 μm (Chapter 6). The mesotheliomagenic datasets also have an elevated level of specific surface area (Korchevskiy & Wylie, 2022).	The term is important to be introduced into the toxicological and analytical practice because not every particle longer than 5 μm with an aspect ratio greater than 3:1 is carcinogenic.

mesotheliomagenic potential. The dimensional coefficient of carcinogenicity (DCC) is a new metric allowing for the forecast of mesothelial carcinogenicity for both EMPs and CNTs (Korchevskiy & Wylie, 2025a).

6. The rigidity of elongate mineral particles is a necessary condition for their biological activity. Biopersistence, rigidity index, DCC, and EMPA parameters can be combined to quantify the full process of toxicokinetics and toxicodynamics of elongate particles.
7. Particles with definite mesotheliomagenic potency (including carbon nanotubes and elongate mineral particles) appear to have a width in the range from 30 nm to 0.2 μm and a length from 5 to 30 μm.
8. Generally, the unified asbestos terminology (or more precisely, the terminology for elongate mineral particles) is feasible if the mineralogical and toxicological meanings of the terms are well understood and reconciled. The need for such terminology is obvious for practical purposes, with health protection of workers and communities being a priority.

REFERENCE LIST

BAuA. (2021). *CLH report: Proposal for harmonized classification and labelling. Multi-walled carbon tubes (synthetic graphite in tubular shape) with a geometric tube diameter range ≥30 nm to <3 μm and a length ≥ 5 μm and aspect ratio 3:1, including multi-walled carbon nanotubes, MWC(N)T.* https://echa.europa.eu/et/registry-of-clh-intentions-until-outcome/-/dislist/details/0b0236e18195a284

Berman, D. W., & Crump, K. S. (2008a). Update of potency factors for asbestos-related lung cancer and mesothelioma. *Critical Reviews in Toxicology*, *38*(Suppl 1), 1–47. https://doi.org/10.1080/10408440802276167

Berman, D. W., & Crump, K. S. (2008b). A meta-analysis of asbestos-related cancer risk that addresses fiber size and mineral type. *Critical Reviews in Toxicology*, *38*(Suppl 1), 49–73. https://doi.org/10.1080/10408440802273156

Bernstein, D. M. (2022). The health effects of short fiber chrysotile and amphibole asbestos. *Critical Reviews in Toxicology*, *52*(2), 89–112. https://doi.org/10.1080/10408444.2022.2056430

Cook, P. M., Swintek, J., Dawson, T. D., Chapman, D., Etterson, M. A., & Hoff, D. (2016). Quantitative structure-mesothelioma potency model optimization for complex mixtures of elongated particles in rat pleura: A retrospective study. *Journal of Toxicology and Environmental Health, Part B*, *19*(5–6), 266–288. https://doi.org/10.1080/10937404.2016.1195326. PMID: 27705548

Darnton, L. (2023). Quantitative assessment of mesothelioma and lung cancer risk based on Phase Contrast Microscopy (PCM) estimates of fibre exposure: An update of 2000 asbestos cohort data. *Environmental Research*, *230*, 114753. https://doi.org/10.1016/j.envres.2022.114753

Davis, J. M., Addison, J., McIntosh, C., Miller, B. G., & Niven, K. (1991). Variations in the carcinogenicity of tremolite dust samples of differing morphology. *Annals of the New York Academy of Sciences*, *643*, 473–490. https://doi.org/10.1111/j.1749-6632.1991.tb24497.x

Gordon, R. E. (2018). Analytic analyses of human tissues for the presence of asbestos and talc. In M. Arita & N. Sakaguchi (Eds.), *Electron microscopy – novel microscopy trends*. https://doi.org/10.5772/intechopen.73375

Gualtieri, A. F., Pollastri, S., Gandolfi, N. B., & Gualtieri, M. L. (2018). In vitro acellular dissolution of mineral fibres: A comparative study. *Scientific Reports*, *8*, 7071. https://doi.org/10.1038/s41598-018-25531-4

Hodgson, J. T., & Darnton, A. (2000). The quantitative risks of mesothelioma and lung cancer in relation to asbestos exposure. *Annals of Occupational Hygiene*, *44*(8), 565–601.

Jurinski, J., & Rimstidt, J. (2001). Biodurability of talc. *American Mineralogist*, *86*, 392–399. https://doi.org/10.2138/am-2001-0402

Korchevskiy, A. A., Rasmuson, J. O., & Rasmuson, E. J. (2019). Empirical model of mesothelioma potency factors for different mineral fibers based on their chemical composition and dimensionality. *Inhalation Toxicology*, *31*(5), 180–191. https://doi.org/10.1080/08958378.2019.1640320

Korchevskiy, A. A., & Wylie, A. G. (2021). Dimensional determinants for the carcinogenic potency of elongate amphibole particles. *Inhalation Toxicology*, *33*(6–8), 244–259. https://doi.org/10.1080/08958378.2021.1971340

Korchevskiy, A. A., & Wylie, A. G. (2022). Dimensional characteristics of the major types of amphibole mineral particles and the implications for carcinogenic risk assessment. *Inhalation Toxicology*, *34*(1–2), 24–38. https://doi.org/10.1080/08958378.2021.2024304

Korchevskiy, A. A., & Wylie, A. G. (2025a). Habit of elongate amphibole particles as a predictor of mesothelial carcinogenicity. *Toxicology Reports*, *14*, 101908. https://doi.org/10.1016/j.toxrep.2025.101908

Korchevskiy, A. A., & Wylie, A. G. (2025b, April 24). The empirical metric of mesothelial carcinogenicity for carbon nanotubes and elongate mineral particles. *Inhalation Toxicology* (online). https://doi.org/10.1080/08958378.2025.2486087

Lowers, H., & Meeker, G. (2002). *Tabulation of asbestos-related terminology* (USGS Open-File Report 02-458). https://jifsan.umd.edu/files/wordpress/wp-content/uploads/2018/11/Asbestos-Symposium-2018-Meeker-General-Reference-01.pdf

Mossman, B. T. (2008). Assessment of the pathogenic potential of asbestiform vs. nonasbestiform particulates (cleavage fragments) in in vitro (cell or organ culture) models and bioassays. *Regulatory Toxicology & Pharmacology*, *52*(1 Suppl), S200–S203. https://doi.org/10.1016/j.yrtph.2007.10.004

National Institute for Occupational Safety and Health (NIOSH). (2011). *Current intelligence bulletin 62: Asbestos fibers and other elongate mineral particles: State of the science and roadmap for research* (DHHS (NIOSH) Publication No. 2011-159). Asbestos Fibers and Other Elongate Mineral Particles | NIOSH | CDC.

Roggli, V. L. (2015). The so-called short-fiber controversy: Literature review and critical analysis. *The Archives of Pathology & Laboratory Medicine*, *139*(8), 1052–1057. https://doi.org/10.5858/arpa.2014-0466-RA. PMID: 26230599

Schiller, J. E., Payne, S. L., & Khalafalla, S. E. (1980). Surface charge heterogeneity in amphibole cleavage fragments and asbestos fibers. *Science*, *209*, 4464. https://doi.org/10.1126/science.209.4464.1530

U.S. Environmental Protection Agency (U.S. EPA). (2014). *IRIS toxicological review of Libby amphibole asbestos* (Final Report, EPA/635/R-11/002F). U.S. Environmental Protection Agency.

Wylie, A. G., & Korchevskiy, A. A. (2023). Dimensions of elongate mineral particles and cancer: A review. *Environmental Research*, *230*, 114688. https://doi.org/10.1016/j.envres.2022.114688

Wylie, A. G., Korchevskiy, A. A., Segrave, A. M., & Duane, A. (2020). Modeling mesothelioma risk factors from amphibole fiber dimensionality: Mineralogical and epidemiological perspective. *Journal of Applied Toxicology*, *40*(4), 515–524. https://doi.org/10.1002/jat.3923

Wylie, A. G., Korchevskiy, A. A., Van Orden, D. R., & Chatfield, E. J. (2022). Discriminant analysis of asbestiform and non-asbestiform amphibole particles and its implications for toxicological studies. *Computational Toxicology*, *23*, 100233. https://doi.org/10.1016/j.comtox.2022.100233

14 Regulatory priorities for elongate mineral particles in the new era

A. Korchevskiy & A. Wylie

Historically, regulations and standards have played a pivotal role in improving the environment and occupational conditions worldwide. Because of the great efforts of medical doctors, toxicologists, and hygienists, regulatory measures to protect against respiratory hazards, including carcinogenic commercial asbestos fibers, have been put in place. Efficient limitations imposed on asbestos production and an asbestos ban have reduced the risks of asbestosis, mesothelioma, and lung cancer, saving the lives of thousands of workers, their families, and community members.

However, it should be noted that current regulatory policies for asbestos face significant methodological issues because the crossroads of science and regulations are not in order. First, the mineralogy of asbestos is generally ignored for regulatory purposes. This has brought us to the current situation: almost worldwide, the most hazardous asbestiform amphiboles are regulated at the same level as much less dangerous chrysotile fibers.

Second, the regulations ignore the differences in fiber sizes, except for the very general acceptance of the inclusion of asbestos fibers being longer than 5 μm, with an aspect ratio greater than 3:1. The need for more specific size characterization of fibers has not been addressed, in spite of the U.S. EPA's long-term efforts to develop the so-called bin-specific methodology of risk assessment in the early 2000s (U.S. EPA, 2008).

Third, no unified approach has been established for the regulation of elongate particles of the same mineral with different habits, even though habit certainly affects the biological activity of particles. Only the U.S. OSHA has attempted to regulate asbestiform fibers differently from cleavage fragments, requiring the exclusion of non-asbestiform varieties from compliance counting for asbestos, but without guidance on how to do so. However, the U.S. EPA has not accepted the need to regulate asbestiform and non-asbestiform amphiboles differently.

The last controversy causes a significant issue related to the widespread presence of non-asbestiform amphibole, a common rock-forming mineral. Small amounts of elongate particles, mostly cleavage fragments, can be emitted from many earth-moving operations in construction or mining. Regulating this type of dust in the same way as the emission of commercial asbestos is detrimental because it will put industries in a complicated position without an obvious reason. Cleavage fragments of amphibole minerals are not equivalent to commercial asbestos, and there is no sense

DOI: 10.1201/9781003424277-15

in applying strict requirements to the emission of nuisance dust that many massive amphiboles produce by comminution.

The most recent studies summarized in this book demonstrate once again that elongate mineral particles of amphibole, serpentine, and other silicates are not homogeneous populations that can be regulated in a uniform way. Even though the banning of asbestos in the United States is not expected to change the current situation significantly because the effective elimination of commercial asbestos from industrial practices happened long ago, it requires a refocus on how to regulate asbestos effectively because it is not possible to ban common rock. In a nutshell, diversified principles should be applied to elongate particles of various types.

The following framework is proposed.

ASBESTOS MINERALS SHOULD BE REGULATED DIFFERENTLY

Chrysotile, amphiboles, and zeolites should have different standards and exposure limits. Table 14.1 shows potency factors for mesothelioma and corresponding occupational exposure levels for 45 years of exposure that would not exceed a 1 in 10,000 and 1 in 1,000 risk.

In 2024, the U.S. EPA established a so-called existing chemical exposure limit (ECEL) for chrysotile asbestos at 0.005 f/cc (PCM) as an eight-hour time-weighted average (TWA) (U.S. EPA, 2024). Based on Darnton (2023, 2024), the exposure at 0.005 f/cc PCM to chrysotile every day for 45 years would yield 1.4 cases of mesothelioma and 7 cases of lung cancer per 1,000,000. This level cannot be interpreted as a statistically significant risk increase, comprising just a fraction of the baseline rate of respiratory cancers in non-exposed populations.

VARIOUS SIZES OF ELONGATE PARTICLES SHOULD BE REGULATED DIFFERENTLY

One of the important conclusions from scientific studies during the last decade is that amphibole particles longer than 5 μm with width ≤0.15 to 0.20 μm (EMPA category)

TABLE 14.1
Possible estimations of levels of occupational exposure corresponding to specific risk benchmarks (onset age 18 years, duration 45 years).

Mineral type	Mesothelioma potency factor R_M (%), based on Darnton, 2023	Level of exposure to not exceed risk of 1 per 10,000 (f/cc)	Level of exposure to not exceed risk of 1 per 1,000 (f/cc)
Non-textile chrysotile	0.0011	0.38	3.8
Textile chrysotile	0.010	0.041	0.41
Crocidolite	0.52	0.0008	0.008
Amosite	0.11	0.0038	0.038
Libby amphiboles	0.03	0.014	0.14

can be used as a surrogate for the total exposure in mesothelioma regulations. EMPA is predictive for mesothelioma risk, and the absence of this category in the size distribution signifies negligible mesothelioma potency. According to our studies of CNTs and EMPs, the range of diameters from 0.03 to 0.20 μm includes the necessary components of an exposure to produce mesothelioma in humans. Therefore, a regulatory limit can be established specifically for amphibole EMPs.

The following example can be applied for risk assessment purposes by using the model of mesothelioma potency factor from Wylie et al., 2020. According to the model by Wylie et al., the mesothelioma potency factor R_M can be estimated from the EMPA fraction (%) as

$$R_M = -0.012 + 0.011\text{EMPA}\cdot$$

If *y* (f/cc) were an airborne concentration of EMPA amphibole particles with a known EMPA fraction (%), the risk per 10,000 workers during 45 years of full-time work can be approximated as

$$\begin{gathered}\text{RISK (per 10,000 per lifetime)} = \\ (-0.012 + 0.011\text{EMPA})^{*}\, y/\text{EMPA}^{*}45^{*}10{,}000. \end{gathered} \quad (14.1).$$

From this equation, the risk level can be approximated for amphibole particles, and the acceptable exposure calculated. The relationship in Equation 14.1 is illustrated in Figure 14.1.

For example, for Libby amphiboles with an EMPA fraction of about 4%, the risk level can be assessed as

$$\text{RISK}\left(\text{Libby amphiboles}\right) = 4590\text{y} \quad (14.2).$$

If the target risk level is one case of mesothelioma per 10,000 workers (the target risk level in NIOSH carcinogenic policy), the level of EMPA exposure *y* should be less than 0.0002 (f/cc EMPA). However, if the historical OSHA risk acceptability level of 1 per 1,000 were followed, the regulations could be set with a maximum exposure at the level of 0.002 (f/cc EMPA).

The relationship shown in Equation 14.1, however, is suitable for amphiboles but not for other classes of minerals that vary in biopersistence. For chrysotile asbestos, the risk level should be decreased proportionally to the biopersistence coefficient that was discussed in other chapters of this book. For example, the biopersistence of chrysotile can be assumed to be 0.3 years, and Libby amphiboles (as tremolite) as 49 years (Gualtieri, 2018). From here, the relative coefficient of biopersistence between Libby amphiboles and chrysotile would be about 169.

If the EMPA fraction were 4% for a chrysotile sample, Equation 14.2 can be substituted by

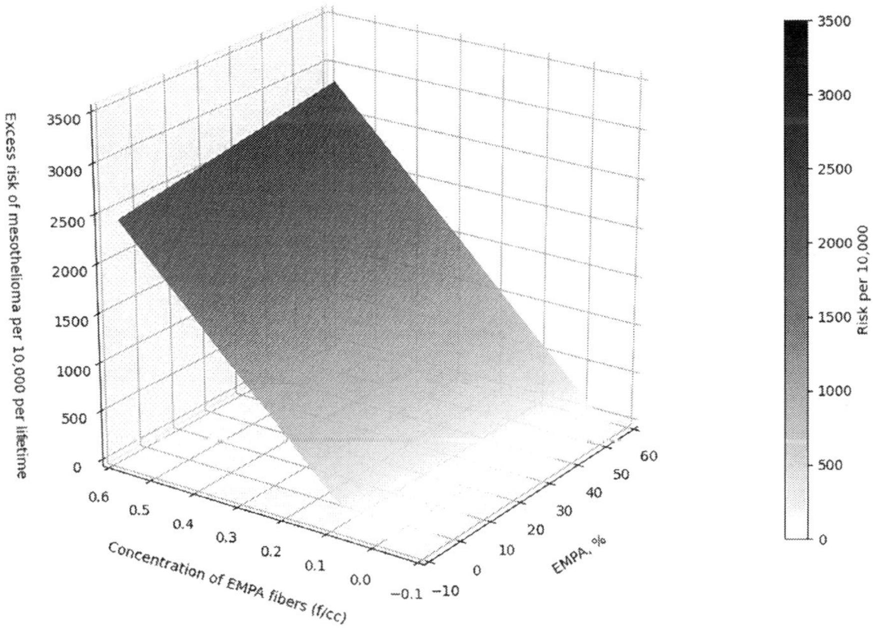

FIGURE 14.1 The model of excess mesothelioma risk depending on EMPA concentration (f/cc) and EMPA fraction in the exposure (%).

$$\text{RISK}\left(\text{Chrysotile}\right) = 27.8\text{y} \qquad (14.3).$$

SAMPLING METHODOLOGY SHOULD BE SUPPORTED BY TOXICOLOGICAL INFORMATION

While scientific studies may benefit from the collection of full dimensional information when aerosolized asbestos samples are collected, the environmental and occupational monitoring process would benefit from limiting the collected fibers by specific toxicologically based criteria.

In particular, the development of sampling methods that would specifically address airborne mesotheliomagenic EMPA particles would be beneficial. In this case, the samples should contain elongate particles longer than 5 μm, with a diameter less than or equal to 0.15 to 0.20 μm.

Figure 14.2 demonstrates the relationship between the width of particles in the dimensional database as related to aerodynamic diameter, calculated by Timbrell's method (Timbrell, 1965). The red squares (the part of the graph to the left of the dividing line) correspond to EMP-5 width≤0.20 μm, and the blue circles (the part of the graph to the right from the dividing line) correspond to EMP-5 particles with width>0.20 μm.

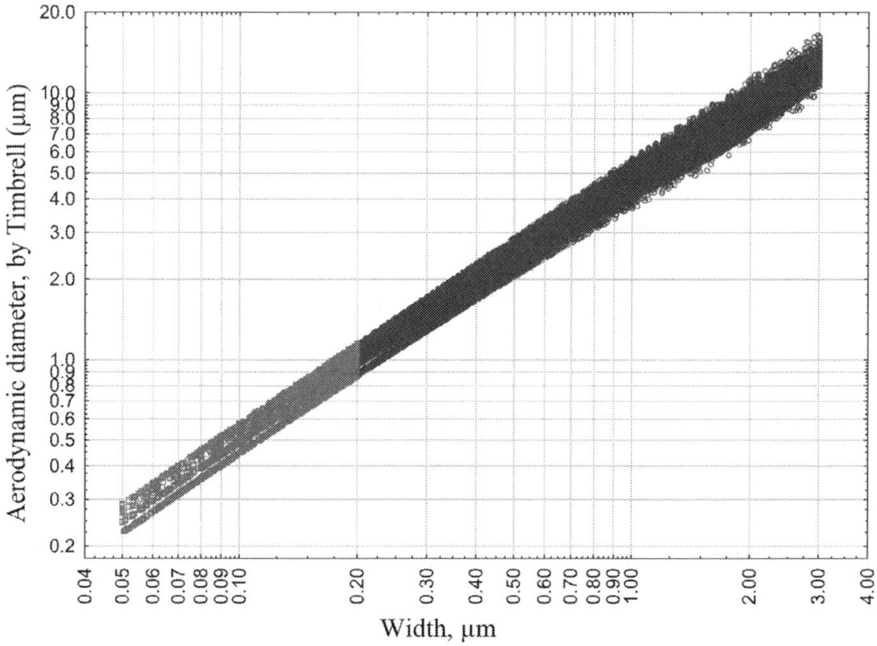

FIGURE 14.2 The relationship between the width of EMP-5 particles in the dimensional database as related to aerodynamic diameter, calculated by Timbrell's method (Timbrell, 1965). The red squares (the part of the graph to the left of the dividing line) correspond to particles with width≤0.20 μm, and the blue circles (the part of the graph to the right of the dividing line) correspond to particles with width>0.20 μm.

As we can see, all EMPA particles (100%) and a small fraction of non-asbestiform particles (3.4%) have an aerodynamic diameter of less than 1.2 μm. Sampling devices that limit the aerodynamic diameter to the upper threshold of 1.2 μm should be sufficient to select mesotheliomagenic particles from the air samples.

IMPORTANCE OF COUNTING CRITERIA

Counting criteria for elongate mineral particles is an important part of asbestos regulations. As a rule, current methodologies require the counting of EMPs longer than 5 μm (EMP-5).

Substituting electron microscopy for phase contrast microscopy in asbestos fiber counting opens unique opportunities for precise asbestos analysis. In particular, the mineral type making up elongate particles can usually be determined by TEM to estimate the risk level for a given exposure concentration, especially if the source is known.

It is important, however, to remember that quantitative values of risk in mesothelioma and/or lung cancer per unit of asbestos exposure were estimated in terms of optical microscopy (if not by earlier methods, like midget impinger, with subsequent recalculation to phase-contrast microscopy concentrations). Changes in the microscopic method used to count asbestos fibers that affect the visibility of the fibers would result in the need to revise health standards (0.1 f/cc would not be equal to 0.1 f/cc anymore).

Whether or not PCM microscopy is able to visualize very thin fibers has been a point of discussion in the literature. Some authors have argued that fibers with a width of less than about 0.2 μm could not be visualized by PCM (Havics, 2010). Accordingly, a so-called PCM equivalent was introduced for electron microscopy, requiring the counting of only fibers with a width greater than 0.25 μm (see NIOSH method 7402; 2022). Recently, NIOSH recognized that PCM was much more efficient than suggested. The new version of the method, NIOSH 7400, states that chrysotile fibers as thin as 0.15 μm and amphibole fibers as thin as 0.05 μm can be counted by PCM by trained microscopists. This is a significant change in the counting rules. For example, for chrysotile, 18.6% of all particles longer than 5 μm will have a width between 0.15 and 0.25 μm. For amphiboles, 27.4% of EMPs longer than 5 μm will be in this width range.

Therefore, it should be acknowledged that TEM measurements of asbestos exposure are comparable with the risk-based standards and potency factors derived from PCM concentration units in terms of dimensional structure and composition. Other factors may impact the difference between TEM and PCM concentrations, for example, differences in sample preparation.

We also believe that for practical purposes, counting only fibers longer than 5 μm is sufficient for monitoring methodology. Wylie and Korchevskiy (2023) reviewed the available data on the length threshold for asbestos carcinogenicity. It should be recognized that the majority of evidence confirms that only fibers longer than 5 μm are toxicologically relevant. Also, as we noted above, only fibers not thicker than 0.15 μm appear to be mesotheliomagenic. Obviously, this statement should be adjusted to the precision of dimensional measurements, as the category of 0.15 μm may include fibers with a true width of up to 0.2 μm. New methods, including artificial intelligence techniques, should bring additional value to the dimensionality-based assessment of exposure and in-depth risk analysis because of measurement uncertainty.

HABIT OF ELONGATE MINERAL PARTICLES AND REGULATORY PRACTICES

Non-asbestiform amphibole particles (cleavage fragments) should be excluded from regulatory consideration as asbestos and treated like dust in specific size categories. Non-asbestiform particles longer than 5 μm in the dimensional database (described elsewhere in this book) have an average aerodynamic diameter of 5.5 μm, with a median of 5.1 μm. For regulatory purposes, most are expected to be characterized as PM10 rather than PM2.5. To the contrary, asbestiform particles have the average aerodynamic diameter of 1.9 μm with median of 1.5 μm, putting them into the ultrafine PM2.5 category. The argument that cleavage fragments can form asbestos-sized fibers is simply incorrect; EMPA particles are extremely rare among fragments.

For PM10 dust, the current National Ambient Air Quality Standard (NAAQS) is 150 μg/m^3, assuming lifetime exposure of 24 hours per day. This level corresponds to an occupational exposure of about 700 μg/m^3 (8 hours per day, 5 days per week, 45 years). The average weight of non-asbestiform fibers in our database is 28 x 10^{-12} g. Therefore, the level of 700 μg/m^3 corresponds to about 25 f/cc, or 1125 f/cc-years, which can serve as a provisional benchmark for any corresponding effects of non-asbestiform amphibole dust exposure.

In general, the regulatory environment should serve as a support for best practices in risk assessment, allowing prioritization of hazards and not mixing up dangerous and non-dangerous agents. Asbestos is a hazardous, carcinogenic agent. However, the asbestos hazard arises from a specific type of fiber, one with biological rigidity and very small width. Asbestos should not be equated with fine and ultrafine dust, and cleavage fragments, even those close to the size of some asbestos fibers, should not be mistaken for true asbestos. Dust is unable to produce mesothelioma in humans if it does not contain an asbestiform fraction that is thin enough to produce cascading effects leading to rare but extremely invasive mesothelial cancers.

REFERENCE LIST

CDC/NIOSH (NIOSH). (2019). *Asbestos and other fibers by PCM, method 7400, issue 3: NIOSH manual of analytical methods (NMAM)* (5th ed.). https://www.cdc.gov/niosh/nmam/pdf/7400.pdf

Darnton, L. (2023). Quantitative assessment of mesothelioma and lung cancer risk based on phase contrast microscopy (PCM) estimates of fibre exposure: An update of 2000 asbestos cohort data. *Environmental Research*, *230*, 114753. https://doi.org/10.1016/j.envres.2022.114753

Darnton, L. (2024). The Hodgson and Darnton approach to quantifying the risks of mesothelioma and lung cancer in relation to asbestos exposure. In A. Korchevskiy, J. Rasmuson, & E. Rasmuson (Eds.), *Health risk assessment for asbestos and other fibrous minerals* (pp. 233–269). John Wiley & Sons, Inc. ISBN: 978-1-119-43843-4, https://doi.org/10.1002/9781119438397

Gualtieri, A. F. (2018). Towards a quantitative model to predict the toxicity/pathogenicity potential of mineral fibers. *Toxicology and Applied Pharmacology*, *361*, 89–98. https://doi.org/10.1016/j.taap.2018.05.012

Havics, A. (2010). Asbestos fiber counting by different optical contrast techniques. *The Microscope*, *58*(2), 51–62.

National Institute for Occupational Safety and Health (NIOSH). (2022, August 1). *Asbestos by TEM: Method: 7402, issue 3*. https://www.cdc.gov/niosh/nmam/pdf/7402.pdf

Timbrell, V. (1965). The inhalation of fibrous dusts. In *Biological Effects of Asbestos: Annals of the New York Academy of Sciences*, *132*(1), 255–273. https://doi.org/10.1111/j.1749-6632.1965.tb41107.x

U.S. Environmental Protection Agency (U.S. EPA). (2008). *Proposed approach for estimation of BIN-specific cancer potency factors for inhalation exposure to asbestos, risk assessment*. https://19january2021snapshot.epa.gov/sites/static/files/2015-11/documents/2008_prop_asbestos_approach.pdf

U.S. Environmental Protection Agency (U.S. EPA). (2024). *Asbestos part 1; chrysotile asbestos; regulation of certain conditions of use under the toxic substances control act (TSCA)* (40 CFR 751, 2024-05972, 89 FR 21970). https://www.federalregister.gov/

documents/2024/03/28/2024-05972/asbestos-part-1-chrysotile-asbestos-regulation-of-certain-conditions-of-use-under-the-toxic

Wylie, A. G., & Korchevskiy, A. A. (2023). Dimensions of elongate mineral particles and cancer: A review. *Environmental Research*, *230*, 114688. https://doi.org/10.1016/j.envres.2022.114688

Wylie, A. G., Korchevskiy, A., Segrave, A. M., & Duane, A. (2020). Modeling mesothelioma risk factors from amphibole fiber dimensionality: Mineralogical and epidemiological perspective. *Journal of Applied Toxicology*, *40*(4), 515–524. https://doi.org/10.1002/jat.3923

Index

Made in the USA
Las Vegas, NV
19 September 2026

81e4d061-c4a0-43f2-b48c-1c0654d720bcR01